Cardiac Cell and Gene Transfer

METHODS IN MOLECULAR BIOLOGY™

John M. Walker, SERIES EDITOR

METHODS IN MOLECULAR BIOLOGY™

Cardiac Cell and Gene Transfer

Principles, Protocols, and Applications

Edited by

Joseph M. Metzger

Department of Physiology, Department of Internal Medicine, and Director, Center for Integrative Genomics, University of Michigan, Ann Arbor, MI

Humana Press 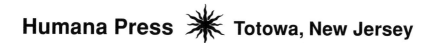 Totowa, New Jersey

© 2003 Humana Press Inc.
999 Riverview Drive, Suite 208
Totowa, New Jersey 07512

www.humanapress.com

The content and opinions expressed in this book are the sole work of the authors and editors, who have warranted due diligence in the creation and issuance of their work. The publisher, editors, and authors are not responsible for errors or omissions or for any consequences arising from the information or opinions presented in this book and make no warranty, express or implied, with respect to its contents.

This publication is printed on acid-free paper. ∞
ANSI Z39.48-1984 (American Standards Institute) Permanence of Paper for Printed Library Materials.

Production Editor: Adrienne Howell.

Cover design by Joseph M. Metzger and Patricia F. Cleary.

For additional copies, pricing for bulk purchases, and/or information about other Humana titles, contact Humana at the above address or at any of the following numbers: Tel: 973-256-1699; Fax: 973-256-8341; E-mail: humana@humanapr.com, or visit our Website at www.humanapress.com

Photocopy Authorization Policy:

Printed in the United States of America. 10 9 8 7 6 5 4 3 2 1

Library of Congress Cataloging in Publication Data

Cardiac cell and gene transfer : principles, protocols, and applications / edited by Joseph M. Metzger.
    p. cm. -- (Methods in molecular biology ; 219)
    Includes bibliographical references and index.
    ISBN 0-89603-994-3 (alk. paper)   1-59259-350-X (ebook)
      1. Heart--Diseases--Gene therapy. 2. Genetic transformation. 3. Heart cells. 4. Myoblast transfer therapy.
    I. Metzger, Joseph Mark, 1957-. II. Methods in molecular biology (Totowa, N.J.) ; v. 219.

RC684.G44 C37 2003
616.1'206--dc21

                                                                    2002027345

Preface

Heart disease is the leading cause of death in developed countries. Recent experimental advances featuring cellular, molecular, and genetic tools and technologies offer the potential for new therapeutic strategies directed toward remediation of inherited and acquired heart diseases. Whether these recent basic science advances will ultimately translate to clinical efficacy for patients with heart disease is unknown and is important to ascertain. *Cardiac Cell and Gene Transfer: Principles, Protocols, and Applications* is designed to provide the reader with up-to-date coverage of a myriad of specific methodologies and protocols for gene and cell transfer to the myocardium. Each chapter features a "Notes" section that provides useful "how to" problem-solving insights that are often left unstated in standard published protocols.

Cardiac Cell and Gene Transfer: Principles, Protocols, and Applications addresses principles and applications of cell and gene transfer to the heart, including protocols for vector production and purification. Detailed step-by-step methods and applications for first/second-generation adenoviral vectors, adeno-associated vectors, gutted adenoviral vectors, and lentiviral vectors are included. Additionally, detailed methods for cardiac cell grafting and transplantation are provided, and these chapters highlight the prospects of cell-based therapies for cardiac repair. The book also covers specific in vivo techniques for cardiac gene transfer, and specifies subsequent cellular and organ-level physiological assessment techniques and protocols. Accordingly, this book is designed for basic science and clinical researchers in the academic, pharmaceutical, and biotechnology sectors of the cardiovascular community.

Joseph M. Metzger

Contents

Contributors

FARIS P. ALBAYYA • *Department of Physiology, University of Michigan, Ann Arbor, MI*

LEORA B. BALSAM • *Falk Cardiovascular Research Center, Department of Cardiothoracic Surgery, Stanford University School of Medicine, Stanford, CA*

D. KEITH BISHOP • *General Surgery, University of Michigan Medical Center, Ann Arbor, MI*

ANDREA R. BORTON • *Department of Cardiac Surgery and Department of Physiology, University of Michigan, Ann Arbor, MI*

ADA BUVOLI • *Department of Molecular, Cellular and Developmental Biology, University of Colorado at Boulder, Boulder, CO*

MASSIMO BUVOLI • *Department of Molecular, Cellular and Developmental Biology, University of Colorado at Boulder, Boulder, CO*

BARRY J. BYRNE • *Departments of Pediatrics and Molecular Genetics and Microbiology, University of Florida School of Medicine, Gainesville, FL*

KEVIN S. CAHILL • *Departments of Pediatrics and Molecular Genetics and Microbiology, University of Florida School of Medicine, Gainesville, FL*

JEFFREY S. CHAMBERLAIN • *Department of Neurology, University of Washington School of Medicine, Seattle, WA*

KENNETH R. CHIEN • *Institute of Molecular Medicine, University of California, San Diego, La Jolla, CA*

GEIR CHRISTENSEN • *Institute for Experimental Medical Research, University of Oslo, Ullevaal University Hospital, Oslo, Norway*

WILLIAM C. CLAYCOMB • *Department of Biochemistry and Molecular Biology, Louisiana State University Health Sciences Center, New Orleans, LA*

FEDERICA DEL MONTE • *Cardiovascular Research Center, Massachusetts General Hospital, Charlestown, MA*

J. KEVIN DONAHUE • *Institute of Molecular Cardiobiology, Johns Hopkins University School of Medicine, Baltimore, MD*

DONGSHENG DUAN • *Department of Molecular Microbiology and Immunology School of Medicine, University of Missouri, Columbia, MO*

JOHN F. ENGELHARDT • *Department of Anatomy and Cell Biology, University of Iowa College of Medicine, Iowa City, IA*

DIMITRIOS GEORGAKOPOULOS • *Cardiology Division, Johns Hopkins School of Medicine, Baltimore, MD*

PETER J. GRUBER • *The Cardiac Center, Children's Hospital of Philadelphia, Philadelphia, PA*

ROGER J. HAJJAR • *Cardiology Laboratory of Integrative Physiology and Imaging, Cardiovascular Research Center, Harvard Medical School, Massachusetts General Hospital, Charlestown, MA*

JENNIFER C. HIRSCH • *Department of Surgery, University of Michigan Health System, Ann Arbor, MI*

NORIYUKI KASAHARA • *Institute for Genetic Medicine and Department of Pathology, Keck School of Medicine, University of Southern California, Los Angeles, CA*

DAVID A. KASS • *Cardiology Division, Johns Hopkins University School of Medicine, Baltimore, MD*

LARRY KEDES • *Institute for Genetic Medicine and Department of Biochemistry and Molecular Biology, Keck School of Medicine, University of Southern California, Los Angeles, CA*

PAUL D. KESSLER • *Peter Belfer Laboratory, Division of Cardiology, Johns Hopkins University School of Medicine, Baltimore, MD*

WALTER J. KOCH • *Department of Surgery, Duke University Medical Center, Durham, NC*

STEPHAN E. LEHNART • *Institute of Molecular Cardiobiology, Johns Hopkins University School of Medicine, Baltimore, MD*

LESLIE A. LEINWAND • *Department of Molecular, Cellular and Developmental Biology, University of Colorado at Boulder, Boulder, CO*

DAMIEN LOGEART • *Division of Cardiology, Hôpital Beaujon AP-HP, Clichy France and INSERM U460, Faculté de Médecine X Bichati, University of Paris 7, Paris, France*

GUANYI LU • *Department of General Surgery, University of Michigan Medical Center, Ann Arbor, MI*

JEAN-JACQUES MERCADIER • *Departments of Physiology and Cardiology, Faculté de Médecine X Bichat, University of Paris 7, Paris, France*

JOSEPH M. METZGER • *Department of Physiology, Department of Internal Medicine, and Center for Integrative Genomics, University of Michigan, Ann Arbor, MI*

DOUGLAS N. MINIATI • *Department of Cardiothoracic Surgery, Falk Cardiovascular Research Center, Stanford University School of Medicine, Stanford, CA*

CHARLES E. MURRY • *Department of Pathology, University of Washington School of Medicine, Seattle, WA*

MARK F. PITTENGER • *Osiris Therapeutics Inc., Baltimore, MD*

HANS REINECKE • *Department of Pathology, University of Washington School of Medicine, Seattle, WA*

ROBERT C. ROBBINS • *Department of Cardiothoracic Surgery, Falk Cardiovascular Research Center, Stanford University School of Medicine, Stanford, CA*

TSUYOSHI SAKODA • *Institute for Genetic Medicine, Keck School of Medicine, University of Southern California, Los Angeles, CA*

JEANNINE M. SCOTT • *Department of Neurology, University of Washington School of Medicine, Seattle, WA*

MICHAEL L. SZATKOWSKI • *Albert Einstein Medical Center, Philadelphia, PA*

HENDRIK T. TEVAEARAI • *Department of Surgery, Duke University Medical Center, Durham, NC*

CATALIN TOMA • *Division of Cardiology, Peter Belfer Laboratory, Johns Hopkins University School of Medicine, Baltimore, MD*

YIBIN WANG • *Department of Physiology, University of Maryland School of Medicine, Baltimore, MD*

MARGARET V. WESTFALL • *Cardiac Surgery Section, University of Michigan School of Medicine, Ann Arbor, MI*

STEVEN M. WHITE • *Department of Biochemistry and Molecular Biology, Louisiana State University Health Sciences Center, New Orleans, LA*

YONGPING YUE • *Department of Molecular Microbiology and Immunology School of Medicine, University of Missouri, Columbia, MO*

I

VECTORS FOR CARDIAC GENE TRANSFER

PRODUCTION, PURIFICATION, AND APPLICATIONS

1

Adenoviral Vectors

Production and Purification

Faris P. Albayya and Joseph M. Metzger

1. Introduction

Current methodologies in first-generation adenoviral gene transfer, however novel their approach to vector delivery, are ultimately limited by the purity of the vector being delivered. Purity in this case is defined both from the standpoint of genetic homogeneity, and from the absence of any toxic elements that may jeopardize cellular homeostasis and/or virion-cell receptor interactions. The evolution from plasmid to recombinant adenoviral vector, therefore, necessitates the orchestration of production and purification. In vector development there is a constant need for confirmation stemming from the many vulnerabilities that may be imposed on the system in the cascade of events linking plasmid endocytosis to viral genomic encapsidation. The propensity with which wild-type virions tend to outgrow any engineered competitors is a primary concern in an effort to package and propagate a recombinant adenoviral genome.

This chapter details protocols for cotransfection assays, viral DNA preparations, Southern blot analyses, plaque purification assays, small- and large-scale viral preparations, and the CsCl purification of recombinant virus. The first aspect of development is that of the isolation of infectious viral particles by means of cotransfection assays *(1)*. Recovered from these assays are crude lysates, very often composed of a mixture of recombinant and wild-type viral particles. Identification of lysates bearing recombinant virus is performed by means of Southern blot analysis to determine the best candidate from which to perform plaque purification *(2)*. The plaques harvested and amplified into plaque lysates from the cotransfection samples are themselves applied to a sec-

From: *Methods in Molecular Biology, vol. 219: Cardiac Cell and Gene Transfer*
Edited by: J. M. Metzger © Humana Press Inc., Totowa, NJ

ond round of plaque purification. The second group of plaques is amplified and verified, yielding a candidate from which a relay of expansion assays will be performed and CsCl purified.

2. Materials

2.1. Cell Culture Media and Passaging Solutions

1. Dulbecco's modified Eagle's medium (DMEM, 1X solution; GibcoBRL, Rockville, MD) containing 4500 mg/L D-glucose, L-glutamine, pyridoxine hydrochloride, phenol red, and sodium bicarbonate, but without sodium pyruvate. Supplement 445 mL DMEM with 5 mL of penicillin-streptomycin stock solution (P/S; Gibco-BRL), which contains 5000 U/mL penicillin G (sodium salt) and 5000 μg/mL streptomycin sulfate in 0.85% saline, and also 50 mL fetal bovine serum (FBS, ES cell-qualified; Gibco-BRL). This is stored at 4°C for up to 21 d.
2. Trypsin-EDTA stock solution (T/E, 1X solution; Gibco-BRL) containing 0.5 g/L trypsin (1:250) and 0.2 g/L EDTA (tetrasodium) in Hank's balanced salt solution without calcium chloride, magnesium chloride (hexahydrate), or magnesium sulfate (heptahydrate). Thaw, realiquot, and freeze down as 5-mL samples at –20°C for up to 2 yr.

2.2. Cotransfection Solutions

1. 2X HEPES-buffered saline (2X HBS): Into 80 mL ddH$_2$O, combine 1.6 g NaCl, 0.0215 g Na$_2$HPO$_4$ (anhydrous), 1.0 g HEPES (sodium salt), 0.074 g KCl, and 0.20 g D-(+)-glucose (anhydrous). Adjust to pH 7.05 with 1 *M* HCl. Bring volume up to 100 mL. Sterilize by membrane filtration through a 0.22-μm-membrane filter. Store as 5-mL aliquots at –20°C for up to 1 yr.
2. 2 *M* Calcium chloride stock solution: Into 20 mL ddH$_2$O, add 7.35 g CaCl$_2$ (dihydrate). Bring volume up to 25 mL. Sterilize by membrane filtration through a 0.22-μm-membrane filter. Store as 1-mL aliquots at –20°C for up to 1 yr.

2.3. Viral DNA Isolation Solutions

1. 1 *M* Tris-HCl, pH 8.0: Into 800 mL ddH$_2$O, add 53.0 g Trizma Base (Sigma) and 88.8 g Trizma-HCl (Sigma). Verify the pH to be 8.0. Bring the solution up to 1 L. Sterilize by membrane filtration through a 0.22-μm-membrane filter and store at room temperature for up to 1 yr.
2. Lysis buffer: Into 80 mL ddH$_2$O, add 1 mL of 1 *M* Tris-HCl, pH 8.0, and 6 mL of 10% (w/v) sodium dodecyl sulfate (SDS) stock solution. Bring volume up to 100 mL. Sterilize by membrane filtration through a 0.22-μm-membrane filter and store at room temperature for up to 6 mo. Proteinase K (resuspended in ddH$_2$O and stored as a 10 mg/mL stock solution in 100-μL aliquots at –20°C) is added to yield a final working concentration of 100 μg/mL.
3. 5 *M* Sodium chloride stock solution: Into 80 mL ddH$_2$O, add 29.22 g NaCl (*see* **Note 1**). Bring volume up to 100 mL. Autoclave to sterilize. Store at room temperature for up to 1 yr.

4. 3 *M* Sodium acetate stock solution: Into 80 mL ddH$_2$O, add 40.83 g sodium acetate (trihydrate). Adjust pH to 5.2 with glacial acetic acid. Bring volume up to 100 mL. Autoclave to sterilize. Store at room temperature for up to 1 yr.

5. 0.5 *M* EDTA, pH 8.0: Into 800 mL ddH$_2$O, add 186.1 g of EDTA (disodium salt, dihydrate; Sigma-Aldrich, St. Louis, MO). Adjust the pH to 8.0 using NaOH (~20 g of NaOH pellets; *see* **Note 2**). Bring volume up to 1 L. Sterilize by membrane filtration through a 0.22-μm-membrane filter. Store at room temperature for up to 1 yr.

6. Tris-HCl/EDTA + RNase A solution: Into 80 mL ddH$_2$O, add 1 mL of 1 *M* Tris-HCl, pH 8.0, and 200 μL 0.5 *M* EDTA, pH 8.0, stock solutions. Bring volume up to 100 mL. Sterilize by membrane filtration through a 0.22-μm-membrane filter. Add 1 μL of 10 mg/mL RNase A stock solution (RNase A resuspended in sterile ddH$_2$O and stored in 250-μL aliquots at −20°C) per 1 mL Tris-HCl/EDTA pH 8.0, stock solution. Store at 4°C for up to 3 mo.

2.4. Nonilsotopic Southern Blotting Solutions

1. 20X SSC solution: To make up 1 L, stir 175.32 g NaCl and 88.2 g sodium citrate into 800 mL ddH$_2$O. Adjust the pH to 7.0 with 1 *M* HCl solution and bring volume up to 1 L. Autoclave to sterilize. Store at room temperature for up to 1 yr.

2. 3 *M* NaCl solution: To make up 1 L, stir 175.32 g NaCl into 800 mL ddH$_2$O. Adjust volume to 1 L and sterilize by autoclaving. Store at room temperature for up to 1 yr.

3. 1 *M* Tris-HCl, pH 7.0: To make up 1 L, stir 149.72 g Trizma-HCl and 6.06 g Trizma base into 800 mL ddH$_2$O. Check to make sure pH is ~7.0. Bring up to 1 L and sterilize by membrane filtration through a 0.22-μm-membrane filter. Store at room temperature for up to 1 yr.

4. Hybridization solution (w/o dry milk): To make up 180 mL, add 50 mL 20X SSC, 2 mL of 10% (w/v) *N*-laurylsarcosine solution, and 0.4 mL 10% (w/v) SDS solution to 127.6 mL ddH$_2$O. Filter-sterilize through a 0.22-μm-membrane filter and store at room temperature for up to 1 yr.

5. Maleic acid buffer (pH 7.5): To make up 1 L, stir 11.6 g maleic acid and 8.76 g of NaCl into 800 mL ddH$_2$O. To bring the solution to the proper pH, slowly add ~7.9 g of NaOH pellets, the last few pellets being added while the pH is being read by a pH meter. Bring up to 1 L and autoclave to sterilize. Store at room temperature for up to 1 yr.

6. Standard hybridization solution: To make up 40 mL: Dissolve 1 g of non-fat dry milk in 10 mL of maleic acid buffer (pH 7.5). This may require heating to get the milk into solution. Add 4 mL of the dry-milk solution to 36 mL of hybridization solution.

7. 2X SSC/0.1% SDS solution: To make up 500 mL, bring 50 mL of 20X SSC solution and 5 mL of 10% (w/v) SDS solution up to 500 mL using ddH$_2$O. Filter-sterilize and store at room temperature for up to 1 yr.

8. 1X SSC/0.1% SDS solution: To make up 500 mL, bring 25 mL of 20X SSC solution and 5 mL of 10% (w/v) SDS solution up to 500 mL using ddH$_2$O. Filter-sterilize and store at room temperature for up to 1 yr.

9. 0.1X SSC/0.1% SDS solution: To make up 500 mL, bring 2.5 mL of 20X SSC solution and 5 mL of 10% (w/v) SDS solution up to 500 mL using ddH$_2$O. Filter-sterilize and store at room temperature for up to 1 yr.

10. 10X Washing buffer: Make up a 3% (v/v) polyoxyethylene (20) sorbitan monolaurate solution by adding 3 mL of polyoxyethylene (20) sorbitan monolaurate (Tween-20; Sigma) into a 100 mL volumetric flask, bringing up to volume using maleic acid buffer (pH 7.5). Filter-sterilize and store at room temperature for up to 1 yr. Use maleic acid buffer when diluting to make the 1X working solution. Store at room temperature for up to 1 yr.

11. Detection buffer: To make up 1 L, stir 5.84 g of NaCl and 12.1 g of Trizma base into 800 mL of ddH$_2$O. Adjust the pH to 9.5 using 1 M HCl, and then bring up to 1 L. Autoclave to sterilize. Store at room temperature for up to 6 mo.

12. Blocking buffer: To make up 50 mL: Stir 1.5 g non-fat dry milk into 50 mL of maleic acid buffer, yielding a 3% dry milk blocking buffer solution.

2.5. Plaque Purification Solutions for Overlay

1. 1.6% Noble agar solution: Prepared in 50 mL aliquots by combining 50 mL ddH$_2$O and 0.8 g Noble agar (Becton-Dickinson, Sparks, MD) in a 100-mL bottle to be autoclaved into solution. Cool and store at room temperature for up to 3 mo. When ready to use, microwave to a boil and swirl into solution. Incubate in a 50°C H$_2$O bath to bring the temperature back down to 50°C until ready to mix with MEM-based component for overlay.

2. Modified Eagle's medium (MEM, 2X solution; Gibco-BRL) containing sodium bicarbonate and L-glutamine, but without phenol red (*see* **Note 3**).

3. MEM-based component of plaque assay overlay: Volumes to follow are for the preparation of 80 mL of overlay; combine 40 mL MEM, 3.2 mL FBS, 984 µL of 1 M MgCl$_2$, and 360 µL of P/S. Sterilize by membrane filtration through a 0.22-µm-membrane filter. Incubate in a 37°C H$_2$O bath until ready to mix with 1.6% Noble agar component for overlay.

2.6. CsCl Purification and Dialyzing Solutions

1. 10 mM Tris-HCl/1 mM MgCl$_2$, pH 8.0 stock solution: Into 450 mL ddH$_2$O, add 5 mL 1 M Tris-HCl, pH 8.0 solution, and 500 µL 1 M MgCl$_2$. Bring volume up to 500 mL. Sterilize by membrane filtration through a 0.22-µm-membrane filter and store at room temperature for up to 1 yr.

2. CsCl solutions for viral banding: For 1.1 g/mL CsCl solution, add 11.93 g CsCl (Roche; MB grade, Indianapolis, IN) to a tared beaker on a balance. Using 10 mM Tris-HCl/1 mM MgCl$_2$, pH 8.0, bring weight up to 100 g. Stir into solution. Store at room temperature for up to 1 yr. For 1.3, 1.34, and 1.4 g/mL CsCl solutions, add 31.24, 34.41, and 38.83 g, respectively, bringing each sample weight up to 100 g using 10 mM Tris-HCl/1 mM MgCl$_2$, pH 8.0.

3. Dialyzing solution is composed of solutions A, B, and C (*1*). Solution A: Into 800 mL ddH$_2$O, add 80 g NaCl, 2 g KCl, 11.5 g Na$_2$HPO$_4$ (anhydrous) and 2 g

KH_2PO_4 (anhydrous). Bring volume up to 1 L and sterilize by 0.22-μm-membrane filtration. Solution B: Into 80 mL ddH_2O, add 1 g $CaCl_2$ (dihydrate). Bring volume up to 100 mL and sterilize by 0.2-μm-membrane filtration. Solution C: Into 80 mL ddH_2O, add 1 g $MgCl_2$ (hexahydrate). Bring volume up to 100 mL and sterilize by 0.2-μm-membrane filtration. Solutions A, B, and C can all be stored at room temperature for up to 1 yr. The dialysis solution is then made by sequentially adding 100 mL of solution A, 10 mL of solution B, and 10 mL of solution C to 700 mL ddH_2O. Bring volume up to 1 L and sterilize by 0.2-μm-membrane filtration into a sterilized bottle. This solution should be made up the day before dialyzing and allowed to chill to 4°C.
4. Glycerol is used as the cryogenic agent in the final dialysis solution. Into a sterile bottle, add 100 mL sterilized glycerol (99+%; Sigma). By 0.2-μm-membrane filtration, add 900 mL of dialysis solution. Store at 4°C until ready for dialyzing.

3. Methods
3.1. Passage and Maintenance of Cell Cultures

The cell line utilized in the methods to follow, HEK 293 (American Type Culture Collection, ATCC# CRL-1573), is a human embryonic kidney cell line transformed with adenovirus 5 (Ad 5) DNA in the laboratory of Frank L. Graham *(1)*. All of these procedures are to be performed within a laminar flow hood.

1. For general passaging, following aspiration of the confluent dish, add trypsin-EDTA (1 mL per 60-mm dish, 3 mL per 100-mm dish, or 6 mL per 150-mm dish) and return to the 5% CO_2/37°C-incubator for 3–5 min.
2. Dissipate the cell layer by tapping the side of the dish, and add DMEM w/10% FBS + P/S (3 mL per 60-mm dish, 9 mL per 100-mm dish, or 18 mL per 150-mm dish). Transfer contents to a centrifuge tube. Centrifuge at 201g for 5 min at room temperature.
3. Aspirate off the supernatant. Resuspend the pellet in DMEM w/10% FBS + P/S, diluting 1:3 to 1:12, depending on when cells will be needed. Plate on tissue culture-treated dishes, and incubate in 5% CO_2/37°C incubator. Passing at 1:3 allows for ~90–100% confluence, usually in 2 d; passing at 1:12 allows such confluence within 4–6 d (*see* **Note 4**).

3.2. Cotransfection

The construction of recombinant adenoviral vectors is accomplished by seeding HEK 293 cells with two plasmids enveloped together by means of calcium phosphate precipitation. The first plasmid, pJM17 (Bioserve Biotechnology, Laurel, MD), contains a derivative of the Ad5 genome with a partial deletion in the E1 region, restricting viral propagation to the HEK 293 cell line, which expresses the deleted E1 region *in trans*. In addition, there is a partial deletion in the E3 region, allowing for the incorporation of a pBRX insert. The insert allows for plasmid replication in bacteria but renders the viral genome too large for encapsidation *(3)*. The second plasmid bears an expression cassette containing a cytomegalovirus (CMV) promoter, the protein coding sequence, and the SV40 polyadenylation signal. Two fragments of the Ad5 genome flank the cassette. The homologous architecture of both plasmids allows for the replacement of the pBRX insert with the expression cassette, yielding a packageable, replication-deficient, recombinant genome. All these procedures are to be performed within a laminar flow hood.

1. Passage cells into six to eight 60-mm dishes per sample 2–3 d prior to being assayed, to yield optimal cotransfecting conditions of ~80–85% confluency.
2. Thaw and chill on ice the components of the cotransfection overlay, including 2X HBS, the shuttle vector containing the cDNA cassette, pJM17, and 2 M $CaCl_2$.
3. To a sterile 2-mL tube, add 500 µL 2X HBS, 10 µg shuttle vector, and 10 µg pJM17. Bring the volume up to 937.5 µL using sterile ddH_2O. Mix components by inversion. Add 62.5 µL of 2 M $CaCl_2$ and mix by inversion.
4. Incubate cotransfection mixtures at room temperature for 1 h.
5. Aspirate plates (two plates per reaction mixture) and replenish with 3.5 mL of DMEM w/10% FBS + P/S per dish during the 1-h mixture incubation period.
6. Add 500 µL of each mixture, in a drop-wise fashion, to each designated plate. With minimal swirling, return to the 5% CO_2/37°C-incubator for 4 h.
7. Gently aspirate each plate. Wash each dish with 4 mL PBS prewarmed to 37°C. Aspirate plates and replenish each with 4 mL DMEM w/10% FBS + P/S. Return to incubator for 16–24 h.
8. Aspirate and replenish each dish with 3 mL DMEM w/10% FBS + P/S. Return to incubator.
9. The plates should be fed 1–2 mL DMEM w/10% FBS + P/S every 2–3 d until ~d 7, being mindful not to exceed a total dish volume of ~8 mL *(see* **Note 5***)*.
10. Cytopathic effect (CPE) is visualized 6–11 d post-cotransfection. The plate should be allowed to reach 100% CPE with ~100% cell layer detachment, usually 5–10 d after initial plaque formation. Collect contents and freeze down at –20°C.
11. Release and rescue of the viral particles is dependent on the lysing of the cells. This is accomplished by a series of four freezing and thawing cycles by means of a 37°C H_2O bath and a dry-ice/EtOH bath. Try to minimize the duration of time past completion of each thaw (i.e., the visual observation of no ice) in the 37°C H_2O bath to reduce the chance of the lysate temperature increasing to a virus-deactivating level.
12. Spin down the samples for 10 min at 1258g and 4°C. Recover the supernatant and aliquot as 1.5-mL samples in cryogenic vials to be frozen down at –20°C.

3.3. Viral DNA Isolation

To verify both the presence of recombinant virions and the correct cDNA insertion location and orientation within these particles, viral DNA must be acquired for Southern blot analyses.

1. Passage HEK 293 cells into 60-mm dishes, one plate needed per cotransfection sample, 2–3 d before, to yield a confluency of 95–100%.
2. Add 50–200 µL of each cotransfection crude lysate to 1 mL DMEM w/10% FBS + P/S. Aspirate the plates, inoculate, and incubate for 1 h in a 5% CO_2/37°C incubator. For optimal viral distribution, rocking the plates every 10 min during the incubation is recommended (*see* **Note 6**).
3. Overlay each plate with an additional 3 mL DMEM w/10% FBS + P/S. Return to the incubator overnight.
4. Check CPE development after 24 h. The plates should exhibit ~50–75% CPE with minimal cell detachment. Return to the incubator overnight.
5. At 36–48 h post infection, the cell layers should reveal ~100% CPE, with most of the cells still adhering to the plate. Gently aspirate each dish. Carefully apply, swirl, and aspirate 4-mL PBS rinse (*see* **Note 7**).
6. Add 800 µL of lysis buffer (fortified with Proteinase K) to each plate and incubate in 5% CO_2/37°C-incubator for 1 h.
7. Add 200 µL of 5 M NaCl to each plate in a dropwise fashion. Swirl each plate to thoroughly mix. Incubate on ice for 1 h.
8. Collect the viscous contents of each plate into a microcentrifuge tube. Spin down in the centrifuge at 20,800g and 4°C for 1 h.
9. Using a flame-sterilized inoculation loop, remove and discard the pelleted cellular debris from each tube. Divide each remaining supernatant into two microcentrifuge tubes of equal volume.
10. Add an equal volume of phenol/chloroform/isoamyl alcohol (25:24:1; Fisher Scientific, Pittsburgh, PA) to each tube. Invert 5–6 times until the aqueous layer (top) appears cloudy. Centrifuge at 20,800*g* and 4°C for 15 min.
11. Carefully recover the aqueous layer, which at this point should appear clear, into another tube. Be sure to record the volume. Add 2 vol of absolute ethanol (200 proof) and 1/10 vol of 3 M sodium acetate. Incubate at –20°C for at least 30 min. The samples may remain incubated for up to a month, if necessary.
12. Spin down samples at 20,800*g* and 4°C for 20 min.
13. Aspirate off the supernatant, add 1 mL of 70% ethanol per sample, and spin down at 20,800*g* and 4°C for 10 min.
14. Aspirate off the supernatant and allow the pellets, which should appear white at this point, to air-dry. The pellets will appear transparent once they are dry, usually within 5–10 min. Do not overdry, which may inhibit resuspension.
15. Resuspend each pellet in 15 µL of TE + RNase A and incubate in a 37°C water bath for 1 h.
16. Combine like samples and freeze down at –20°C.

3.4. Nonisotopic Southern Blot

This assay is derived from the Southern hybridization protocol described in **ref. 2**. Set up digests that will verify the correct location and orientation of the desired DNA fragment.

1. Perform restriction endonuclease digestions on the viral DNA samples, usually between 8 and 10 μg.
2. In a separate digestion of 1–2 μg of the shuttle vector, isolate and gel-purify the cDNA fragment. Bring 30 ng of the purified cDNA up to 16 μL using sterile ddH_2O
3. Heat-denature sample by submerging in boiling ddH_2O for 10 min. Quick chill in a dry ice/EtOH bath for 30 s while adding 4 μL of 5X DIG High Prime labeling mix (Roche). Remove and thaw on ice. Mix and incubate in 37°C H_2O bath for 20 h. Terminate reaction with labeling mix by adding 4 μL of 100 mM EDTA solution (pH 8.0). Store at –20°C.
4. Separate fragments on a 0.8% agarose gel run at 80–90 V along with the isolated cDNA fragment, functioning as the positive control. Capture UV pictures of the banding patterns accompanied by a fluorescent ruler to assist in manipulation of the transfer membrane in the steps to follow.
5. Transfer DNA from the agarose gel to a nylon membrane by means of a standard capillary action transfer.
6. Prehybridize the membrane by incubating in standard hybridization solution for 1 h at 68°C in a hybridization oven.
7. Add 5X DIG High Prime-labeled probe to 20 mL of standard hybridization solution. Heat-denature the sample by submerging in boiling ddH_2O for 10 min. Discard prehybridization solution and replace with probed-hybridization solution. Incubate overnight at 68°C in hybridization oven.
8. Pour off and freeze-down probed-hybridization solution at –20°C, which may be used up to 4 more times. Perform duplicate 15-min washes with 2X SSC/0.1% SDS solution at 68°C in the hybridization oven.
9. Continue with duplicate 1X SSC/0.1% SDS solution washes for 15 min at 68°C, followed by one wash in 0.1X SSC/0.1% SDS solution, also at 68°C in the hybridization oven for 15 min.
10. Wash membrane in 1X washing buffer for 1 min at room temperature. Transfer membrane to 25 mL of blocking solution. Incubate on rocking platform for 1 h at room temperature.
11. Dilute 2.5 μL of anti-digoxigenin-AP conjugate (FAB fragments; Roche) in 25 mL of blocking solution. Discard first wash and add blocking/antibody solution. Incubate on rocking platform for 30 min at room temperature.
12. Set up autoradiography cassette with a tapered sheet protector or Saran wrap to act as an envelope in the developing process. Incubate at 37°C for 15 min prior to loading film.
13. Discard blocking solution. Perform two 15-min 1X washing buffer solution washes.
14. Rinse in detection buffer for 2 min at room temperature.
15. Lay the transfer membrane flat on top of the taped-down flap of the sheet protector or Saran wrap. In a dropwise manner, add 10–20 evenly distributed CSPD Ready-To-Use (Roche) solution drops to the membrane. Fold the other flap down. In a circular motion, wipe a paper towel over the top flap to push out any bubbles or excess solution to the Whatman paper that should line the bottom of the cassette.

16. Load film. Incubate at 37°C for 10–15 min. Develop film, reexposing for longer or shorter durations as needed.

3.5. Plaque Purification of Viral Lysates

The objective of the plaque purification assay is to isolate virions derived from a single plaque. A single plaque is the end result of the replication and packaging of a single viral particle's genome, eventually causing the lysis of that cell and dispersion of virions infecting the neighboring cells, leading to the formation of the plaque. Since the lysate harvested from the cotransfection assay very likely possesses both recombinant and wild-type virions, this purification is a means of isolating either recombinant or wild-type virus.

1. HEK 293 cells need to be plated 2–3 d before to yield a confluency of ~85–90%.
2. Make up the MEM component of the overlay and incubate at 37°C. Microwave 1.6% Noble agar and incubate in 50°C H_2O bath.
3. The initial inoculation is in DMEM with 2% FBS + P/S. Dilute DMEM w/10% FBS + P/S 1:5 in serum-free DMEM + P/S. Incubate in 37°C H_2O bath.
4. Viral dilutions of a cotransfection lysate or plaque lysate of the sample begin with a 1:10 dilution by adding 120 µL of the lysate to 1.080 mL DMEM with 2% FBS + P/S. The next dilution, 1:1000, is prepared by adding 12 µL of the prepared 1:10 dilution into 1.188 mL of DMEM w/2% FBS + P/S. The 10^{-5} dilution is prepared by adding 12 µL of the 10^{-3} dilution into 1.188 mL of DMEM w/2% FBS + P/S, and the 10^{-6} is prepared by adding 120 µL of the 10^{-5} dilution into 1.080 mL of DMEM w/2% FBS + P/S. The final two dilutions to be prepared are the 10^{-7} and 10^{-8}, the first by adding 120 µL of the 10^{-6} into 1.080 mL of DMEM w/2% FBS + P/S and the second by adding 120 µL of the 10^{-7} into 1.080 mL of DMEM w/2% FBS + P/S. The rationale for making greater than 1 mL of each dilution is to ensure that a 1-mL inoculant will be able to be delivered.
5. Aspirate four 60-mm dishes and infect with 1 mL of the 10^{-5}, 10^{-6}, 10^{-7}, and 10^{-8} dilutions. Incubate for 1 h, rocking the plates every 10 min to ensure uniform infection.
6. Aspirate plates. Combine overlay components. Gently add 8 mL of overlay to each plate *see* **Note 8**). Let the plates sit in the hood at room temperature for 30 min to allow the overlay to polymerize. Return the plates to the incubator.
7. Plaques should become visible 4–7 d post infection. Circle plaques on the bottom of the plate. Using a 10–100-µL pipettor set at 50 µL, depress the pipettor and plug the plaque, easing the button up after the tip touches the bottom, and then pulling the tip out after the entire contents have been taken up.
8. Deposit each plaque/agar plug into 1 mL of DMEM w/10% FBS + P/S. The samples are then frozen down at –20°C.
9. Plaque expansion assays are performed to yield a plaque lysate from each collected plaque. This is accomplished by infecting an 85%-confluent 60-mm dish with the thawed, collected 1 mL-sample, incubating for 1 h, and then overlaying with 3 mL of DMEM w/10% FBS + P/S. Allow the plate to reach 100% CPE with 100% cell layer detachment from the plate.

10. The plaque lysates, once having gone through the freeze–thaw (four times) process, can then be used to inoculate plates for viral DNA isolations to be digested and assayed by means of Southern blotting, verifying the presence and correct orientation of the cDNA. This is termed the first-round plaque purification. From these results, one of the plaque lysates that tests positive is used to seed a second set of plaque assays, from which plaques are once again picked, expanded, and verified by Southern blotting. This is the second-round plaque purification.

3.6. Small-Scale Viral Preparation

Having isolated a lysate possessing the cDNA in the correct orientation and location within the viral genome, the next step involves the serial expansion of this sample to the point at which a large-scale preparation may be seeded for isolation and purification of a concentrated viral stock.

1. With the lysate recovered in the conclusion of the second-round plaque purification assay, five 60-mm dishes at a cellular confluence of 90–95% are inoculated with 500 µL of recovered lysate/dish. Using serum-free DMEM + P/S, dilute 2.5 mL of the recovered lysate in 2.5 mL of media. Aspirate the plates and administer a 1 mL inoculation volume per dish. Incubate for 1 h in a 5% CO_2/37°C-incubator, rocking the plate every 10 min.
2. Overlay each plate with an additional 3 mL of DMEM w/10% FBS + P/S. Incubate overnight.
3. At the 24-h postinfection time point, the plates should be exhibiting approx 100% CPE (*see* **Note 9**). Usually, an additional 24-h incubation period will bring the plates to harvestable conditions, namely at 80–100% of the rounded-up cells are detached from the plate surface. Harvest, perform routine freeze/thaw (4X) protocol, aliquot into one tube, and freeze down at –20°C.
4. The next serial infection calls for the inoculation and harvesting of five 100-mm dishes, similar to the previous infection, except 10 mL of the previously recovered lysate is diluted in 5 mL of serum-free DMEM + P/S allowing for 3 mL-inoculation volumes to be administered to each dish. Following the 1-h incubation period, an additional 7 mL of DMEM w/10% FBS + P/S is overlaid on each dish. Incubate, harvest, freeze-thaw, and store as performed in the previous expansion assays.
5. The final serial infection requires ten 150-mm dishes. The entire recovered volume of lysate from the five 100-mm dish expansion assay is brought up to a total volume of 60 mL using serum-free DMEM. Each plate is inoculated with 6.0 mL of diluted lysate. Following the 1-h incubation, an additional 14 mL of DMEM w/10% FBS + P/S is overlaid on each dish. Incubate, harvest, and freeze-thaw as performed in the previous expansion assays. Freeze down the sample at –20°C.

3.7. Large-Scale Viral Preparation

The lysate rescued in this assay will go on to be purified via CsCl gradient purification methods.

1. Plate 100 150-mm dishes 5–6 d prior to infection to yield a confluency of 90–95%.
2. Into three sterilized tissue-culture bottles, divide the recovered lysate from the 10 150-mm dish expansion assay into three equal volumes. Bring each volume up to 200 mL with serum-free DMEM + P/S. Since cell adherence to the plates is temperature-dependent, only 10–14 dishes should be infected at one time.
3. Aspirate 11 dishes. Infect each plate with 6 mL of diluted recovered lysate. Return plates to the incubator for a 1-h incubation. Infect the next set of 10 plates. Upon returning the second set of plates, rock the first set of dishes. Before the third set of plates is aspirated, place the second 200 mL of diluted lysate in a 37°C H_2O-bath. As the third set of inoculated plates is returned to the incubator, rock the first and second sets.
4. Remove the second 200 mL of diluted lysate and follow the same procedure as dictated for the first 33 dishes, followed by the third set.
5. Allow the plates to incubate for 48 h, checking for proper infection progression at the 24-h time point.
6. Deposit the rescued lysate of two plates into a 50-mL centrifuge tube, harvesting 10 dishes at a time. Incubate tubes at 37°C in a 5% CO_2 incubator. Harvest the remaining dishes in the same manner, transferring each set to the incubator.
7. Spin down tubes at 201g for 5 min and 4°C. This step may require the tubes to be divided depending on the capacity of the centrifuge.
8. Into a bleach bucket, carefully dump off the supernatant of each tube. Dispense 16.5 mL of 10 mM Tris-HCl,1 mM $MgCl_2$ pH 8.0 solution into the first tube (or 0.5 mL/plate harvested). Resuspend the pellet. Transfer the resuspension volume to the second tube and continue down the line. Continue through all 17. The final tube containing the resuspended pellets from all 33 plates is frozen down at –80°C.
9. Repeat the procedure for the next two sets of 33 (or 34) plates.
10. Freeze-thaw samples 4 times, stopping at the fourth freeze-down. Store tubes at –80°C.

3.8. CsCl Purification and Dialysis of Large-Scale Viral Preparation

These procedures are all to be performed in a laminar flow hood, except for 4°C dialysis incubations, which should be sealed to prevent any airborne contamination.

1. Thaw resuspended pellet solutions from the large preparation in a 37°C H_2O bath. Spin down tubes in Eppendorf 5810R for 10 min at 1811g and room temperature.
2. Transfer supernatants to new tubes, being careful to record the recovered volumes. Add 5 µL/mL of recovered supernatant of both 10 mg/mL RNase A and 10 mg/mL DNase I stock solutions (RNase A and DNase I resuspended in sterile ddH_2O and stored in 250-µL aliquots at –20°C) yielding final concentrations of 50 µg/mL. Incubate in a 37°C H_2O bath for 15 min (swirling every 2–3 min).
3. Weigh out 0.135 g of CsCl/mL of recovered supernatant and add to each tube. Dissolve CsCl into solution by inverting the tube 8–10 times.

4. Spin down samples in Eppendorf 5810R for 10 min at 3220g and 4°C. This is a clarifying spin to remove any residual cellular debris.

5. Transfer supernatants to new tubes, being careful to record the recovered volumes. Place samples on a bed of ice.

6. Pour CsCl gradients: With X equaling the volume of recovered supernatant, dispense (31-X) mL of 1.3 g/mL CsCl solution into each of the three Beckman Ultra-Clear centrifuge tubes. Carefully add 7 mL of 1.4 g/mL CsCl solution under 1.3 g/mL CsCl solution to form a step gradient (*see* **Note 10**). Mark a dot at the interface of the two layers to be used as a reference point later in the assay.

7. Carefully add each lysate on top of the step gradient (**Fig. 1**). Load tubes into the swing buckets of the Beckman SW28 rotor. Create a balance using the same volumes used to create the step gradient, as well as the volume of lysate overlaid on the gradient using 1.1 g/mL CsCl solution, which is approximately the same density as the recovered lysate (fortified with CsCl).

8. Spin in a Beckman L8-80M Ultra-Centrifuge for 4 h at 80,800g and 5°C.

9. Carefully remove the tubes and place in tube holder of band-pulling apparatus (**Fig. 2**). Using an 18GA short-beveled needle attached to a 5-mL syringe, puncture the tube approx 2–3 mm below the banded virus, which will appear at the interface of the step gradient indicated by the dot previously marked (*see* **step 6**). With the bevel facing upward, coming into contact with the bottom of the band, draw the syringe plunger up, collecting as much of the opaque band as possible.

10. Load the band into an OptiSeal centrifuge tube. Fill the remainder volume of the tube with chilled 1.34 g/mL CsCl solution up to the base of the neck, avoiding any droplets on the neck surface. Tap out any bubbles. Seal tubes. Weigh and balance as needed. It is imperative that the weights of the opposing sample or balance be as close to equal as possible (within 0.05 g).

11. Load the Beckman NVT65 rotor. Spin in a Beckman L8-80M Ultra-Centrifuge for 16–20 h at 378,000g and 5°C.

12. Remove tubes and load in band-pulling setup. Gently remove the OptiSeal tube cap. Using an 18-gauge short-beveled needle attached to a 5-mL syringe, puncture the tube 1–2 mm below the band and draw out with minimal amount of excess CsCl solution. Load into a 10000 MWCO Slide-A-Lyzer cassette (Pierce, Rockford, IL).

13. With the buoy attached, float cassette in 1 L of chilled, sterilized PBS solution (glassware/ stir bar sterilized as well). On a stir plate in a 4°C cold room, start solution stirring at a very slow rate for 1–2 h.

14. Transfer cassette to 1 L of chilled, sterilized PBS w/10% glycerol solution (glassware/stir bar sterilized as well) for 16–20 h.

15. Draw 2 mL of air into a 5-mL syringe with an 18-gauge needle. Entering from a new hole, puncture the cassette and dispense the 2 mL of air. Holding the syringe with the needle pointing upward, the cassette still attached, draw up the band and deposit into sterile tube. The band can be diluted with sterile PBS w/10% glycerol solution, if needed.

16. Aliquot into cryovials as 25, 50, and/or 100 µL-sized samples. Freeze down at –80°C.

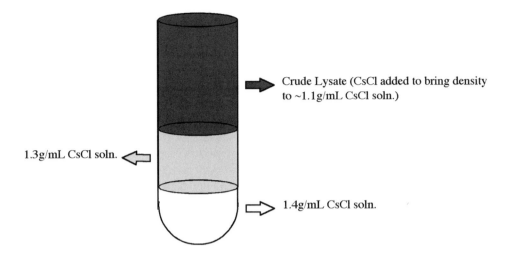

Fig. 1. Crude lysate/CsCl step gradient layout.

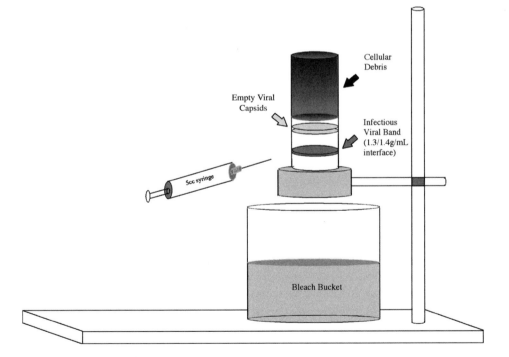

Fig. 2. Viral band-pulling apparatus.

4. Notes

1. The solution may need to be heated to solubilize the NaCl.
2. The disodium salt of EDTA will not go into solution until the pH has been adjusted to ~8.0.
3. Because the MEM utilized in this protocol does not contain phenol red, it is often difficult to gauge the pH of the solution visually. Since the pH is critical in the overlay used for the plaque purification assays, it is essential that the freshness of the MEM be monitored, usually by discarding any opened MEM older than 21 d.
4. For larger dilution passages, i.e. 1:8–1:12, it is a good idea to aspirate and replenish the media on each dish every 2–3 d to maintain optimum physiologic pH conditions.
5. The reason for the cutoff point in the addition of media is twofold. The more media added, the greater the titer of the developing lysate is diluted, thus prolonging harvestable conditions. The problem this may pose is that as the virus is made and propagated, the pH of the media often decreases, threatening the integrity of the viral capsids and ultimately the titer. Second, by limiting the volume, an attempt is made to maximize the titer of the rescued lysate, facilitating the steps to follow.
6. Depending on the time that was required to reach harvesting conditions in the cotransfection assay, the volume of stock virus used to inoculate the plates for viral DNA isolation assay should be adjusted accordingly. For instance, a lysate harvested by d 11 probably bears a higher titer than a lysate harvested at d 21. Therefore, 35–50 µL should be used for higher titer stocks and 150–500 µL used for lower titer lysates. These suggested volumes are approximations in order to retain the 48-h time frame needed for optimal viral DNA recovery.
7. If the cells appear to be loose, it is often recommended to skip the PBS rinse in order to preserve the intact nature of the cell layer. Most of the residual impurities will be filtered out in the phenol/chloroform/isoamyl alcohol extraction.
8. Be sure to add the overlay to the inside wall of the plate, rather than directly onto the cell layer. Since the overlay temperature is going to be greater than 37°C, this could cause the cells to come up off the plate and should be avoided.
9. Depending on the titer of the recovered plaque lysate, 36–48 h may be needed to reach these CPE conditions. Unlike the cotransfection lysate titer issue, an additional 24–48 h should not alter the prescribed inoculation volumes in the small-scale preparation protocol seeding with the plaque lysate.
10. The calculated volume of 1.3 g/mL CsCl solution should be added first. Draw up the 7 mL volume of 1.4 g/mL CsCl and submerge the pipet all the way to the bottom of the centrifuge tube. Very gently release the solution, which should stack under the 1.3 g/mL CsCl layer. Be sure to hold the tube up to the light afterwards to check for a sharply defined interface between the two layers. This is the position that should be marked for banding/collection reference.

References

1. Graham, F. L. and Prevec, L. (1991) Manipulation of adenovirus vectors, in *Gene Transfer and Expression Protocols*, vol. 7 (Murray, E. J., ed.), Humana, Totowa, NJ, pp. 109–128.
2. Sambrook, J., Fritsch, E. F., and Maniatis, T. (1989) Analysis of genomic DNA by Southern hybridization in, *Molecular Cloning-A Laboratory Manual*, 2nd ed. (Irwin, N., ed.), Cold Spring Haprbor Laboratory, Cold Spring Harbor, NY, pp. 9.31–9.62.
3. Westfall, M. V., Rust, E. M., Albayya, F., and Metzger, J. M. (1998) Adenovirus-mediated myofilament gene transfer into adult cardiac myocytes, in *Methods in Muscle Biology*, vol. 52 (Emerson, C. P. and Sweeney, H. L., eds.), Academic, San Diego, CA, pp. 307–322.

2

Gutted Adenoviral Vectors for Gene Transfer to Muscle

Jeannine M. Scott and Jeffrey S. Chamberlain

1. Introduction

Adenoviral vectors are a popular choice for gene transfer protocols because they are well characterized, have a relatively large cloning capacity (up to 36 kB), and can be grown to high titers (10^{13} particles/mL) *(1)*. Despite these attributes, first-generation adenoviral vectors retain many viral genes that can elicit a strong immune response, severely limiting their utility for studies in vivo *(2)*. Our laboratory and others have been developing "gutted" or helper-dependent adenoviruses, which lack all viral coding sequences and therefore should greatly enhance the persistence of the vector in vivo *(3,4)*. We have used this technology to deliver to muscle full-length cDNAs of the largest known gene, dystrophin, under control of the mouse muscle creatine kinase enhancer plus promoter *(4–6)*.

By design, gutted adenoviral vectors must be grown in the presence of a helper virus to supply *in trans* all the viral proteins required for growth and replication of the gutted genome. Consequently, the gutted vector must then be purified away from the helper virus that is simultaneously produced. Specific packaging cell lines may be very useful for limiting the production of infectious helper virus while promoting the growth of the gutted virus. This chapter describes the methods used by our laboratory for generating, expanding, and titering gutted adenoviral vectors for gene transfer to muscle.

1.1. General Features of Gutted Adenoviral Vectors

The structure of a gutted adenovirus is a double stranded DNA genome that has at its termini the adenoviral inverted terminal repeat (ITR) sequences. These sequences, along with the covalently attached adenoviral terminal pro-

From: *Methods in Molecular Biology, vol. 219: Cardiac Cell and Gene Transfer*
Edited by: J. M. Metzger © Humana Press Inc., Totowa, NJ

tein, serve as the natural origin of replication *(4,7,8)*. Adjacent to the left ITR is the viral packaging sequence, which is made up of seven A/T-rich pseudo-repeats normally located between 240 and 375 bp from the left end of the adenovirus 5 (Ad5) genome *(9)*. The remaining length of the sequence is comprised of the desired expression construct(s) including regulatory elements, reporter genes, and "stuffer" sequences. Although the maximum length of an adenoviral genome can be 37.6 kB *(10)*, for the purpose of purification from helper virus (see below), we recommend that the total length of the gutted virus genome be 27–30 kB. Smaller genome sizes have been observed to rearrange, necessitating the inclusion of a noncoding stuffer DNA fragment if the expression cassette being studied is too small *(11)*.

1.2. Role of the Helper Virus

The ideal helper virus provides robust adenoviral gene expression yet does not compete with or interfere with packaging of the gutted virus. We use helper viruses that are replication-deficient owing to deletion of viral sequences in the Ad early region 1 (E1A and B genes). These gene products are supplied by the packaging cell line. This strategy ensures that any helper virus that escapes negative selection and is copurified with the gutted virus cannot replicate in a nonpermissive cell. To restrict amplification of the helper virus, we use helper viruses that contain "floxed" packaging signals, i.e., the packaging signal is flanked by *lox*P sites. One of our packaging cell lines, C7-cre, constitutively expresses cre recombinase, which recognizes the *lox*P sites and excises sequences between them. This cell line is capable of selecting against expansion of the helper virus by removing the packaging signal from >99% of the helper virus genomes *(12)*, conferring to the gutted virus a competitive advantage for packaging proteins and ultimately producing higher yields.

1.3. Construction of Viral Genomes in Plasmid Backbones

Although construction of the large plasmids that contain the gutted or helper virus genomes can be problematic, we have had good success using a method of homologous recombination in *E. coli*. With this method, expression cassettes and/or stuffer fragments are inserted into the gutted virus shuttle vector that contains the adenoviral ITRs and packaging signals. Unique restriction sites are inserted just outside of the ITRs and are used for template preparation prior to viral rescue (*see* **Subheading 3.1.**). This digestion releases the viral genome from the bacterial origin of replication and antibiotic resistance gene of the plasmid backbone.

1.4. Rescue, Amplification, and Purification of Gutted Viruses

To initiate the production of a gutted virus, linear templates of both the gutted and helper viruses are cotransfected into an E1A/E1B-complimenting cell line, such as 293 cells *(13)*. We use the C7 cell line, which was derived from 293 cells and stably expresses the adenoviral polymerase and preterminal proteins *(14,15)*. These proteins improve the conversion of DNA templates to viral genomes, a process we refer to as viral "rescue" *(16)*. If a plasmid-embedded helper virus is not available, one can also initiate gutted virus production using protease-digested viral DNA in the cotransfection, or simply by adding purified helper virus 16–20 h following transfection of the gutted virus template *(3,4)*. When viral cytopathic effects (CPEs) are observed in all cells, the cells are harvested with their growth medium and the viral titer is amplified on larger monolayers of cells through three to six passages until the desired titer is achieved, usually 10^{11} particles per 150-mm dish. The virus from the final cell lysate is purified through two CsCl gradients: the first gradient separates the viruses from cellular components and debris, whereas the second gradient separates the gutted virus from the helper virus. The virus is then dialyzed, titered, and stored in aliquots at –70°C.

2. Materials

1. 293 Cells (or derivatives such as C7 or C7-cre cells).
2. Tissue culture dishes (60, 100, and 150 mm) and 24-well plates.
3. DMEM + FBS: Dulbecco's modified Eagle's medium with L-glutamine supplemented with 10% Fetal bovine serum (FBS) and 100 µg/mL each penicillin G and streptomycin (all from GibcoBRL, Rockville, MD).
4. Phenol/chloroform (1:1) mixture.
5. Ethanol.
6. 0.1X TE: 1 mM Tris-HCl, 0.1 mM EDTA, adjust pH to 8 with 1 M HCl.
7. 2X HEPES-buffered saline (HBS): 20 mM HEPES, 150 mM NaCl, pH 7.03, 0.22-µm filter sterilized.
8. CaCl$_2$, 2 M.
9. Chloroquine, 100 mM.
10. Phosphate-buffered saline (PBS), pH 7.4 (Gibco-BRL).
11. 30% Glycerol in water, 0.45-µm filter sterilized.
12. 10% NP-40 in sterile water.
13. 250-mL Centrifuge bottles (Kendro Laboratory Products, Newtown, CT).
14. 20% (w/v) polyethylene glycol (PEG) 8000, 2.5 M NaCl (0.45 µm filtered).
15. Cell scraper (Sarstedt, Newton, NC).
16. DNase I (10 mg/mL).
17. RNase A (10 mg/mL).
18. 20 mM Tris-HCl, pH 8.0, 1 mM MgCl$_2$.
19. CsCl (density 1.3 g/mL) in 20 mM Tris-HCl, pH 8.0 (0.45 µm filtered).
20. CsCl (density 1.34 g/mL) in 20 mM Tris-HCl, pH 8.0 (0.45 µm filtered).
21. CsCl (density 1.4 g/mL) in 20 mM Tris-HCl, pH 8.0 (0.45 µm filtered).
22. CsCl (powder).
23. Dialysis membrane or cassettes (10,000 mw cutoff; Slide-a-Lyzer, Pierce, Rockford, IL).

24. 20 mM HEPES, pH 7.4.
25. 20 mM HEPES, pH 7.4 with 5% sucrose.
26. Virion lysis solution: 0.1% sodium dodecyl sulfate (SDS), 10 mM Tris-HCl, pH 7.4, and 1 mM EDTA.
27. EcR-293 cells (Invitrogen, Carlsbad, CA) .
28. Ponasterone A (Invitrogen) in 100% ethanol.
29. 24-Well culture dish coated with poly-L-lysine (Becton Dickinson, Bedford, MA).
30. PBS with 0.5% glutaraldehyde.
31. NBT/BCIP tablets (Sigma, St. Louis, MO).
32. X-gal substrate solution: 1 mg/mL X-gal, 41 mg/mL $K_3Fe(CN)_6$, 52 mg/mL $K_4Fe(CN)_6 \cdot 3H_2O$, 1 mM $MgCl_2$ in PBS.
33. Taqman Universal PCR Master mix (Applied Biosystems, Foster City, CA).
34. PCR primers.
35. Taqman probe (Applied Biosystems).
36. Real-time polymerase chain reaction (PCR) thermocycler/detector.

3. Methods

3.1. Rescue of Gutted Viruses by Cotransfection

To initiate a gutted virus preparation, linear gutted and helper virus templates are cotransfected into C7 cells. After 6–10 d, when all the cells have been infected, the titer of the gutted virus will be between 10^5 and 10^7 transducing units (tu)/mL, and the helper virus titers will be between 10^8 and 10^9 tu/mL. Ideally, the gutted virus titer following rescue will be $>10^6$ tu/mL, allowing for a multiplicity of infection (MOI) of 1 for the gutted virus during the next passage. It has been reported that optimal titers of gutted virus are obtained when the termini of the gutted and helper input DNA are identical *(17)*. When one uses purified viral DNA as the source for helper virus rescue, the termini are covalently linked to terminal protein, making this an ideal substrate for replication. In this case, the gutted virus template is an inferior competitor for replication by the C7 cells and will ultimately be produced at much lower titers.

1. Seed a 60-mm tissue culture dish with approx 10^6 C7 cells in 5 mL of DMEM + FBS. Incubate until these cells reach approx 80% confluency, usually overnight (*see* **Note 1**).
2. Digest 5 µg each of the gutted and helper plasmid DNAs to release the viral genome templates completely from the plasmid backbone (*see* **Note 2**).
3. Extract the digested DNA with phenol/chloroform 1 time and then ethanol-precipitate, using caution to avoid shearing the long DNA fragments during these steps. Resuspend the DNA pellet in 220 µL 0.1X TE, pH 8.0.
4. Add 250 µL of 2X HBS and mix (*see* **Note 3**).
5. Precipitate the DNA by slowly adding 31 µL of 2 M $CaCl_2$ with gentle and constant mixing. Incubate the solution for 20 min at 22°C.

6. Add 5.5 µL of 100 m*M* chloroquine to the culture medium, gently rock the plate, and then add the DNA dropwise to the cells. Incubate at 37°C for 4.5 h in a tissue culture incubator (*see* **Note 4**).
7. Glycerol shock the cells by aspirating the medium from the cells and gently washing the monolayer with prewarmed PBS. Aspirate the PBS and then add 1.5 mL of 15% glycerol/1X HBS solution to the cells. After 40 s, remove the glycerol solution and rinse the cells twice with PBS.
8. Re-feed the plates with fresh DMEM + FBS. Incubate at 37°C until viral CPE reaches 100%, usually 8–12 d (*see* **Note 5**).
9. Collect the cells and medium from the plate and freeze/thaw 3 times in a dry ice-ethanol bath and a 37°C water bath. Store at –70°C. This is referred to as P0.

3.2. Amplification and Purification of Gutted Adenovirus

The titer and absolute amount of gutted virus is increased through several rounds of infection (passages). Below is a general outline of how the gutted virus can be expanded on C7-cre cells. This procedure may be modified based on empiric data for each unique gutted virus.

3.2.1. Amplification Through Serial Passages

1. Prepare a 100-mm tissue culture dish with an 80% confluent monolayer of C7-cre cells.
2. Inoculate the cells with 1.3 mL of infected cell lysate (P0) obtained from the co-transfection procedure (*see* **Subheading 3.1.** and **Note 6**). Incubate until CPE is complete, usually 2–4 d. Harvest the lysate and freeze/thaw as described in **Subheading 3.1., step 9**. Store at –70°C.
3. Titer the gutted and helper viruses in this lysate (P1) using one of the procedures described in **Subheading 3.3.**
4. Prepare a 150-mm tissue culture dish with an 80% confluent monolayer of C7-cre cells.
5. Inoculate the plate with 2 mL of infected cell lysate (P1) supplemented with the appropriate amount of purified helper virus. The additional amount required (if any) should be based on the titer of the helper virus in P1. The final helper virus MOI should be 5–10 tu per cell. Incubate the cells until CPE is complete, usually 2–4 d. Harvest the lysate and freeze/thaw as above. Store at –70°C.
6. Titer the helper and gutted viruses produced in this passage (P2) as described in **Subheading 3.3.**
7. The final 2 rounds of amplification are carried out as in **steps 5–6**, using 10 and, then 50–100 × 150-mm dishes of C7–cre cells (*see* **Note 7**).
8. When CPE is complete in the final round of infection, harvest the cells and medium by adding 1 mL of 10% NP–40 to dissolve all cell membranes and transfer the lysate into 250 mL centrifuge bottles. Freeze the lysate in a dry ice–ethanol bath and store at –70°C, or begin the purification procedure (*see* **Subheading 3.2.2.**).

3.2.2. Purification of Gutted Adenoviral Vector

Gutted adenoviruses can be purified using protocols available for conventional adenovirus vectors, except that additional centrifugation steps are required to separate the gutted from the helper virus. We have found that the methods of Graham and Prevec *(1)* and Gerard and Meidell *(18)* both work well. A modified version of the latter is presented below.

1. Centrifuge the virus-containing lysate at 12,000*g* for 10 min at 4°C to remove cellular debris.
2. Transfer the supernatant to fresh, sterile 250-mL bottles, 160 mL per bottle, and add 80 mL PEG/NaCl solution. Mix well and place bottles in ice for 1 h to precipitate the virus particles.
3. Collect the virus particles by centrifugation at 12,000*g* for 20 min at 4°C. Promptly pour off the supernatant and keep the bottles inverted to allow the liquid to drain. Using a tissue, carefully wipe out the neck of the bottle to remove all traces of solution (*see* **Note 8**).
4. Resuspend the virus in a small volume (usually 5 mL per 2 pellets) of 20 mM Tris-HCl, pH 8.0, 1 mM MgCl$_2$. This procedure is most easily accomplished using a flexible cell scraper to ensure that all the virus is retrieved. Transfer the virus solution to a 50-mL conical tube.
5. Add DNase I and RNase A to a final concentration of 50 µg/mL each. Incubate at 37°C for 30 min to remove any genomic or unpackaged nucleic acids that were coprecipitated with the virus particles.
6. To the virus solution, add CsCl to a final density of 1.1 g/mL (0.135 g CsCl per mL). When completely dissolved, pellet any residual debris by centrifuging at 8000*g* for 5 min at 4°C. Collect the supernatant and note the volume (*x*).
7. Prepare CsCl gradients in Beckman Ultra-Clear SW28 centrifuge tubes as follows: First, pipet (31-*x*) mL 1.3 g/mL CsCl solution into the empty tube. Second, slowly pipet 7 mL 1.4 g/mL solution *under* the 1.3 g/mL solution. Mark the interface of the CsCl solutions. Finally, overlay the virus-containing solution on the gradient.
8. Centrifuge at 53,000*g* for 4–16 h at 5°C.
9. After centrifugation, the viruses will appear in the gradient as a double opalescent band near the interface of the 1.4 and 1.3 g/mL solutions. Using an 18-gauge needle attached to a 5-mL syringe, pierce the side of the tube just below these bands and slowly collect this region of the gradient, usually 0.5–0.9 mL.
10. Transfer this solution directly into a quick-seal ultracentrifuge tube. Fill the tube with 1.34 g/mL CsCl, seal and centrifuge at 320,000*g* for 12 h followed by 73,000*g* for an additional 12 h at 5°C in a Beckman NVT65 rotor (or equivalent).
11. The band of gutted virus will be 4–5 mm above the helper virus. Use a dark background and strong, direct light to visualize the bands clearly. Pierce the top of the tube with a 16-gauge needle to prevent formation of a vacuum, then carefully insert an 18-gauge needle between the two bands, and slowly pull the gutted virus band. Repeat **steps 10–11** if desired, keeping in mind that, although addi-

tional gradients will increase the purity of the gutted virus prep, there will be a decrease in the overall yield.

12. Dialyze the gutted virus in 20 mM HEPES, pH 7.4, with three changes of buffer. For the last change, add 5% sucrose to the buffer.

13. Aliquot in small tubes and freeze in a dry ice/ethanol bath. Store at –70°C (*see* **Note 9**).

3.3. Assessing Gutted and Helper Virus Titers During Expansion and Following Purification

If the gutted and helper viruses each contain reporter genes, analysis of the titer of these viruses can be accomplished by a simple transduction experiment in a permissive cell line, followed by an assay for the reporter gene product. We typically include a β-galactosidase gene in our gutted viruses and a human alkaline phosphatase gene in the helper viruses, both under the control of an inducible promoter. If one or both of the viruses lack reporter genes, it will be necessary to estimate the viral titers according to genome copy number by Southern analysis or real-time PCR. Both these methods involve comparing dilutions of the virus preparation with a standard curve of known quantity of reference material, i.e., plasmid DNA. We routinely use real-time PCR to estimate the viral genome copy number in infected cell lysates. Finally, to assay the amount of replication competent helper virus, one can perform an adenovirus plaque assay in a complementing cell line, according to standard protocols (*1*), although this assay requires up to 14 d to complete. These assays are described below.

3.3.1. Colorimetric Assay for Transducing Units

The reporter genes in our viruses are driven by the ecdysone-responsive promoter from pIND (Invitrogen), which is induced when EcR-293 cells are treated with ponasterone A, an analog of ecdysone.

1. Plate approx 10^6 EcR-293 cells in 1 mL of complete medium per well of a 24-well cell culture plate. Incubate overnight to produce a monolayer of 100% confluence.

2. Dilute infected cell lysates in medium containing 5 µL/mL Ponasterone A. Typical dilutions are $10^{-4} - 10^{-2}$ for titering virus in a C7–cre cell lysate, and $10^{-8} - 10^{-6}$ for purified virus.

3. Replace culture medium on cells with 300 µL diluted virus solution. Incubate for 16 h at 37°C.

4. Remove medium, wash cells once with PBS, and then fix cells with 0.5% glutaraldehyde in PBS for 10 min at room temperature. Wash twice with PBS.

5. For alkaline phosphatase assays, inactivate the endogenous enyzme by incubating the cells in PBS at 65°C for 1 h.

6. Add 0.5 mL substrate solution (NBT/BCIP for alkaline phosphatase or X-gal for β-galactosidase) and incubate overnight at 37°C.

7. Count positively stained cells and calculate the number of transducing units per mL of lysate.

3.3.2. Real-Time PCR Assay for Genome Copy Number

Primer pairs and probe to detect gutted or helper viruses must not amplify endogenous sequences from the packaging cell line. (C7-cre cells contain adenovirus sequences from the left end of the genome, as well as the polymerase and terminal protein genes). For helper virus detection, we use a sequence found in the L2 region of the virus defined by the following primer sequences: forward, 5'-CGCAACGAAGCTATGTCCAA-3'; reverse, 5'-GCTTGTAA TCCTGCTCTTCCTTCTT-3'; and probe, 5'- VIC-CAGGTCATCGCGCC GGAGATCTA-TAMRA-3'. The gutted virus is detected using a primer/probe set made from a region of the murine MCK promoter.

1. Dilute the reference plasmid in PCR-grade water such that the samples contain decreasing copies of the target sequence, e.g. 10,000, 1000, 100, 10 copies/μL, etc.
2. Dilute infected cell lysate 10^{-3} in PCR-grade water (*see* **Note 10**).
3. To assay purified virus stocks, dilute the virus fivefold in virion lysis solution and incubate at 56°C for 10 min. Make additional 10-fold dilutions in water before performing the PCR assay.
4. Using the standard curve, calculate the genome copy number per mL (*see* **Note 11**).

4. Notes

1. It is helpful to achieve a very even distribution of cells over the entire surface of the plate. Uneven plating will lead to insufficient lysis in some areas and total CPE in others.
2. The plasmids can be digested together if the same enzyme is being used.
3. Prepare and test the efficiency of 2X HBS solutions as described *(19)*, as commercial stocks often perform poorly. Store the 2X HBS at –20°C for up to 6 mo.
4. During this incubation time, dilute the 30% glycerol solution with an equal volume of 2X HBS and equilibrate it, the PBS, and the culture medium to 37°C.
5. Viral CPE is considered 100% when all cells are round and mostly detached from the tissue culture dish.
6. Because this lysate was prepared in C7 cells, in which the helper virus growth is unrestricted, it contains ample amounts of helper virus to support a second round of gutted virus growth. Later passages in the amplification procedure, which are prepared in C7-cre cells, will not contain sufficient amounts of helper virus and will need to be supplemented to support production of the gutted virus.
7. Following the infection of 10×150-mm dishes, it is prudent to determine the titer of the gutted virus. If the genome copy number is $>10^9$ copies/mL, proceed with the large-scale expansion of 50–100 dishes; otherwise, repeat the 10-plate infection until the titer reaches its maximum, and then inoculate the final set of plates.
8. The pellet will be a widely dispersed, opaque region that covers most of the side of the bottle. There may also be a small pellet of debris at the bottom of the bottle.
9. Prepare aliquots according to the volume required for the planned experimental

procedure, as freeze/thawing purified virus will cause a decrease in the infectious titer. Estimate the particle count prior to aliquoting by incubating 5 µL of virus solution in virion lysis solution at 56°C for 10 min. Particle number per mL is equivalent to $[(A_{260} \times 21)/0.909] \times 10^{12}$ P/mL *(20)*.

10. Crude lysates must be diluted at least 1000-fold to eliminate quenching of fluorescence by components of the culture medium.
11. The calculated genome number is used to evaluate only the relative expansion of the virus in each passage since all genomes, packaged and unpackaged, are detected with this assay. For purified virus, however, we have found that the copy number correlates with the particle number as determined by A_{260} spectrophotometry.

Acknowledgments

We thank Catherine Barjot, Dennis Hartigan-O'Connor, Giovanni Salvatori, Michael Hauser, and Rajendra Kumar-Singh for many helpful discussions and for assistance in developing these protocols. This work was supported by NIH grant AG 015434 to J.S.C.

References

1. Graham, F. L. and Prevec, L. (1991) Manipulation of Adenovirus Vectors, in *Methods in Molecular Biology*, Vol. 7: *Gene Transfer and Expression Protocols.* (Murray, E. J., ed.), Humana, Totowa, pp. 109–128.
2. Yang, Y., Nunes, F. A., Berencsi, K., Furth, E. E., Gonczol, E., and Wilson, J. M. (1994) Cellular immunity to viral antigens limits E1-deleted adenoviruses for gene therapy. *Proc. Natl. Acad. Sci. USA* **91,** 4407–4411.
3. Kochanek, S., Clemens, P. R., Mitani, K., Chen, H.-H., Chan, S., and Caskey, C. T. (1996) A new adenoviral vector: Replacement of all viral coding sequences with 28 kb of DNA independently expressing both full-length dystrophin and β-galactosidase. *Proc. Natl. Acad. Sci. USA* **93,** 5731–5736.
4. Kumar-Singh, R. and Chamberlain, J. S. (1996) Encapsidated adenovirus minichromosomes allow delivery and expression of a 14 kb dystrophin cDNA to muscle cells. *Hum. Mol. Genet.* **5,** 913–921.
5. Dello Russo, C., Scott, J., Hartigan-O'Connor, D., et al. (2002) Functional reversal of dystrophy in adult mdx mouse muscle using gutted adenoviral vectors expressing full-length dystrophin. In press.
6. Hauser, M. A., Amalfitano, A., Kumar-Singh, R., Hauschka, S. D. and Chamberlain, J. S. (1997) Improved adenoviral vectors for gene therapy of Duchenne muscular dystrophy. *Neuromusc. Disord.* **7,** 277–283.
7. Temperley, S. M. and Hay, R. T. (1992) Recognition of the adenovirus type 2 origin of DNA replication by the virally encoded DNA polymerase and preterminal proteins. *EMBO J.* **11,** 761–768.
8. Schaack, J., Ho, W. Y., Freimuth, P., and Shenk, T. (1990) Adenovirus terminal protein mediates both nuclear matrix association and efficient transcription of adenovirus DNA. *Genes Dev.* **4,** 1197–1208.
9. Grable, M. and Hearing, P. (1990) Adenovirus type 5 packaging domain is

composed of a repeated element that is functionally redundant. *J. Virol.* **64,** 2047–2056.

10. Bett, A. J., Prevec, L., and Graham, F. L. (1993) Packaging capacity and stability of human adenovirus type 5 vectors. *J .Virol.* **67,** 5911–5921.

11. Parks, R. J. and Graham, F. L. (1997) A helper-dependent system for adenovirus vector production helps define a lower limit for efficient DNA packaging. *J. Virol.* **71,** 3293–3298.

12. Barjot, C., Hartigan-O'Connor, D. O., Scott, J. M., Salvatori, G., and Chamberlain, J. S. (2002) Packaging cell lines for gutted adenoviral vector growth using E1, E2b, and E3-deleted helper viruses. In press.

13. Graham, F. L., Smiley, J., Russell, W. C., and Nairn, R. (1977) Characteristics of a human cell line transformed by DNA from human adenovirus type 5. *J. Gen. Virol.* **36,** 59–72.

14. Amalfitano, A., Begy, C. R., and Chamberlain, J. S. (1996) Improved adenovirus packaging cell lines to support the growth of replication-defective gene-delivery vectors. *Proc. Natl. Acad. Sci. USA* **93,** 3352–3356.

15. Amalfitano, A. and Chamberlain, J. S. (1997) Isolation and characterization of packaging cell lines that co-express the adenovirus E1, DNA polymerase, and preterminal proteins: implications for gene therapy. *Gene Ther.* **4,** 258–263.

16. Hartigan-O'Connor, D., Amalfitano, A., and Chamberlain, J. S. (1999) Improved production of gutted adenovirus in cells expressing adenovirus preterminal protein and DNA polymerase. *J. Virol.* **73,** 7835–7841.

17. Hartigan-O'Connor, D., Barjot, C., Crawford, R. and Chamberlain, J. (2002) Efficient rescue of gutted adenovirus genomes allows rapid production of concentrated stocks without negative selection. *Hum. Gene Ther.* **13,** 519–531.

18. Gerard, R. D. and Meidell, R. S. (1995) Adenovirus vectors, in *DNA Cloning: a Practical Approach.* (Hames, B., and Glover, D., eds.), Oxford University Press, Oxford, pp. 285–307.

19. Sambrook, J., Fritsch, E. F., and Maniatis, T. (1989) *Molecular Cloning: A laboratory manual.* Cold Spring Harbor Laboratory Press, Cold Spring Harbor, NY.

20. Mittereder, N., March, K. L., and Trapnell, B. C. (1996) Evaluation of the concentration and bioactivity of adenovirus vectors for gene therapy. *J. Virol.* **70,** 7498–7509.

3

Dual Vector Expansion of the Recombinant AAV Packaging Capacity

Dongsheng Duan, Yongping Yue, and John F. Engelhardt

1. Introduction

Adeno-associated virus (AAV) as a vector for gene therapy of cardiovascular diseases has received much recent attention *(1–6)*. This enthusiasm is based on the success of numerous proof of principal gene transfer experiments. Stable high-level expression has been achieved following a variety of delivery methods (direct cardiac muscle injection, coronary vascular or carotid artery infection) and in a wide range of animal models from rodents to pigs *(7–12)*. A side-by-side comparison between viral and nonviral vectors in rabbit heart suggests that rAAV is much more efficient than nonviral vectors such as naked or liposome-complexed DNA. At the same time, rAAV also displays the least inflammatory response in comparison with other viral vectors such as adenovirus and herpes simplex virus *(13)*. Regulated myocardial transgene expression has also been demonstrated with an AAV vector containing glucocorticoid response elements in rat heart *(14)*.

Recently, several therapeutic genes have been tested for AAV-mediated gene therapy in animal models of cardiovascular diseases such as ischemic heart attack, hypertension, and congenital cardiomyopathy. For example, rAAV-mediated gene delivery of vascular endothelial growth factor (VEGF), a potent angiogenic protein, has been shown to induce significant neovascular formation in ischemic mouse heart in the absence of angioma formation *(15)*. Furthermore, expression of angiotensinogen antisense RNA using an rAAV vector led to a significant attenuation of hypertension and recovery of left ventricular hypertrophy in hypertensive rats *(16,17)*. In a TO-2 strain of hamster, a model for dilated cardiomyopathy owing to δ-sarcoglycan deficiency, an rAAV

From: *Methods in Molecular Biology, vol. 219: Cardiac Cell and Gene Transfer*
Edited by: J. M. Metzger © Humana Press Inc., Totowa, NJ

vector carrying the δ-sarcoglycan gene has been used to correct pathophysi-
ologic changes. In association with robust and persistent δ-sarcoglycan gene
expression following rAAV transfer, morphologic and hemodynamic studies
demonstrated substantial functional correction *(18)*. However, in all these successful applications of rAAV, the size of the therapeutic genes was less than
4.5 kb, which enables the entire expression cassette to be cloned in a single
AAV vector.

In wild-type AAV-2 (serotype 2 AAV), a 4681-nucleotide-long, single-
stranded DNA genome is packaged in mature virions. However, when the size
of the recombinant viral genome reaches 110% of the wild-type virus (~5.1 kb),
the efficiency for packaging infectious viral particles drops sharply *(19)*. This
small packaging capacity is one of the most challenging barriers in AAV-based
gene therapy technologies. Many larger therapeutic genes such as factor VIII
in hemophilia A and the mini-dystrophin gene in Duchenne's muscular dystrophy, cannot be packaged into a single AAV virion without further truncations
to the therapeutic genes.

Several recent research breakthroughs have made rAAV-mediated gene
therapy for larger genes (therapeutic genes larger than 5 kb) a viable reality.
Studies on AAV transduction biology demonstrate that AAV genomes can form
large circular concatamers through inverted terminal repeat (ITR) mediated
intermolecular recombination *(20–22)*. Interestingly, most junctions are orga-
nized in a head-to-tail orientation. *trans*-splicing dual vector method effectively doubles the size of genes that can be delivered by a single AAV virion
(23–25,27). *Trans*-splicing in this context is defined as the reconstruction of an
intact transcript by splicing in "Trans" between two covalently linked vector
genomes, each carrying separate parts of the transgene (**Fig. 1**; *see* **Note 1**).
This technology involves dividing a large therapeutic gene or cDNA into two
portions at an exon-exon junction. Each part of the gene, which is now small

---

Fig. 1. Schematic illustrations of three different strategies to overcome rAAV packaging size limitations. Two different dual vector approaches based on AAV intermolecular heterodimerization are currently used to increase the packaging capacity of
rAAV vectors. (**A**) The *trans*-splicing method. In this approach, the promoter and the
5' half of the transgene are included in one vector (AV.Donor). A splicing donor (SD)
signal is also inserted between the transgene and the 3' inverted terminal repeat (ITR)
in AV.Donor. A second rAAV vector (AV.Acceptor) contains the splicing acceptor
signal (SA), the 3' half of the transgene, and the polyA sequence. Following coinfection
with both vectors, head-to-tail intermolecular recombination between the vectors
physically links the 5' half and the 3' half of the transgene together in circular (as
shown) and/or linear (not shown) heterodimers. In circular dimers (as shown), one of
the two junctions contains the splicing donor signal, a junctional ITR sequence, and
the splicing acceptor signal. The hnRNA transcript initiated from the promoter is

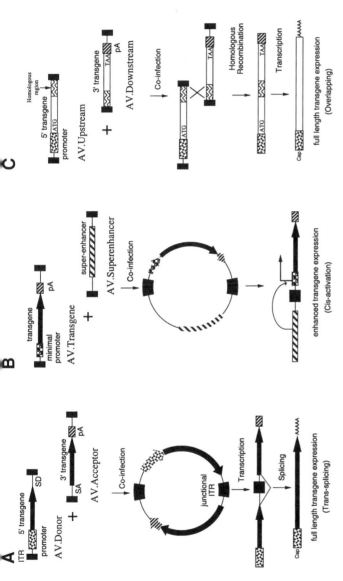

Fig. 1. (*continued*) spliced in the nucleus to generate the full-length mRNA. Finally, a functional protein is translated from the spliced mRNA. (**B**) The *cis*-activation method. This technique is especially useful to boost the level of expression from transgenes (such as CFTR) that can just fit into a single AAV virion. The transgene (with or without a minimal promoter) is cloned in AV.Transgene. A second vector contains multiple enhancer elements (AV.Superenhancer). Following coinfection, ITR-mediated intermolecular recombination places enhancers either upstream or downstream of the transgene. Finally, the level of transgene expression is exponentially increased by the juxtaposed enhancer elements. (**C**) A mechanistically different approach to express oversized transgenes with rAAV vectors. This method is based on homologous recombination between independent transgene-containing segments encoded in independent viral vectors. The promoter and the 5′ portion of the transgene are cloned into an AV.Upstream vector. The 3′ portion of the transgene and the polyA sequence is cloned into an AV.Downstream vector. The DNA sequence at the end of the AV.Upstream and the beginning of the AV.Downstream is identical. Following coinfection, the overlapping homologous regions in these two vectors recombine and reconstitute a functional expression cassette.

enough for a single AAV virion, is then cloned into independent AAV viruses. The first AAV vector (usually called the AV.Donor) contains a promoter, the first half of the gene, and an engineered splicing donor (SD) sequence. The second AAV vector (usually called the AV.Acceptor) starts with a splicing acceptor (SA) signal and the second part of the transgene followed by a polyA sequence. Coinfection with both AV.Donor and AV.Acceptor vectors leads to head-to-tail heterodimer and concatamer formation between these two vectors. A heterogeneou (hn)RNA molecule is produced from the heterodimer in a *trans*-vector fashion and the full-length protein is produced from the *cis*-spliced mRNA (**Fig. 1**).

The *cis*-activation dual vector method also takes advantage of AAV vector heterodimer formation (**Fig. 1B**) *(26)*. Many therapeutic transgenes including the cystic fibrosis transmembrane regulator (CFTR) can just fit into a single AAV virus (with or without a minimal promoter). In these cases, low transgene expression driven by the AAV ITR or a minimal promoter often falls short of therapeutic requirements. In the *cis*-activation approach, multiple enhancers (termed superenhancer) are incorporated into a single rAAV vector (AV.Superenhancer), and following coinfection and intermolecular recombination with a second transgene containing rAAV vector (AV.Transgene), transgene expression can be significantly enhanced. Importantly, substantial increases in AAV-mediated transgene expression can be achieved irrespective of the orientation of the enhancer elements and transgene.

The most recently developed rAAV dual vector approach includes the mechanistically distinct use of overlapping dual vectors for delivering large transgenes *(27)*. This method is based on the homologous recombination between two rAAV vectors that share a common DNA segment. The foundation of this approach was first suggested by early studies with AAV proviral plasmids demonstrating that homologous recombination between AAV genomes can be highly efficient *(28)*. This indicated the possibility that cloning truncated 5' and 3' regions of a large therapeutic gene, with an overlapping segment, into two AAV vectors might result in homologous recombination and reconstitute the full-length transgene (*see* **Note 1**).

The protocols described in this chapter are limited to the design and generation of the *trans*-splicing and overlapping AAV vectors for expressing an intact, functional transgene. The production of *cis*-activation vectors is not discussed.

2. Materials

2.1. Cell Culture

1. 293 cells (ATCC #CRL-1573). This is a hypotriploid human fetal kidney cell line transformed by sheared human adenovirus type 5 DNA *(29)*. Sequence analy-

sis suggested that about 4.3 kb of adenoviral DNA (nt 1–4344) is inserted in chromosome 19 (19q13.2) *(30)* (*see* **Note 2**). Constitutive expression of adenoviral E1a and E1b gene products provides the helper function for AAV genome replication. These cells are split 1:6 every 3 d and should not be allowed to overgrow. We recommend routinely testing the cell culture for mycoplasma contamination. Cells infected with mycoplasma generally grow much slower and do not attach to tissue culture plates well (*see* **Note 3**).

2. DMEM (Dulbecco's modified Eagle's medium), high glucose with L-glutamine (Gibco-BRL, Grand Island, NY, cat. no. 11965-092). Store at 4°C.
3. Fetal bovine serum (FBS) with a high plating efficiency (Gibco-BRL, cat. no. 26140079). Store at –20°C.
4. PBS (phosphate-buffered saline): 137 mM NaCl, 2.7 mM KCl, 8.0 mM Na$_2$HPO$_4$, 1.5 mM KH$_2$PO$_4$. Sterilize by filtration (0.2 µm) and keep at 4°C.
5. Penicillin G: 100 U/mL DMEM culture medium (Gibco-BRL, cat. no. 15140-122). Store at –20°C.
6. Streptomycin: 100 µg/mL DMEM culture medium (Gibco-BRL, cat. no. 15140-122). Store at –20°C.
7. 1X Trypsin-EDTA: 0.05 % Trypsin, 1 mM EDTA/4Na (Gibco-BRL, cat. no. 25200-056). Store at 4°C.

2.2. Proviral Plasmid Cloning and Large-Scale Propagation

1. High-fidelity polymerase chain reaction (PCR) kit. Taq DNA polymerase has a relatively high error rate. To decrease PCR-related mutations, we recommend using the Expand High Fidelity PCR System from Roche (Indianapolis, IN, #1-732-641). The 5'-3' exonuclease proofreading activity of the Pwo DNA polymerase in this system results in DNA synthesis with a much higher fidelity. Store at –20°C. (*see* **Note 4**).
2. Electroporation-competent *E. coli* SURE cells (>5 × 10^9 transformants/µg DNA; Stratagene, La Jolla, CA, #200227): Genotype (e14- (McrA-) D(mcrCB-hsdSMR-mrr)171 endA1 supE44 thi-1 gyrA96 relA1 lac recB recJ sbcC umuC::Tn5 (Kanr) uvrC [F' proAB lacIqZD(M15 Tn10 (Tetr)]). Eukaryotic genes containing inverted repeats are quite unstable when they are propagated in bacterial cells. The inverted repeats can be rearranged or deleted by *E. coli* DNA repair systems. SURE cells contain mutations in the genes involved in DNA repair and recombination pathways (such as uvrC, umuC, SbcC, RecJ, recB, and recJ). These modifications have greatly increased the stability of AAV proviral plasmids during cloning and subsequent large-scale preparation. However, it should be pointed out that SURE cells are a kanamycin-resistant strain, so a kanamycin-resistant gene should not be used as a selection marker in the proviral plasmid. Store at –80°C.
3. *E . coli* Pulser (Bio-Rad, cat. no. 1652102).
4. Gene Pulser cuvets, 0.1-cm gap (Bio-Rad, cat. no. 165-2089).
5. 14-mL polypropylene round-bottomed tubes, 17 × 100 mm (Becton Dickinson Labware, Franklin Lakes, NJ, Falcon 4059).
6. S.O.C. medium (Gibco-BRL, #15544-034). Store at room temperature.

7. Amp selection LB agar plates (100 µg/mL ampicillin). Store at 4°C.
8. Standard materials for large-scale plasmid preparation. To achieve the best transfection efficiency for AAV production, we recommend preparing the *cis* proviral plasmids and helper plasmids by CsCl/ethidium bromide equilibrium centrifugation. A detailed protocol is given in *Current Protocols in Molecular Biology* (**Subheading 1.7.6.**) *(31)*.

2.3. Recombinant AAV Production and Purification

1. Helper virus: Ad.CMVLacZ (or Ad.CMVEGFP), an E1 deleted recombinant adenovirus (available from the Vector Core Facility, The University of Iowa) (*see* **Note 5**).
2. Helper plasmid for type 2 AAV: pTrans *(32)* (ATCC, #68066). This plasmid provides the Rep and Cap gene required for rAAV propagation (*see* **Note 6**).
3. Helper plasmid for type 1 and type 5 AAV: p5E18(2/1) for rAAV-1 packaging *(33)*. pAV2-Rep and pAV5-Trans for rAAV-5 packaging *(34)*. These plasmids provide viral replication and structural proteins for pseudo-packaging a type 2 rAAV genome into type 1 and type 5 capsids (*see* **Note 7**).
4. 2.5 M CaCl$_2$. Sterilize by filtration and store at –20°C.
5. 2X HBS buffer: 0.3 M NaCl, 1.5 mM Na$_2$HPO$_4$, and 40 mM HEPES, pH 7.05. Sterilize by filtration and store at –20°C. It is very important to keep the pH of 2X HBS buffer in the range of 7.05 ± 0.05 in order to achieve high transfection efficiency.
6. DNAse I (Sigma D4513, 11 mg protein/vial, total 33 K [kuniz] units) (*see* **Note 8**).
7. 0.5% Trypsin (10×). Store at –20°C.
8. 10% Sodium deoxycholate. Store at room temperature.
9. Beckman Biosys 2000 Workstation (semipreparative high-performance liquid chromatography [HPLC] system).
10. Poros HE/M heparin column (bed volume 1.7 mL) (PerSeptive, Applied Biosystems, Cambridge, MA, #1-5222-26).
11. Viral lysate dilution buffer: 20 mM Tris-HCl, pH 8.0, 150 mM NaCl, and 0.5% sodium deoxycholate (fresh made). The viral lysate from 10×150-mm plates is resuspended in about 100 mL dilution buffer.
12. Low salt HPLC buffer: 20 mM Tris-HCl, pH 8.0/100 mM NaCl. Store at room temperature.
13. High salt HPLC buffer: 20 mM Tris-HCl, pH 8.0/1 M NaCl. Store at room temperature.
14. HEPES AAV dialysis buffer: 20 mM HEPES, 150 mM NaCl, pH 7.8. Filter-sterilize and store at 4°C.
15. Dialysis tubing: 12,000 MW cutoff. (Gibco-BRL, #15961-014). Store at 4°C.
16. Bio-Dot SF manifold microfiltration apparatus (Bio-Rad, Hercules, CA, #BIO-DOT SF).
17. Alkaline AAV digestion buffer: 0.4 M NaOH, 20 mM EDTA (freshly made prior to use).
18. Slot blot hybridization solution (5X SSC, 5X Denhardt's Solution, 1% sodium dodecyl sulfate [SDS], and 50 % formamide, add 100 µg/mL denatured salmon sperm DNA just before use).

3. Methods

3.1. *Generating* Trans-*Splicing Vectors*

Although an endogenous intron sequence might provide an ideal splicing signal for a given transgene, the size of endogenous introns is often too large for the *trans*-splicing approach. Therefore, a small heterologous intron or a synthetic intron is usually more appropriate for *trans*-splicing vectors. In this protocol, we will use the prokaryotic β-galatosidase (LacZ) gene as a template to exemplify the procedure of generating AV.Donor and AV.Acceptor *trans*-splicing vectors for a given cDNA.

3.1.1. *Vector Design and Cloning*

3.1.1.1. SELECTION OF THE *TRANS*-SPLICING SITE

The consensus nucleotide sequences at exon-intron-exon junctions are used as guidelines for selecting the position in a transgene cDNA for division into two *trans*-splicing vectors (**Fig. 2A**). The most conserved motif between two exons is NAAG (exon 1)//GNNN (exon 2) or NCAG (exon 1)//GNNN (exon 2) *(35)*. To divide the *LacZ* gene, we have chosen to insert the splicing signals between nucleotides 2742 and 2743 (**Fig. 2B**) *(27)*. The DNA sequence in this region matches the definition of a standard exon-exon junction. Several additional regions in the LacZ coding sequence also meet this requirement; all these regions could potentially serve as division sites. In fact, Xiao and colleagues *(24)* have used a putative exon-exon junction site between nucleotides 1761 and 1762 and successfully generated a set of LacZ *trans*-splicing vectors. For a given therapeutic transgene, if the information on its genomic structure is available, we recommend choosing an endogenous exon-exon boundary for division of the gene.

3.1.1.2. SELECTION OF THE SPLICING SIGNALS

Only approx 6 nucleotides at the 5' end of the intron and 30 nucleotides at the 3' end of the intron are necessary for correct splicing (**Fig. 2A**). Small endogenous and heterologous introns have been tested in the *trans*-splicing of the erythopoietin (Epo) and LacZ genes, respectively *(23,24)*. To increase further the flexibility in cloning *trans*-splicing vectors, we have tested a small synthetic intron for facilitating *trans*-splicing of the LacZ gene. This 132-bp chimeric intron is from the commercially available plasmid pCI (Promega, #E1731). The donor splicing signal is from the first intron of the human β-globulin gene, and the splicing acceptor sequence is from an intron in the human immunoglobulin heavy chain gene.

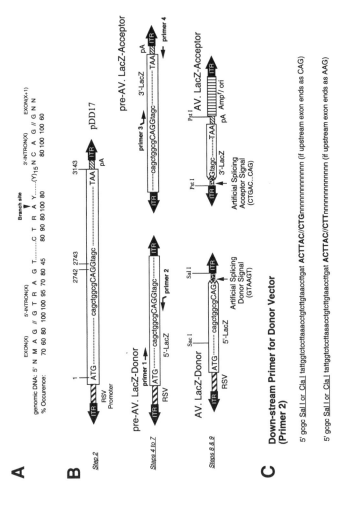

Fig. 2. Construction of *trans*-splicing AAV vectors. (**A**) The consensus sequences at exon/intron boundaries in a genomic DNA. The numbers below the nucleotides indicate the probability of a specific nucleotide in a particular position. M, adenine or cytosine; R, adenine or guanine; Y, cytosine or thymidine. (**B**) PCR-mediated stepwise division of a LacZ transgene is presented as an example (*see* **Subheading 3.1.1.4.** for details). (**C**) Specific primers for introducing a splicing donor signal (primer 2: downstream primer for the AV.Donor vector) and a splicing acceptor signal (primer 3: upstream primer for the AV.Acceptor vector) into proviral plasmids. A synthetic intron from pCI (Promega, #E1731) was used as the template for creating splicing signals. The conserved nucleotides in both the intron and the exon are in bold uppercase (*see* **Subheading 3.1.1.4.**; **steps 4** and **5** for detail). N, transgene-specific nucleotide. Plasmid backbone sequences are not shown in this diagram.

3.1.1.3. OUTLINE OF CLONING STRATEGY FOR CONSTRUCTION OF INTERMEDIATE VECTORS

An intron splicing signal can be inserted into the selected splicing site in the transgene by a PCR-mediated approach. This will generate a cDNA with one intron. This modified cDNA is then divided into two parts within the intron region, and each part is separately cloned into two rAAV vectors. This strategy has been successfully used to generate dual AAV vectors for both the Epo and LacZ genes *(23,24)*. An alternative, more flexible approach is to introduce splicing signals into AAV vectors after the transgene is split and inserted into two AAV vectors. This can be achieved by cutting the transgene into two parts using restriction sites close to the targeted exon-exon boundary. The 5' and the 3' portions of the transgene are then separately cloned into the multiple cloning site (MCS) of two AAV proviral cloning vectors to generate the intermediate vectors (pre-Donor vector and pre-Acceptor vector; **Figs. 2B** and **3**). Finally, a PCR mediated approach is used to add the splicing donor signal into the pre-Donor vector to produce the AV.Donor vector. Similarly, the branching site and splicing acceptor signals are cloned into the pre-Acceptor vector to produce AV.Acceptor.

Several AAV proviral plasmids with different features useful for inserting transgenes have been constructed. These include pDD188, pDD293, and pDD295. Both pDD188 and pDD293 can be used as the pre-Donor cloning vector. The difference between these two vectors is that pDD188 contains a strong viral promoter from the Rous sarcoma virus 3' long terminal repeat (RSV promoter), whereas in pDD293, investigators can insert the promoter of their choice between *Kpn*I and one of the downstream cloning sites (**Fig. 3**). pDD295, which has a second MCS followed by a polyA sequence just upstream of the 3' ITR, is intended for use in cloning the 3' end of the divided transgene to generate the pre-Acceptor vector (**Fig. 3**).

3.1.1.4. PROVIRAL PLASMID CONSTRUCTION

1. The first step in construction of *trans*-splicing vectors is to clone the therapeutic gene of choice into a eukaryotic expression vector. This plasmid will be used as a template for dividing the transgene into the pre-Donor and the pre-Acceptor vectors. In vitro transfection of this plasmid can also serve as a positive control for the subsequent functional evaluation of transgene expression from the *trans*-splicing vectors. In our example, the LacZ gene was obtained from pCMVβ (Clontech, #6177-1).

2. The 5' portion of the transgene including the translation start site is cloned into the MCS sites of either of the AAV pre-Donor cloning vectors pDD188 or pDD293. If RSV is to be utilized as the promoter, the *Sal*I restriction site in pDD188 will be selected for introducing the splicing donor sequence. Alterna-

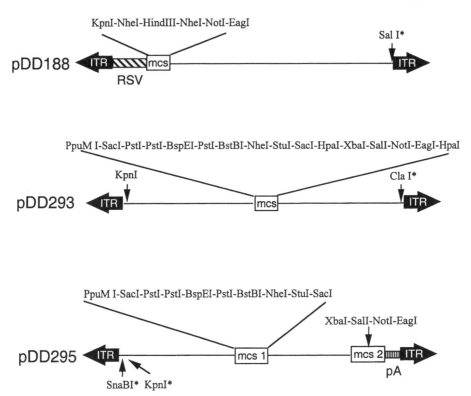

Fig. 3. Schematic diagram of three AAV proviral cloning plasmids for generating *trans*-splicing vectors. These proviral cloning plasmids have been engineered with multiple cloning sites. Unique cloning restriction sites are listed for each vector. Placement of restriction enzyme sites in the multicloning site (MCS) is not drawn to scale. The restriction sites marked with an asterisk are used for introducing splicing sequences. Both pDD188 and pDD293 can be used for cloning the AV.Donor proviral plasmid (i.e., *cis* plasmid). The pDD295 plasmid is used for cloning the AV.Acceptor proviral plasmid (*see* **Subheading 3.1.1.3.** for details). Plasmid backbone sequences are not shown in this diagram.

tively, if a unique promoter is to be used for expression, we suggest choosing pDD293 as the pre-Donor cloning vector. In this case, the *Cla*I site should be reserved for introducing the splicing donor sequence (**Fig. 3**). No matter which MCS vector is used, it is always very important to double check whether *Sal*I or *Cla*I cuts within the cloned 5' portion of the transgene. If a *Sal*I restriction site exists in this region, then pDD293 should be used as the pre-Donor cloning vector. Alternatively, if the *Cla*I restriction site exists in this region, then pDD188 should be used as the pre-Donor cloning vector. In the case of LacZ *trans*-splicing vectors, the entire LacZ gene was cloned into an RSV-containing AAV vector (pDD17), as previously described (**Figs. 2B**, **4A**) *(36)*.

3. The 3' portion of the transgene including its translational stop codon is then cloned between the MCS 1 and MCS 2 sites in the pre-Acceptor cloning vector pDD295 (**Fig. 3**). An SV40 polyA sequence is included in this plasmid to facilitate the expression of the *trans*-spliced gene product. The *KpnI/SnaBI* sites in pDD295 are designed for introducing the splicing acceptor signal.

4. PCR is used to introduce the splicing donor sequence into the pre-Donor vector. The upstream primer (primer 1) for cloning the AV.Donor vector is composed of a 20–25-mer oligonucleotide located upstream of a unique restriction site in the cDNA used for cloning the final product. The design of this primer should follow the general PCR primer designing principles. In the LacZ *trans*-splicing example, the primer 1 (EL752) sequence is: 5'-GTCATAGCGATAAC<u>GAGCTC</u>CT GCAC-3'. This primer contains a unique *SacI* restriction site (underlined nucleotides) for inserting the PCR product into a pre-AV.LacZ-Donor. The downstream primer (primer 2) for the PCR reaction is composed of a unique *SalI* (or *ClaI*) site at the 5' end followed by nucleotides complementary to the splicing donor signal in the intron of pCI. Finally, a stretch of 30 nucleotides complementary to the 3' end of the last exon in AV.Donor is added to the primer 2 (**Fig. 2C**; *see* **Note 9**). In the LacZ *trans*-splicing example, the primer 2 (EL753) sequence is: 5' GCGCgtcgac<u>TATTGGTCTCCTTAAACCTGTCTTGTAACCTTGATA</u> **CTTACCTG**CGCCAGCTGGCAGTTCAGGCCAATCCGCGCCGG-3'. The lowercase "gtcgac" indicates the unique *SalI* restriction site. The underlined nucleotides represent the intron donor sequence, and the splice site consensus nucleotides are in bold.

5. A similar principle is applied for designing the PCR primers for cloning the AV.Acceptor vector. The upstream primer (primer 3) is composed of a unique restriction site, splicing acceptor signals, and the first 30 nucleotides from the downstream exon in the transgene. **Figure 2C** outlines a general upstream primer based on pDD295. In the LacZ *trans*-splicing example, the primer 3 (EL751) sequence is 5' GCGCctgcag<u>CTCTTGCGTTTCTGATAGGCACCTATTGGTC TTA**CTGAC**</u>ATCCACTTTGCCTTTCTCTCCA**CAGG**TAGCAGAGCGGGT AAACTGGCTCGGATTAGGGCCGC-3'. The underlined nucleotides represent the intron acceptor sequence, and the consensus nucleotides are in bold. In order to generate LacZ *trans*-splicing vectors capable of rescuing circular intermediates, the AV.LacZ-Acceptor is not generated from the MCS vector pDD295. Instead, the splicing acceptor sequence and the second part of the LacZ gene are cloned in a previously described shuttle vector, AV.EGFPori3 (pDD29) *(20)*. This vector contains a bacterial replication origin and an ampicillin resistance gene and can be used to retrieve the circular concatamers from AV.LacZ-Donor and AV.LacZ-Acceptor coinfected cells. Therefore, the unique restriction site (lowercase "ctgcag") in EL751 is *PstI* instead of *SnaBI* or *KpnI*, as in pDD295. In the example of the LacZ *trans*-splicing vectors, the downstream primer (primer 4) for AV.LacZ-Acceptor (EL 688) is 5'-GCGCctgcagCATACCACATT TGTAGAGGTTTTAC-3'. Again, the lowercase "ctgcag" represents a *PstI* restriction site.

6. The PCR products are generated with the Expand High Fidelity PCR System (Roche) according to the manufacturer's instructions (*see* **Note 4**).

7. The donor PCR product is digested with *Sal*I (or *Cla*I) and the unique restriction site within the transgene. In the case of AV.LacZ-Donor, the splicing donor signal PCR fragment is digested with *Sac*I and *Sal*I. The acceptor PCR product is digested with the *Sna*BI (or *Kpn*I) and the unique restriction site in the transgene. In generating AV.LacZ-Acceptor, the PCR fragment is digested with *Pst*I. Finally, the digested fragments are gel-purified (*see* **Note 10**).

8. The pre-Donor and pre-Acceptor plasmids will serve as the backbone for inserting the PCR fragments. These two intermediate plasmids are also digested with the appropriate restriction enzymes. For example, the pre-Donor plasmid can be digested with *Sal*I (or *Cla*I) and the unique restriction site within the transgene. The pre-Acceptor plasmid can be digested with *Sna*BI (or *Kpn*I) and the second unique restriction site within the transgene (if pDD295 is used as the MCS vector for pre-Acceptor cloning). In the example of the LacZ *trans*-splicing vector, the pre-Donor plasmid is digested with *Sac*I and *Sal*I, and the AV.LacZ-Acceptor backbone plasmid pDD29 is digested with *Pst*I. After digestion, the backbone fragments are also gel-purified.

9. Ligations are performed using standard protocols for T4 DNA ligase from Gibco-BRL (#15224-017) at 15°C overnight.

10. Transformations are performed with SURE competent cells using one-fifth of each ligation reaction. Higher transformation efficiency is achieved by electroporation using electroporation-competent cells (Stratagene, #200227) instead of heat-shock SURE competent cells (Stratagene, #200238).

11. Individual clones are picked for plasmid minipreparation and are analyzed by restriction digestion and sequencing. We recommend using miniprep kits that yield sequencing quality plasmids, such as the Wizard Plus SV Minipreps DNA Purification System (Promega, Madison WI, #A1460). It is important to make sure that the PCR-amplified DNA sequences have no mutations. It is similarly important to validate that the viral ITR in each individual clone is intact. The ITR is the only viral element retained in recombinant AAV vectors. The ITR sequence carries information critical for rAAV packaging and transduction. For type 2 AAV ITR, we recommend performing restriction analysis with *Sma*I (cuts within the C and C' arm in the ITR), *Bss*HII, and *Msc*I (cuts within the A and A' arm's in the ITR).

3.2. Generating Overlapping Vectors

The approach for generating overlapping AAV vectors is much more simple and straightforward than that for *trans*-splicing AAV vectors (*see* **Note 1**). In this section, we will use the LacZ gene to illustrate procedures for constructing Upstream and Downstream AAV overlapping vectors (**Fig. 4A**). An alternative generic approach is also presented (**Fig. 4B**).

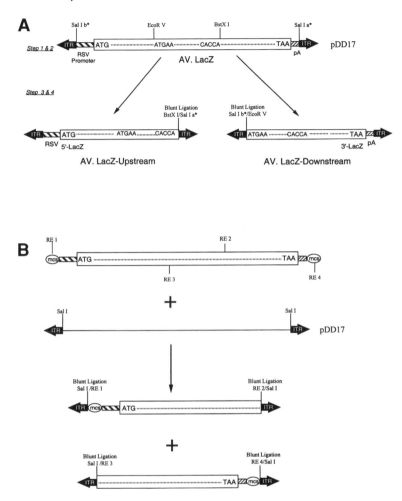

Fig. 4. Schematic outline of rAAV overlapping vector cloning strategies. (**A**) Construction of AAV LacZ overlapping vectors. To generate the AV.LacZ-Upstream and AV.LacZ-Downstream proviral plasmids, either the 3' end of the entire expression cassette (including the 3' one-third of the LacZ gene and the polyA) or the 5' end of the entire expression cassette (including the RSV promoter and the 5' one-third of the LacZ gene) is removed from pDD17 by restriction digestion, and the remaining parts are self-religated (*see* **Subheading 3.2.2.1.** for details). The asterisk indicates that only one of the *Sal*I sites is functional, whereas the other *Sal*I site is inactivated. (**B**) An alternative generic overlapping vector cloning strategy. In this method, the entire expression cassette is first cloned into an eukaryotic expression cassette. The 5' portion of the expression cassette and the 3' portion of the expression cassette are then separately cloned into AAV backbone vectors. The length of overlap will be determined by the distance between restriction enzymes RE 2 and RE 3 (*see* **Subheading 3.2.2.2.** for details). Plasmid backbone sequences are not shown in this diagram.

3.2.1. Principle of Vector Design

The key issue for generating functional overlapping vectors is to have sufficient overlap between the AV.Upstream and AV.Downstream vectors. Insufficient length will decrease the probability of homologous recombination between two vectors and result in low-level transgene expression. However, if the overlap between the two vectors is too long, then we will lose the advantage of this approach in conforming to the packaging capacity of AAV.

3.2.2. Proviral Plasmid Cloning

Two different strategies can be used to generate overlapping AAV vectors. In the first strategy (as is shown below in the LacZ overlapping vectors), the entire expression cassette is cloned into an AAV proviral plasmid. The promoter and 5' end of the transgene (or the 3' end of the transgene and polyA sequence) are removed at a later step with specific restriction enzymes (**Fig. 4A**). Alternatively, in the second strategy, a therapeutic transgene can also be cloned into an eukaryotic expression cassette first. Subsequently, the first half of the expression cassette to be encoded in AV.Upstream vector is released by restriction digestion and then inserted into the AAV proviral plasmid. The AV.Downstream vector is produced in a similar manner (**Fig. 4B**).

3.2.2.1. LacZ Overlapping Vector Construction

1. As described above, a complete RSV-AAV LacZ plasmid (pDD17) is constructed first (**Figs. 2B** and **4A**) *(36)*.
2. A partial *Sal*I digestion is then performed. The linearized DNA fragment is gel-purified (*see* **Note 10**) and blunted with T4 DNA polymerase to inactivate either one of the two *Sal*I sites. The 5' *Sal*I (*Sal*Ib) inactivated plasmid is designated pDD327. The 3' *Sal*I (*Sal*Ia) inactivated plasmid is designated pDD323.
3. To generate AV.LacZUpstream, pDD327 is double-digested with *Bst*XI and *Sal*I. The smaller fragment containing the 3' end of LacZ and the polyA is discarded. The larger fragment is then religated by blunt end ligation.
4. To generate AV.LacZDownstream, pDD323 is double-digested with *Sal*I and *Eco*RV. The smaller fragment containing the promoter and 5' end of the LacZ is discarded, and the larger fragment is then religated by blunt end ligation.

3.2.2.2. Construction of Overlapping AAV Vectors for Any Given Gene

1. First, the gene of interest is cloned into a commercially available eukaryotic expression vector such as pcDNA3.1 (Invitrogen, #V790-20), pREP4 (Invitrogen, #V004-50), pCI (Promega, #E1731), or pSI (Promega, #E1721).
2. The AAV backbone for cloning overlapping vectors is generated by *Sal*I digestion of pDD17 (**Figs. 2B** and **4A**) *(36)*. After digestion, the larger fragment containing the ITR is blunted with T4 DNA polymerase and gel-purified (*see* **Note 10**). To decrease the background from self-ligation, the AAV backbone

fragment is dephosphorylated with calf intestinal alkaline phosphatase (New England Biolabs, #M0290).

3. The transgene insert for the upstream vector is released by double digestion with restriction enzymes RE 1 and RE 2. The isolated insert fragment is then blunted with T4 DNA polymerase. Finally, the insert is ligated to the AAV backbone prepared in **step 2** to generate the pAV.Upstream proviral plasmid.

4. The insert for the downstream vector is released by double digestion with restriction enzymes RE 3 and RE 4. The isolated insert fragment is then blunted with T4 DNA polymerase. Finally, the insert is ligated to the AAV backbone prepared in **step 2** to generate the pAV.Downstream proviral plasmid.

3.3. Recombinant AAV Preparation

1. Human 293 cells free of wild-type AAV are cultured in high-glucose DMEM containing 10% FBS and 1% penicillin G/streptomycin. Split 293 cells 1:6 onto 150-mm dishes 2 d prior to viral production. For a given rAAV construct, 40 150-mm dishes are usually seeded for one preparation. If HeLa based producer cell lines are used for rAAV preparation, we recommend following the culture conditions described in the original publications (*see* **Note 3**).

2. When E1-deleted recombinant adenovirus (first-generation recombinant adenovirus) is used as helper virus for rAAV production, 293 cells are usually infected with adenovirus at a multiplicity of infection (MOI) of 5 particles/cell in 2% FBS/DMEM for 1 h prior to proviral plasmid and Rep/Cap helper plasmid transfection. The helper adenovirus should be carefully selected. It should not express the same transgene as the AAV proviral plasmid. For example, in the preparation of AV.LacZ vectors, we recommend using Ad.CMVEGFP instead of Ad.CMVLacZ. The other advantage of using Ad.CMVEGFP is that the adenovirus infection can be easily monitored. However, if the triple-plasmid transfection technique is used for rAAV production (*see* **Notes 5** and **6**), cell culture media should be changed to fresh 10% FBS/DMEM 1–2 h prior to transfection.

3. One hour after infection (if recombinant adenovirus is used as helper virus) or after culture media change (for an adenovirus-free triple-plasmid transfection system), a calcium phosphate transfection cocktail is prepared using an AAV proviral plasmid and the Rep/Cap plasmid (pTrans) in a ratio of 1:3. For each 150-mm plate, 12.5 µg rAAV proviral plasmid is mixed with 37.5 µg of pTrans plasmid in a total volume of 1012 µL H_2O. Then, 113 µL of 2.5 M $CaCl_2$ is added to a final concentration of 0.25 M. Finally, the DNA-calcium mixture is added dropwise to 1125 µL of 2X HBS to produce the DNA-calcium-phosphate precipitate. However, for the adenovirus-free system, the adenoviral helper plasmid (*see* **Note 5**) should also be included in the transfection cocktail, so that the final ratio among the *cis* proviral plasmid, the pTrans plasmid, and the adenoviral helper plasmid is 1:1:3.

4. After the calcium-phosphate transfection cocktail has been incubated at room temperature for about 15–30 min, the cocktail is gently applied dropwise to 293 cells while the culture dish is swirled. The final viral yield is directly correlated

to the transfection efficiency; therefore care should be taken in preparing the transfection cocktail *(31)*. Formation of the calcium phosphate precipitate can be monitored on a coverslip using a phase contrast microscope. Alternatively, for reporter genes such as LacZ or alkaline phosphatase, the transfection efficiency can be directly monitored by cytochemical staining on one of the transfected plates 24 h later.

5. If adenovirus is used as helper, cytopathic effects (CPEs) will be evident at 40–42 h postinfection, and cell lysates are then harvested. However, in the adenovirus-free system, transfected 293 cells will not go to CPE in the same time range. For the triple-plasmid transfection method, cell lysates are usually collected 48–52 h after transfection. Spin the lysate at 500g for 15 min in a benchtop centrifuge and resuspend the cell pellet in 10 mM Tris-HCl (pH 8.0). To help release viral particles from the nuclei, the cell lysate is freeze-thawed three times using dry ice/ethanol and a 40°C water bath. The crude lysate is further broken down by passing it through a 25-gauge needle 3 times. Digest the lysate with DNAse I at 37°C for 30 min followed by a second 30-min digestion with one-tenth volume of 0.5% trypsin and 10% sodium deoxycholate. Normally 1 vial of DNAse I, approx 33 K kuniz units, is used for a 40 150-mm plate viral preparation (*see* **Note 8**). Finally, the lysate is heated at 60°C for 60 min to inactivate contaminating helper adenovirus (*see* **Note 11**). The lysate is then diluted in viral dilution buffer and filtered through a 2-μm pore size disk filter prior to purification.

6. Assemble the Poros heparin column into a Beckman Biosys 2000 Workstation (*see* **Note 12**). Before the virus-containing lysate is loaded, the heparin column should be equilibrated with at least 10 bed volumes of low-salt HPLC buffer. Load the viral lysate at a rate of 4 mL/min. Wash the column with 30 bed volumes of low-salt HPLC buffer.

7. Finally, a linear NaCl gradient (0.1–1 M NaCl) is used to elute the recombinant AAV at a flow rate of 3 mL/min. The rAAV fractions (dominant A_{280} peak fractions) are pooled, dialyzed against HEPES dialysis buffer, and stored in aliquots at –80°C in 5% glycerol (*see* **Note 13**).

8. The physical titer (genomic copy number) of the rAAV stock is determined by slot blotting against plasmid standards (*see* **Note 14**). Duplicate sets of viral stock aliquots (1, 5, and 10 μL) and plasmid copy number controls (10^7, 10^8, 10^9, 10^{10}, 10^{11} molecules/μL) are denatured with 50 μL of alkaline AAV digestion buffer at 100°C for 10 min. Samples are immediately chilled on ice and then brought up to a total volume of 400 μL with digestion buffer. Samples are then loaded onto Hybond-N plus membrane with a Bio-Dot SF manifold microfiltration apparatus. After blotting, DNA is crosslinked to the membrane by UV irradiation. Finally the membrane is prehybridized and then hybridized with a ^{32}P-labeled transgene-specific probe in the slot blot hybridization solution and washed with 1X SSC/1% SDS at 50°C for 15 min, twice. After exposure of the blot to X-ray film, the viral particle titer is determined by comparing the intensity of the viral stock band with that of the plasmid standards.

9. The infectious viral titer can be determined by either histochemical or immunocytologic staining of rAAV-infected cells to detect transgene expression. Alternatively, the replication center assay can be used as a generally applicable method *(37)*.

4. Notes

1. **Advantages and disadvantages of trans-splicing and overlapping approaches.** The main differences between these two methods are their respective maximal packaging capacity and the complexity of cloning the proviral plasmids. The generation of *trans*-splicing vectors has two requirements. First, the transgene must be separated at a particular sequence motif (**Fig. 2A**). Second, an intron sequence has to be introduced into the transgene by a PCR-based approach. This strategy is technically more challenging than generating overlapping vectors. However, the *trans*-splicing method can usually accommodate larger transgenes. For example, in a given expression cassette with a promoter of A kb long and a polyA sequence of B kb long, the maximal transgene size accommodated by the AAV *trans*-splicing approach can be calculated by the following formula:

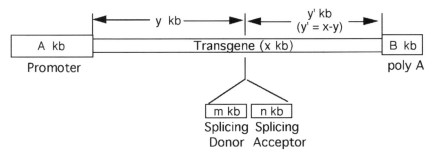

Constants: single virion packaging size = 5 kb, ITR length = 0.15 kb. The maximal size of the foreign sequence in a rAAV = 5 – 0.15 – 0.15 = 4.7.

Maximal length of transgene cDNA for *trans*-splicing vectors (x):

$$x = (4.7 - B - n) + (4.7 - A - m)$$

$$x = 9.4 - (A + B) - (m + n)$$

Calculating the length of donor cDNA segment (y): $y = 4.7 - A - m$ (where A = promoter length, and m = splice donor length). y must be 4.7 kb or less for efficient packaging.

Calculating the length of acceptor cDNA segment (y'): $y' = 4.7 - B - n$ (where y' = maximal length of acceptor cDNA fragment ($y' = x - y$), B = polyA sequence length, and n = splice acceptor length). y' must be 4.7 kb or less for efficient packaging.

Example: A (promoter) = 0.6 kb; B (polyA) = 0.4 kb; m (intron donor signal) = 0.2 kb, n (splicing acceptor signal) = 0.2 kb.

$$x = 9.4 - (0.6 + 0.4) - (0.2 + 0.2)$$

Solution: $x = 8$ kb

∴ The maximum cDNA length for the *trans*-splicing strategy in this example is 8 kb. However, for a similar expression cassette, if the overlapping approach is used, the maximal transgene size can be calculated by the following formula:

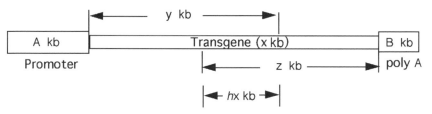

Constants: single virion packaging size = 5 kb, ITR length = 0.15 kb. The maximal size of the foreign sequence in an rAAV = 5 − 0.15 − 0.15 = 4.7 kb.
h is the percentage of overlap in the Upstream and Downstream vectors
Maximal length of transgene cDNA for overlapping vectors (x): $x = y + z - hx$

$$x = (y + z)/(1 + h)$$

$$x = (9.4 - A - B)/(1 + h)$$

Calculating the length of upstream cDNA segment (y): $y = 4.7 - A$ (where $y =$ length of upstream cDNA fragment and A = promoter length). y must be 4.7 kb or less for efficient packaging.
Calculating the length of downstream cDNA segment (z): $z = 4.7 - B$ (where z = length of downstream cDNA fragment and B = polyA sequence length). z must be 4.7 kb or less for efficient packaging.
Example: A (promoter) = 0.6 kb; B (polyA) = 0.4 kb; h (% overlap) = 20%.
Then the maximal length of the transgene

$$x = (9.4 - 0.6 - 0.4)/(1 + 0.2)$$

$$x = 7 \text{ kb}$$

∴ The maximum cDNA length for the overlapping strategy in this example is 7 kb.
2. Interestingly, wild-type AAV-2 preferentially integrates at the human chromosome 19q13.3-qter locus *(38)*. This Rep-facilitated integration does not occur with recombinant AAV.
3. In addition to 293 cells, several HeLa-derived type 2 rAAV packaging cell lines have also been developed recently. In these cell lines, AAV-2 Rep and Cap proteins are expressed from integrated Rep and Cap genes. High-level viral yields have been demonstrated in some of the new producer cell lines with inducible AAV-2 Rep and Cap expression *(39–41)* .
4. Besides the High Fidelity PCR kit from Roche, other PCR polymerases (such as *Pfu* DNA polymerase from Stratagene, #600154) that have the proofreading feature may also be used for cloning AAV *trans*-splicing vectors.

5. To improve biosafety further and eliminate immune reactions to contaminating adenovirus or adenoviral structural proteins, several adenovirus-free systems have been developed. In these protocols, the adenoviral genes required for rAAV preparation are cloned into plasmids. A triple co-transfection of a proviral plasmid, pTrans, and an adenoviral helper plasmid is then used to generate rAAV stock in a virus-free system. Commonly used adenoviral helper plasmids include pXX6-80 *(42)*, pSH3 and pSH5 *(43)*, and pVAE2AE4-2 and pVAE2AE4-5 *(44)*. The pVAE2AE4-2 is commercially available from Stratagene), renamed as pHelper vector (#240071).

6. In addition to pTrans *(32)*, several new helper plasmids have been developed to provide type-2 AAV replication proteins and capsid proteins. These modified helper plasmids, including pACG, pXX2, pCLR1, and pCLV1, have been shown to increase the virus yield *(45,46)*.

7. Eight different serotypes of AAV have been described. Protocols for generating recombinant viral stocks from these serotypes have also been developed. Recent studies suggest that the differences in the capsid structure of these serotypes could offer additional advantages in enhancing transduction efficiency in different cell types *(34,47,48)*. Our studies have indicated that a type 2 rAAV genome packaged in the capsid of another serotype retains the biologic characteristics of the rAAV-2 genome, such as formation of circular transduction intermediates *(34)*. Therefore, depending on the particular application, *trans*-splicing, *cis*-activation, or overlapping rAAV vectors can also be pseudo-packaged in other serotypes to achieve the maximal level of infection and transgene expression.

8. Upon cell death, most progeny AAV virions are retained in the nucleus as paracrystalline aggregates. As a substitute for DNase I, Benzonase (25,000 U; Sigma, #E1014) can also be used to digest nuclear DNA and help release AAV virions.

9. The downstream PCR primer (primer 2, **Fig. 2**) for AV.Donor and the upstream primer (primer 3, **Fig. 2**) for AV.Acceptor are usually longer than 50 nucleotides. Therefore we recommend using PAGE-purified oligonucleotides in the PCR reaction.

10. Gel purification of enzyme-digested PCR fragments can be carried out with commercial kits, such as the QIAquick Gel Extraction Kit from Qiagen (Valencia, CA, #28704) or the GeneClean Kit from Q.BIO gene (Carlsbad, CA, # 1001-200).

11. The step of heat inactivation is not needed if an adenovirus-free triple-plasmid transfection method is used for rAAV production. The purpose of the heat treatment is to inactivate the helper recombinant adenovirus used in the AAV preparation.

12. In addition to the premade heparin column, the Perspective Applied Biosystems (Framingham, MA) also supplies free heparin resin (#1-5228-10) and a self-pack unit for customers to package their own column. A detailed protocol for self-packing a column has been described elsewhere *(49)*.

13. Recent studies suggest that inappropriate storage conditions may decrease the functional titer of rAAV stocks. A divalent cation buffer and minimized heat exposure are recommended for long-term storage *(50)*.

14. Several studies suggest that the HPLC-purified rAAV might have a lower particle-to-infectious unit ratio and perform better than the traditional CsCl-purified rAAV *(51,52)* . However, HPLC-purified rAAV stock tends to contain more empty or partially packaged virions.

Acknowledgments

We gratefully acknowledge Dr. Terry Ritchie for her editorial assistance. Research by the authors' laboratories in the area of this review is funded by NIH grant 2RO1 HL 58340 (to J.F.E.) the Center for Gene Therapy, NIH grant P30 DK54759 (to J.F.E.), and the Muscular Dystrophy Association (to D.D.).

References

1. Lynch, C. M., Aara, P. S., Leonard, J. C., Williams, J. K., Dean, R. H., and Geary, R. L. (1997) Adeno-associated virus vectors for vascular gene delivery. *Circ. Res.* **80,** 497–505.

2. Marshall, D. J. and Leiden, J. M. (1998) Recent advances in skeletal-muscle-based gene therapy. *Curr. Opin. Genet. Dev.* **8,** 360–365.

3. Alexander, M. Y., Webster, K. A., McDonald, P. H., and Prentice, H. M. (1999) Gene transfer and models of gene therapy for the myocardium. *Clin. Exp. Pharmacol. Physiol.* **26,** 661–668.

4. Dedieu, J. F., Mafhoudi, A., Le Roux, A., and Branellec, D. (2000) Vectors for gene therapy of cardiovascular disease. *Curr. Cardiol. Rep.* **2,** 39–47.

5. Phillips, M. I. (2000) Somatic gene therapy for hypertension. *Braz. J. Med. Biol. Res.* **33,** 715–721.

6. Phillips, M. I., Galli, S. M., and Mehta, J. L. (2000) The potential role of antisense oligodeoxynucleotide therapy for cardiovascular disease. *Drugs* **60,** 239–248.

7. Ping, P., Yang, Q., and Hammond, H. K. (1996) Altered beta-adrenergic receptor signaling in heart failure, in vivo gene transfer via adeno and adeno-associated virus. *Microcirculation* **3,** 225–228.

8. Kaplitt, M. G., Xiao, X., and Samulski, R. J. (1996) Long-term gene transfer in porcine myocardium after coronary infusion of an adeno-associated virus vector. *Ann. Thorac. Surg.* **62,** 1669–1676.

9. Gnatenko, D., Arnold, T. E., Zololukhins, S., Nuovo, G. J., Muzyczka, N., and Bahou, W. F. (1997) Characterization of recombinant adeno-associated virus-2 as a vehicle for gene delivery and expression into vascular cells. *J. Investig. Med.* **45,** 87–98.

10. Arnold, T. E., Gnatenko, D., and Bahou, W. F. (1997) In vivo gene transfer into rat arterial walls with novel adeno- associated virus vectors. *J. Vasc Surg.* **25,** 347–355.

11. Maeda, Y., Ikeda, U., Shimpo, M., et al. (1998) Efficient gene transfer into cardiac myocytes using adeno-associated virus (AAV) vectors. *J. Mol. Cell Cardiol.* **30,** 1341–1348.

12. Svensson, E. C., Marshall, D. J., Woodard, K., et al. (1999) Efficient and stable transduction of cardiomyocytes after intramyocardial injection or intracoronary perfusion with recombinant adeno-associated virus vectors. *Circulation* **99,** 201–205.

13. Wright, M. J., Wightman, L. M., Lilley, C., et al. (2001) In vivo myocardial gene transfer: optimization, evaluation and direct comparison of gene transfer vectors. *Basic Res. Cardiol.* **96,** 227–236.

14. Lee, L. Y., Zhou, X., Polce, D. R., et al. (1999) Exogenous control of cardiac gene therapy: evidence of regulated myocardial transgene expression after adenovirus and adeno-associated virus transfer of expression cassettes containing corticosteroid response element promoters. *J. Thorac. Cardiovasc. Surg.* **118,** 26–24, discussion 34–25.

15. Su, H., Lu, R., and . Kan, Y. W. (2000) Adeno-associated viral vector-mediated vascular endothelial growth factor gene transfer induces neovascular formation in ischemic heart. *Proc. Natl. Acad. Sci. USA* **97,** 13,801–13,806.

16. Phillips, M. I. (1997) Antisense inhibition and adeno-associated viral vector delivery for reducing hypertension. *Hypertension* **29,** 177–187.

17. Kimura, B., Mohuczy, D., Tang, X., and Phillips, M. T. (2001) Attenuation of hypertension and heart hypertrophy by adeno-associated virus delivering angiotensinogen antisense. *Hypertension* **37,** 376–380.

18. Kawada, T., Sakamoto, A., Nakazawa, M., et al. (2001) Morphological and physiological restorations of hereditary form of dilated cardiomyopathy by somatic gene therapy. *Biochem. Biophys. Res. Commun.* **284,** 431–435.

19. Dong, J. Y., Fan, P. D., and Frizzell, R. A. (1996) Quantitative analysis of the packaging capacity of recombinant adeno-associated virus. *Hum. Gene Ther.* **7,** 2101–2112.

20. Duan, D., Sharma, P., Yang, J., et al. (1998) Circular intermediates of recombinant adeno-associated virus have defined structural characteristics responsible for long term episomal persistence in muscle. *J. Virol.* **72,** 8568–8577.

21. Duan, D., Yan, Z., Yue, Y., and Engelhardt, J. F. (1999) Structural analysis of adeno-associated virus transduction intermediates. *Virology* **261,** 8–14.

22. Yang, J., Zhou, W., Zhang, Y., Zidon, T., Ritchie, T., and Engelhardt., J. F. (1999) Concatamerization of adeno-associated viral circular genomes ocurs through intermolecular recombination. *J. Virol.* **73,** 9468–9477.

23. Yan, Z., Zhang, Y., Duan, D., and Engelhardt, J. F. (2000) From the Cover: *trans*-splicing vectors expand the utility of adeno-associated virus for gene therapy. *Proc. Natl. Acad. Sci. USA* **97,** 6716–6721.

24. Sun, L., Li, J., and Xiao, X. (2000) Overcoming adeno-associated virus vector size limitation through viral DNA heterodimerization. *Nat. Med.* **6,** 599–602.

25. Nakai, H., Storm, T. A., and Kay, M. A. (2000) Increasing the size of rAAV-mediated expression cassettes in vivo by intermolecular joining of two complementary vectors [see comments]. *Nat. Biotechnol.* **18,** 527–532.

26. Duan, D., Yue, Y., Yan, Z., and Englehardt, J. F. (2000) A new dual-vector approach to enhance recombinant adeno-associated virus-mediated gene expression through intermolecular cis activation. *Nat. Med.* **6,** 595–598.

27. Duan, D., Yue, Y., and Engelhardt, J. F. (2001) Expanding AAV packaging capacity with trans-splicing or overlapping vectors: a Quantitative Comparison. *Mol. Ther.* **4,** 383–396.

28. Senapathy, P. and Carter, B. J. (1984) Molecular cloning of adeno-associated virus variant genomes and generation of infectious virus by recombination in mammalian cells. *J. Biol. Chem.* **259,** 4661–4666.

29. Graham, F. L., Smiley, J., Russell, W. C., and Naim, R., et al. (1977) Characteristics of a human cell line transformed by DNA from human adenovirus type 5. *J. Gen. Virol.* **36,** 59–74.

30. Louis, N., Evelegh, C., and Graham, F. L. (1997) Cloning and sequencing of the cellular-viral junctions from the human adenovirus type 5 transformed 293 cell line. *Virology* **233,** 423–429.

31. Ausubel, F. M., et al. (1995) *Current Protocols in Molecular Biology.* John Wiley, New York.

32. Samulski, R. J., Chang, L. S., and Shenk, T. (1987) A recombinant plasmid from which an infectious adeno-associated virus genome can be excised in vitro and its use to study viral replication. *J. Virol.* **61,** 3096–3101.

33. Xiao, W., Chirmule, N., Berta, S. C., McCullough, B., Gao, G., and Wilson, J. M. (1999) Gene therapy vectors based on adeno-associated virus type 1. *J. Virol.* **73,** 3994–4003.

34. Duan, D., Yan, Z., Yue, Y., Ding, W., and Englehardt, J. F. (2001) Enhancement of muscle gene delivery with pseudotyped AAV-5 correlates with myoblast differentiation. *J. Virol.* **75,** 7662–7671.

35. Senapathy, P., Shapiro, M. B., and Harris, N. L. (1990) Splice junctions, branch point sites, and exons: sequence statistics, identification, and applications to genome project. *Methods Enzymol.* **183,** 252–278.

36. Duan, D., Yue, Y., Yan, Z., Yang, J., and Englehardt, J. F. (2000) Endosomal processing limits gene transfer to polarized airway epithelia by adeno-associated virus. *J. Clin. Invest.* **105,** 1573–1587.

37. Bartlett, J. and Samulski. R. J. (1997) Methods for the construction and propagation of recombinant adeno-associated virus vectors, in *Methods in Molecular Medicine, Gene Therapy Protocols* (P., Robbins, ed.), Humana, Totowa, NJ, pp. 25–40.

38. Kotin, R. M., Siniscalco, M., Samulski, R. J., et al. (1990) Site-specific integration by adeno-associated virus. *Proc. Natl. Acad. Sci. USA* **87,** 2211–2215.

39. Gao, G. P., Qu, G., Faust, L. Z., et al. (1998) High-titer adeno-associated viral vectors from a Rep/Cap cell line and hybrid shuttle virus. *Hum. Gene Ther.* **9,** 2353–2362.

40. Inoue, N. and Russell, D. W. (1998) Packaging cells based on inducible gene amplification for the production of adeno-associated virus vectors. *J. Virol.* **72,** 7024–7031.

41. Liu, X. L., Clark, K. R., and Johnson, P. R. (1999) Production of recombinant adeno-associated virus vectors using a packaging cell line and a hybrid recombinant adenovirus. *Gene Ther.* **6,** 293–299.

42. Xiao, X., Li, J., and Samulski, R. J. (1998) Production of high-titer recombinant adeno-associated virus vectors in the absence of helper adenovirus. *J. Virol.* **72,** 2224–2232.

43. Collaco, R. F., Cao, X., and Trempe, J. P. (1999) A helper virus-free packaging system for recombinant adeno-associated virus vectors. *Gene* **238,** 397–405.

44. Matsushita, T., Elliger, S., and Elliger, C. (1998) Adeno-associated virus vectors can be efficiently produced without helper virus. *Gene Ther.* **5,** 938–945.

45. Li, J., Samulski, R. J., and Xiao, X. (1997) Role for highly regulated rep gene expression in adeno-associated virus vector production. *J. Virol.* **71,** 5236–5243.

46. Cao, L., Lui, Y., During, M. J., and Xiao, W. (2000) High-titer, wild-type free recombinant adeno-associated virus vector production using intron-containing helper plasmids [In Process Citation]. *J. Virol.* **74,** 11,456–11,463.

47. Davidson, B. L., Stein, C. S., Heth, J. A., et al. (2000) Recombinant adeno-associated virus type 2, 4, and 5 vectors: transduction of variant cell types and regions in the mammalian central nervous system. *Proc. Natl. Acad. Sci. USA* **97,** 3428–3432.

48. Chao, H., Lui, Y., Robinowitz, J., Li, C., Samulski, R. J., and Walsh, C. E. (2000) Several log increase in therapeutic transgene delivery by distinct adeno-associated viral serotype vectors. *Mol. Ther.* **2,** 619–623.

49. Yan, Z., Ritchie, T. C., Duan, D., and Engelhardt, J. F. (2002) Recombinant AAV mediated gene delivery using dual vector heterodimerization. *Methods Enzymol.* **346,** 334–357.

50. Turnbull, A. E., Skulimowski, A., Smythe, J. A., and Alexander, I. E. (2000) Adeno–associated virus vectors show variable dependence on divalent cations for thermostability: implications for purification and handling. *Hum. Gene Ther.* **11,** 629–635.

51. Zolotukhin, S., Byrne, B. J., Mason, E., et al. (1999) Recombinant adeno–associated virus purification using novel methods improves infectious titer and yield. *Gene Ther.* **6,** 973–985.

52. Gao, G., Qu, G., Burnham, M. S., et al. (2000) Purification of recombinant adeno-associated virus vectors by column chromatography and its performance in vivo. *Hum. Gene Ther.* **11,** 2079–2091.

4

Lentivirus Vector-Mediated Gene Transfer to Cardiomyocytes

Tsuyoshi Sakoda, Noriyuki Kasahara, and Larry Kedes

1. Introduction

Gene therapy has the potential to reverse the genetic causes and modify the pathophysiology of many innate and acquired diseases *(1–4)*. Transduction of foreign DNA into cardiac myocytes is of potential value for therapeutic applications *(5,6)* and also offers an experimental approach to investigate the roles of individual genes in cardiovascular pathophysiology. Both efficient delivery and long-term expression of transduced genes is required before the full benefit of genetic manipulation strategies can be realized in the cardiovascular system. However, all the current methods of gene delivery have major limitations.

Nonviral methods have been applied to cardiovascular gene therapy in the area of restenosis prevention by transduction of vasculature and by stimulation of collateral circulation through direct injection of naked plasmid DNA encoding angiogenic factors into cardiac muscle. However, these methods are inefficient and can only attain transient expression of the transgene *(7)*, which is suitable and/or desirable for certain applications but insufficient in many others.

Although adenovirus-based vectors allow highly efficient delivery of transgenes and have been frequently employed for cardiac gene transfer both in vitro and in vivo, conventional adenovirus vectors retain 70–80% of the wild-type viral genome, which is expressed at low levels in transduced cells, including cytotoxic viral genes intended to function in host cell lysis. Transgene expression is transient, not only because adenoviruses lack the machinery for integration into the host cell genome, but also because cytotoxic T-cell responses stimulated by presentation of antigenic adenoviral gene products on the surface of transduced cells further attenuate transgene expression; more-

From: *Methods in Molecular Biology, vol. 219: Cardiac Cell and Gene Transfer*
Edited by: J. M. Metzger © Humana Press Inc., Totowa, NJ

over, these cytotoxic and immunostimulatory characteristics of adenovirus vectors represent a significant safety concern *(8)*.

In contrast, standard retrovirus-based vectors, such as the Moloney murine leukemia virus (Mo-MuLV), integrate the transgene into the genome of the target cells and can therefore sustain long-term expression. However such conventional retrovirus-based vectors can transduce only dividing cells *(9)*, thus limiting their use in nonproliferating cells, especially differentiated cardiac myocytes. In addition, silencing of transgene expression over time is a common occurrence.

Recently, the development of lentivirus-based vector systems based on a modified retroviral HIV genome has provided a delivery system that can both transduce nondividing cells and integrate the transgene into the genome of target cells*(10)*. In addition, such lentivirus-based vector particles can be pseudotyped with the glycoprotein envelope of the vesicular stomatitis virus (VSV-G) *(11)*, thus enabling the vector to introduce genes into a broad range of tissues *(10,12,13)*. These features of lentivirus-based vectors, including their relative lack of cytotoxicity, make them useful for delivery of transgenes to cardiac myocytes.

1.1. Advantages of Lentivirus Vectors

Although the life cycle of lentiviruses is similar to that of oncoretroviruses, there are several major differences. Vectors based on oncoretroviruses such as Moloney murine leukemia virus (MLV), which have hitherto been the most popular gene delivery system used in clinical trials, can only transduce cells that divide shortly after infection, because the MLV preintegration complex cannot migrate to the nucleus in the absence of nuclear envelope breakdown during mitosis. However, lentiviruses such as HIV can infect nonproliferating cells, owing to the karyophilic properties of the lentiviral preintegration complex, which allows recognition by the cell nuclear import machinery. Correspondingly, HIV-derived vectors can transduce cell lines that are growth-arrested in culture, as well as terminally differentiated primary cells including neurons, hepatocytes, and cardiomyocytes *(12,14–16)*. In fact, HIV-based vector systems have been described since 1990 *(17–19)* but their efficacy in vivo was first demonstrated only recently *(10)*. Pseudotyped lentiviral vectors have also been shown to mediate efficient delivery, integration, and sustained long-term expression of transgenes into post-mitotic cells such as adult neurons in vivo *(12,14)*.

To replace the HIV gp160 envelope (which would result in a vector that binds only CD4+ cells), lentivirus vectors are pseudotyped (i. e., encoated with a heterologous envelope protein) with VSV-G *(10)*. Such pseudotyping allows efficient transduction of a wide variety of cell types, as the receptor for VSV-G is thought to be a ubiquitous membrane phospholipid such as phosphatidylserine. VSV-G-pseudotyped vectors also exhibit greater stability of virions, as this envelope protein consists of a single transmembrane polypeptide (in contrast to most retrovirus envelopes, which generally consist of an entirely extramembranous surface subunit attached by non-covalent bonds to a transmembrane subunit). This greater degree of structural stability allows efficient concentration of VSV-G-pseudotyped vector preparations simply by ultracentrifugation, without damaging the viral envelope.

Another advantage of lentiviral vector systems is that the promoter inherent in the HIV long terminal repeat (LTR) is critically dependent on the HIV-encoded Tat transactivator protein for transcriptional function. As the sequences encoding Tat are completely removed from the lentiviral vector construct, there is little promoter activity from the LTR, and effective transgene expression is dependent on the addition of an internal promoter. Although our lentiviral constructs all currently contain internal CMV promoters to drive transgene expression (*see* below), this dependence on internal promoters would be particularly advantageous if tissue-specific (e.g., cardiomyocyte-specific) or conditional (e.g., tetracycline-responsive) promoters were to be used. This may also be important for long-term gene expression, as silencing of CMV promoter-driven transgene expression has been described over time in some cells.

1.2. Use of Lentivirus Vectors for Cardiac Gene Transfer

To date there have been few reports regarding application of lentivirus-based vectors to cardiac myocytes (*20,21*). Recently we have compared the efficiency of lentivirus-based vectors with that of murine retrovirus-based vectors for transduction of cultured primary rat cardiac myocytes, cardiac fibroblasts, rat L6 proliferating myoblasts, and differentiated multinucleated myofibers (*16*). Modification of the lentiviral production system enabled us to increase viral particle titers more than 10-fold using sodium butyrate and to generate routinely titers of $>10^8$ TU/mL after one round of concentration. These lentivirus-based vectors carrying reporter genes (bacterial β–galactosidase (LacZ) or jellyfish green fluorescent protein [GFP]) efficiently transduced not only proliferating rat cardiac fibroblasts and L6 myoblasts but also nondividing cardiac myocytes and well-differentiated L6 myofibers. In contrast, murine retrovirus-based vectors transduced only dividing cardiac fibroblasts and L6 myoblasts but did not transduce nonproliferating cardiac myocytes or differentiated myofibers. These findings suggest that lentivirus-based vectors should be useful for delivery of genes to the myocardium in vivo.

2. Materials

2.1. Cardiac Myocyte Preparation

CBFHH 10X stock solution:

	MW	Final conc. (mM)	g per 500 mL 10X stock solution
NaCl	58.44	1370	40.0
KCl	74.56	53.6	2.0
$MgSO_4$ $7H_2O$	246.48	8.1	1.0
KH_2PO_4	136.09	4.4	0.3
Na_2HPO_4 $12H_2O$	358.14	3.4	0.61

To prepare CBFHH (2 L):

a) Dissolve 2.00g dextrose in 1700 mL of distilled water.
b) Add 20 mL of 1 M pH 7.4 HEPES.
c) Adjust to pH 7.4.
d) Dilute to approx 2000 mL.
e) Filter into autoclavable bottles.

2. 2. Virus Production and Transduction

1. 2 M $CaCl_2$.
2. 2X HEPES-buffered saline (HBS):
   140 mM NaCl.
   1.5 mM Na_2HPO_4 $\cdot 12H_2O$.
   50 mM HEPES
   Adjust the pH from 6.9 to 7.2 with NaOH. Select the pH showing the highest transfection efficiency. Note that HBS stored in the refrigerator will yield progressively lower transfection efficiencies over time, and so fresh working stocks should be prepared every month, and HBS stocks should be stored frozen for long-term storage.
3. Polybrene (hexadimethrine bromide) 8 mg/mL stock.
4. Sodium butyrate (*n*-butyric acid sodium salt) 1 M (100X stock).

2. 3. Vector Plasmids

1. Packaging construct pCMVΔR8.2.
2. Envelope construct pCMV-VSV.G.
3. Transfer vector constructs pHR'CMVGFP, pHR'CMVLacZ (**Fig. 1**)

2. 4. β-Galactosidase Staining

1. Fixative solution: 0.5% (v/v) glutaraldehyde in phosphate-buffered saline (PBS).
2. X-gal staining solution: 5 mM Potassium ferricyanide, $K_3Fe(CN)_6$, 5 mM Potassium ferrocyanide, $K_4Fe(CN)_6$ in PBS, 1 mM $MgCl_2$, 1 mg/mL X-Gal (5-bromo-4-chloro-3-indolyl-β-galactoside).

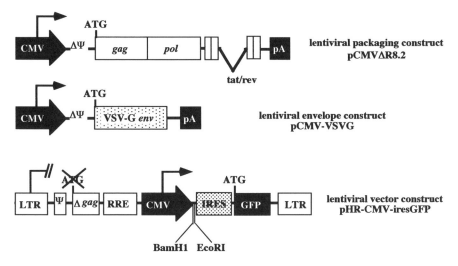

Fig. 1. Schematic maps of the second generation lentivirus transduction system.

2. 5. Immunohistochemical analysis

1. 4% Formaldehyde in PBS.
2. 0.1% Triton X-100 in PBS.
3. Anti-myosin monoclonal antibody MF20 (Developmental Studies Hybridoma Bank, University of Iowa, Iowa City, IA).
4. Fluorescent dye (Texas Red)-conjugated goat anti-mouse immunoglobulin G (IgG) (Jackson ImmunoResearch).

3. Methods

3.1. Cells and Cell Culture

Primary cultures of neonatal rat cardiac myocytes and cardiac fibroblasts were prepared as previously described *(22,23)*. 293T human kidney cells, which were used to produce lentiviruses, were grown in Dulbecco's modified Eagle's medium (DMEM) supplemented with 10% fetal calf serum (FCS) in a 37°C, 5% carbon dioxide humidified environment *(10,12,24)*. The following protocol describes the preparation of cardiac myocytes:

1. Sprague-Dawley rats from 0–3 d after birth.
2. Transfer the animals to a covered container.
3. Flush the container with carbon dioxide, seal, and wait for a few minutes.
4. Sacrifice the animal and expose and isolate the heart.
5. Transfer the heart to a 100-mm tissue culture dish containing 20 mL of cold CBFHH buffer, about 20 hearts per dish. (From now on work in a hood under sterile conditions).

6. Transfer hearts to a 100-mm dish containing 10 mL of CBFHH buffer.
7. Mince the hearts with a scissors. The pieces should be around 2 mm. Do not leave any big pieces.
8. Transfer to a 50-mL beaker and rinse the plate with 7 mL CBFHH.
9. Add 10 mL CBFHH with concentrated trypsin (final 1 mg/mL; CBFHH-Tryp).
10. Incubate in a 5% CO_2 incubator at 37°C for 15 min with stirring.
11. Remove CBFHH-Tryp and suspended cells from the tissue fragments.
12. Add 7 mL CBFHH-Tryp to the remaining heart pieces and incubate in a 5% CO_2 incubator at 37°C for 5 min with stirring.
13. Transfer CBFHH-Tryp (including suspended cardiac cells) into a 50-mL collecting tube.
14. Repeat **steps 12** and **13** about 10–12 times (total 70–80 mL cell solution in 2×50 mL collecting tubes).
15. Spin the collecting tubes at 1000 rpm for 5 min.
16. Aspirate the supernatant with a wide-mouth Pasteur pipet.
17. Add 10 mL DMEM/F12 with 5% FCS each tube and suspend well with gentle aspiration.
18. Collect medium into one 50-mL tube and add 0.4 mL DNAase (1 mg/mL).
19. Pellet the cells at 1000 rpm for 5 min.
20. Aspirate the supernatant and resuspend the cells in 20 mL DMEM/F12 with 5% FCS.
21. Filter the medium through a Swinney filter and wash it with another 20 mL DMEM/F12 with 5% calf serum. (total 40 mL cell solution).
22. Plate the cell solution in 4×100-mm dishes (each 10 mL) and incubate for 30 min to allow adherent fibroblasts to attach.
23. Collect solutions including nonadherent cells (mainly cardiac myocytes) in 50-mL tubes, rinse the dishes with fresh DMEM/F12 with 5% FCS and transfer to the same 50-mL tube.
24. Spin down the cells at 1000 rpm for 5 min.
25. Suspend cells (cardiac myocytes) in a total of 20 mL DMEM/F12 with 5% FCS.
26. Count the cells with a hemocytometer, and plate the cells at the appropriate density.
27. Incubate the cells in a 5% CO_2 incubator at 37°C overnight.
28. Change medium to DMEM/F12 with 5% FCS and 0.1 mM bromodeoxyuridene (BrdU) after 16–20 h.
29. Change medium to DMEM/F12 with 5% FCS without BrdU after 48 h.

3.2. Virus Production and Transduction

Lentivirus-based vectors encoding β-Gal or GFP are generated by transient cotransfection of 293T cells with a three-plasmid combination, as described previously, with slight modifications *(12)*. Our published studies utilized a lentiviral vector system in which the first-generation transfer vector construct pHR'-CMVLacZ or pHR'-CMVGFP was transiently cotransfected along with the second-generation pCMV R8.2 *gag-pol* packaging construct and pMDG *env* construct into 293T cells to produce virus. We are now also employing a third-generation vector system that utilizing a self-inactivating transfer vector and split-genome packaging plasmids that are completely deleted of accessory genes encoding virulence factors (*see* below). These constructs can be used in place of the first- and second-generation plasmids in the same transfection protocol described below. This transient transfection system enables high-level expression of viral proteins and efficient packaging of vector genomes without the need for long-term maintenance of stable packaging cell lines and thus without the attendant risk of recombination leading to generation of helper virus over time. The virus supernatants are then harvested, filtered to remove cell debris, and used to transduce target cells.

1. Transfect, a 100-mm dish of subconfluent 293T cells with 15 µg of pCMVΔR8.2, 15 µg of either pHR'-CMVLacZ or pHR'-CMVGFP, and 15 µg of pMD.G (*see* **Note 1.**) by the calcium phosphate DNA precipitation method *(25,26)*.
2. At 16 h after transfection, adjust the medium to a final concentration of 10 m*M* sodium butyrate (*see* **Note 2**) and incubate the cells for 8 h.
3. Wash the cells and incubate them in fresh medium without sodium butyrate.
4. Harvest conditioned medium 16 h later and filter through 0.45-mm filters.
5. Prepare concentrated viral stocks by one round of ultracentrifugation of the conditioned medium at 50,000*g* at 4°C for 90 min in an SW41 rotor (Beckman Instruments).
6. Resuspend the pellet overnight at 4°C in Hanks' balanced salt solution as described previously *(11)*.
7. For transduction of cardiac myocytes, infect cells overnight with serial dilutions of virus stock in cultured medium supplemented with 8 µg of polybrene per mL.
8. After medium replacement, incubate the cells for 48 h and assess expression of β-Gal or GFP.

Day 1:
9. Make sure 293T cells are at 80–90% confluency and are in an evenly distributed monolayer in the 10-cm plate.
10. In the morning, put 10 mL of fresh medium on the cells. It is essential to have 10 mL medium to avoid toxicity owing to the CaPO$_4$ precipitate.

Late afternoon
11. In one 10-mL Falcon culture tube, add 15 µg of each plasmid and water and mix to a volume of 438 µL. Add 62 µL 2 *M* CaCl$_2$ dropwise to a total volume of 500 µL.
12. Add 2X HBS to the CaCl$_2$/DNA solution slowly, one drop at a time. Vortex the solutions while mixing together.
13. Add solution immediately to the cells, dropwise, slowly, and gently. Place the drops in a circular pattern over the cells to distribute the precipitate evenly. The precipitate tends to clump if agitated immediately; wait 5 min before moving the plate. When moving the plate to the incubator, move it gently to prevent the precipitate from clumping. Leave the cells overnight (for 16 h) in the incubator.

Day 2:
14. In the morning, remove the medium from the cells and replace it with 10 mL of fresh medium containing 10 mM sodium butyrate.
15. Eight hours later, replace the medium with 7 mL fresh medium without sodium butyrate.
16. For titer assays, at this time split HeLa cells so they will be 10% confluent in a 6-well plate.

Day 3:
17. In the morning, harvest the virus from the 293T cells.
18. Take medium from the 293T cells and filter it through a 0.45-μm syringe filter to remove any loose cells.
19. If necessary, fix and stain the 293T cells with X-Gal (for the LacZ transgene) or examine under a UV light microscope (for the GFP transgene) to determine transfection efficiency.
20. Prepare concentrated viral stocks by one round of ultracentrifugation of 7 mL of the conditioned medium at 50,000g at 4°C for 90 min in an SW41 rotor (Beckman Instruments).
21. Resuspend the pellet overnight at 4°C in 70 μL of Hanks' balanced salt solution.

3.3. Analysis of Transduced Cells

Titers (TU/mL) are calculated by dividing the number of LacZ- or GFP-expressing cells counted per dish by the dilution factor. Cells expressing LacZ are fixed and stained with X-Gal as described previously *(27)*. Briefly, the transduced cells are fixed with PBS containing 0.5% glutaraldehyde for 10 min at room temperature. After fixation, LacZ expression is evaluated by histochemical staining with X-Gal in PBS containing 5 mM $K_3Fe(CN)_6$, 5 mM $K_4Fe(CN)_6 \cdot 3H_2O$, 1 mM $MgCl_2$, and 1 mg/mL X-Gal at 37°C for 5–16 h. The following protocol describes β-galactosidase staining:

1. Wash the transduced cells twice with PBS at room temperature.
2. Add fixative solution and fix the cells for 10 min at room temperature.
3. Wash the cells 3 times with 1 mM $MgCl_2$ in PBS.
4. Add X-Gal staining solution and incubate cells for 5–16 h at 37°C.
5. Examine the cells under a light microscope.
6. Note that during X-Gal staining, the pH must be maintained at >7; otherwise endogenous mammalian β-galactosidases (which generally have acidic pH optima) will result in high levels of background staining. Also note that prolonged incubation with the X-Gal substrate will also result in increased levels of background staining over time; to minimize background staining and false-positive results, it is recommended that incubation times be no longer than overnight, that the X-Gal solution be aspirated and the cells washed 1–2× and kept in PBS (with 10% glycerol if desired to delay evaporation) prior to examination, and that an untransduced negative control plate should always be processed for X-Gal staining in parallel for comparison.

3.4. Immunohistochemical Identification of Cardiac Myocytes

Rat cardiac myocytes can be identified by staining with anti-myosin mono-clonal antibody MF20 (Developmental Studies Hybridoma Bank), followed by fluorescent dye (Texas Red)-conjugated goat anti-mouse immunoglobulin G (IgG). Briefly, isolated cardiac myocytes are fixed with 4% buffered formaldehyde for 5 min. The fixed cells are treated with 0.1% Triton X-100 for 5 min. After permeabilization in Triton X-100, cells are incubated for 1 h with MF20, followed by incubation with Texas Red dye-conjugated goat anti-mouse IgG (1:333) for 1 h at room temperature. Finally, the cardiac myocytes are washed several times in PBS and mounted on slides. Texas Red-conjugated anti-mouse IgG can be purchased from Jackson ImmunoResearch.

1. Wash twice with 1X PBS.
2. Fix the cells with 4% formaldehyde in PBS at room temperature for 5 min.
3. Wash 3 times with 1X PBS.
4. Permeabilize with 0.1% Triton X-100 in PBS for 5 min.
5. Wash 3 times with PBS.
6. Add MF20 "neat" (i.e., undiluted) as primary antibody and incubate for 1 h at room temperature.
7. Wash with PBS 3 times.
8. Add Texas-Red (1:333) diluted in PBS with 5% horse serum and 5% albumin as secondary antibody and incubate for 1 h.
9. Wash 3 times with PBS.
10. This method allows simultaneous visualization of both the GFP signal, which is the marker for successful lentiviral transduction, and the Texas Red signal, which identifies α-MHC-positive cardiac myocytes.

4. Notes

1. Vector plasmids. First- and second-generation lentiviral vector constructs are described here; third-generation split-genome packaging constructs and self-inactivating transfer vector constructs can also be used instead, and they are described in a later section. The packaging plasmids and parental transfer vector plasmids were kindly provided by Dr. Luigi Naldini (Institute for Cancer Research and Treatment, University of Torino Medical School, Candiolo, Torino, Italy).
   Packaging construct pCMVΔR8.2. This second-generation packaging construct plasmid (**Fig. 1**) contains the human cytomegalovirus promoter, which drives the expression of HIV-derived lentiviral *gag-pol* proteins. *Env*, *vpu*, and the viral packaging signal are deleted in this plasmid. A polyadenylation site is substituted for the 3' LTR at the end of the *nef* reading frame.
   Envelope construct pCMV-VSV.G. This envelope plasmid encodes the G glycoprotein of VSV-G . As mentioned above, pseudotyping the virion with this envelope has two major advantages. First, entry of VSV into the target cells occurs via binding to ubiquitous phospholipid components of the cell membrane. This

enables VSV-G-pseudotyped vectors to achieve a broad host range. Second, the VSV-G envelope forms highly stable viral particles. This enables virus concentration by ultracentrifugation to achieve high-titer vector solutions.

Transfer vector constructs pHR'CMVGFP and pHR'CMVLacZ. These plasmids contain first-generation transfer vector constructs, which include the *cis*-acting sequences of HIV required for packaging, reverse transcription, and integration. Unique restriction sites are present for the insertion of heterologous cDNAs (LacZ or GFP in this case) to be driven by the CMV promoter. The Rev response element (RRE) flanked by splice signals are included in this plasmid to facilitate efficient nuclear export of the vector mRNA transcript during virus production (**Fig. 1**).

2. Effects of sodium butyrate. To examine the effects of sodium butyrate on virus production, cells were exposed to sodium butyrate at various concentrations and times starting 16 h after transfection. At the end of this treatment, cells were incubated with fresh medium without sodium butyrate and the conditioned medium harvested 16 h later. **Figure 2** shows the effects of various concentrations and incubation times in sodium butyrate on the final viral vector titers. The viral titers are maximally enhanced when 293T cells are exposed to 10 mM sodium butyrate for 8 h as determined by transduction of various cells including cardiac myocytes, 293T cells, and L6 rat myoblasts (**Fig. 2.**). Sodium butyrate routinely increased titers in these cells. Thus, titers derived from 293T cells exposed to sodium butyrate are nearly 1 order of magnitude greater than those obtained without sodium butyrate. After only one round of concentration by ultracentrifugation at 50,000g, titers of $(2.2 \pm 1.0) \times 10^8$ TU/mL on 293T cells are routinely achieved.

We have introduced an efficient system to enhance production of lentivirus-based vectors using sodium butyrate. With respect to the effect of sodium butyrate on virus production, sodium butyrate treatment has been reported to stimulate human CMV gene expression and viral replication in human endothelial cells *(28)*. This enhancing effect by sodium butyrate on virus replication is not specific for human CMV. Similar results have been obtained using other human herpesviruses, Epstein-Barr virus *(29)*, and herpes simplex virus *(30)*. In addition, sodium butyrate has been reported to activate the LTR-directed expression of HIV *(31)*. Therefore, sodium butyrate appears to be associated with a general induction of viruses. In our hands, sodium butyrate treatment at an optimal concentration of 10 mM for an optimal duration of 8 h increased titers by about 9-fold in 293T cells, 11-fold in L6 cells, and 25-fold in cardiac myocytes compared with those obtained without sodium butyrate. Thus, sodium butyrate clearly enhanced viral titers and increased the efficiency of transduction in all cells types tested.

3. Effects of lentivirus and retrovirus-mediated gene transfer into well-differentiated rat neonatal cardiac myocytes. Primary neonatal rat cardiac myocytes and cardiac fibroblasts from the hearts of 2–3-d-old rats were cultured for 3 d and then transduced with lentivirus-based or murine retrovirus-based vectors. The

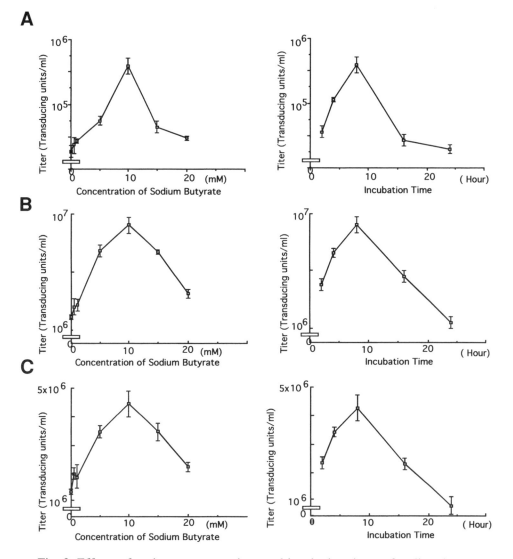

Fig. 2. Effects of various concentrations and incubation times of sodium butyrate on titer (transducing U/mL) of various cells. (**A**) Cardiac myocytes. (**B**) 293T cells. (**C**) L6 cells. Transduction is enhanced when 293T cells were exposed to sodium butyrate after transfection. Lentivirus particles including GFP were generated by transient cotransfection to 293T cells. Conditioned medium was incubated with sodium butyrate at various concentrations and various times. After incubation with sodium butyrate, conditioned medium was harvested and used as virus solution. The values are means ± standard errors of three independent experiments.

cells were stained with X-Gal or processed for immunofluorescence studies 3 d after transduction. **Figure 3A** shows extensive β-Gal staining of cardiac myocytes by lentivirus-mediated LacZ transduction. Although cardiac myocytes were successfully transduced by the lentivirus-based vectors, murine retrovirus-based vectors did not result in detectable levels of cardiac myocyte transduction. The solitary β-Gal-positive cell in **Fig. 3B** is morphologically identified as a contaminating cardiac fibroblast. On the other hand, both lentivirus- and murine retrovirus-based vectors transduced cardiac fibroblasts (**Fig. 3C** and **D**, respectively). Use of lentivirus-based vectors encoding GFP enabled us to assess transduction in living cells without fixation. **Figure 3E** and **F** shows light and fluorescence microscopy of such transduced cardiac myocytes. The GFP-positive cells were beating cardiac myocytes. Finally, GFP-positive cells clearly overlapped the Texas Red dye-positive myosin-expressing cells, indicating viral transduction of cardiac myocytes (**Fig. 3G** and **H**).

The relative efficiencies of murine retrovirus- and lentivirus-based vectors on replicating cardiac fibroblasts and nonreplicating cardicac myocytes are compared in **Fig. 4**. In cardiac fibroblasts, both lentivirus- and murine retrovirus-based vectors effectively transduced and yielded similar titers of $(1.2 \pm 0.6) \times 10^5$ TU/mL and $(2.1 \pm 0.7) \times 10^5$ TU/mL, respectively. However, only lentivirus-based vectors efficiently transduced cardiac myocytes, with a titer of $(6.3 \pm 1.2) \times 10^5$ TU/mL. Furthermore, the GFP expression by lentivirus-based vectors persisted for at least 21 d with no apparent decrease (data not shown). The transduced cardiac myocytes showed no evidence of significant cytotoxicity by microscopic examination, consistent with previous reports *(12,15)*. In contrast, murine retrovirus-based vectors showed low transduction efficiency with titers reaching only $(8.9 \pm 2.1) \times 10^2$ TU/mL. These results demonstrate that efficient long-term transduction of cardiac myocytes in vitro can be achieved by lentivirus-based, but not murine retrovirus-based vectors.

4. Biosafety considerations in the use of lentivirus vectors. As discussed above, lentiviral vectors are generally much less cytotoxic than adenovirus vectors. However, VSV-G pseudotyped vectors can readily be concentrated up to 10^9 infectious particles per mL by ultracentrifugation, and the possible toxicity of concentrated vector preparations containing the highly fusogenic VSV-G protein remains a concern, especially at higher multiplicities of infection. In our experience, the presence of free VSV-G envelope proteins as a contaminant in the vector preparations during transduction of the target cells does appear to reduce target cell viability in certain cell types that are more sensitive to VSV-G toxicity. If this appears to be a problem, as would be indicated if the target cells show cytopathic effects or detach from the plate soon after incubation with the vector preparation, it is useful to clear the free VSV-G protein from the preparation by means of low-speed centrifugation through a 300-kDa MW cutoff filter. Thus, most free proteins including the VSV-G protein will spin through the filter, while the purified virus will remain in the retentate. This procedure also serves to concentrate the vector preparation to a certain extent by volume reduction, without the need

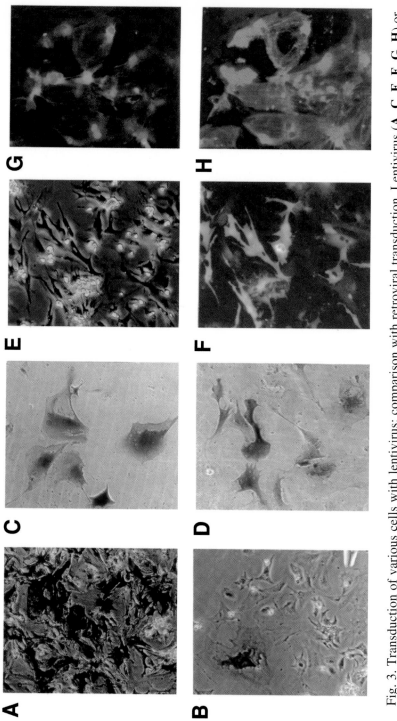

Fig. 3. Transduction of various cells with lentivirus: comparison with retroviral transduction. Lentivirus (**A**, **C**, **E**, **F**, **G**, **H**) or murine retrovirus (**B** and **D**) was used to transduce neonatal cardiac fibroblasts (**C** and **D**) or neonatal cardiac myocytes (**A**, **B**, **E–H**) as described in the text.

to pellet the viruses by ultracentrifugation, if the titers of unconcentrated preparations exhibit inadequate gene transfer efficiency.

The potential toxicity of HIV accessory genes retained in lentiviral vector constructs, as well as the possibility of recombination leading to generation of wild-type virus, has also been raised as a safety concern. Recently, HIV-derived multiply attenuated vector systems deleted of *vif, vpr, vpu, nef,* and *tat* have been reported *(32,33)*. The only remaining auxiliary gene in this system is therefore rev, which, along with the Rev response element (RRE) as its cognate binding sequence, is required for efficient export of the vector and packaging construct RNAs from the nucleus during virus production. Thus the potentials both for toxicity and for recombination leading to the emergence of contaminating replication-competent lentivirus are reduced in these second- and third-generation lentiviral vector systems.

Furthermore, it has previously been found that, despite the lack of significant promoter activity in the absence of Tat, promoter interference between the HIV LTR and the internal CMV promoter can occur, thus significantly attenuating the levels of transgene expression achieved. This has been largely overcome by the use of third-generation self-inactivating (SIN) vectors, in which a portion of the U3 region of the 3' LTR has been deleted *(34)*; thus, after reverse transcription, this deletion will be copied to the 5' LTR and hence result in loss of LTR promoter sequences in the integrated provirus, which therefore prevents interference with the function of the internal promoter. Additionally, this SIN function diminishes the risk that genomic integration of the vector at random sites might lead to activation of adjacent endogenous oncogenes by the LTR promoter in transduced cells.

5. Current improvements in lentivirus vector technology. Recently we have tested third-generation HIV-based packaging systems for the production of lentiviral vectors, using multiply attenuated packaging constructs and SIN vector constructs generously provided by Dr. Luigi Naldini *(10,32,33)*. As discussed above, removal of extraneous accessory gene and *cis* element sequences from the packaging and vector constructs not only reduces the risk of homologous recombination but also results in less cytotoxicity. The lentivirus packaging construct pCMVΔR8.91 (**Fig. 4**) contains the HIV *gag-pol* genes driven by a CMV promoter, with both the packaging signal and most of the *env* gene deleted (except for the RRE and the Tat and Rev coding sequences), and is deleted of *vif, vpr, vpu,* and *nef (32)*.

Further removal of the Tat coding sequence from the packaging plasmid and splitting off the Rev coding sequence to a separate plasmid has also been reported *(33)* and presumably results in a further improvement in safety owing to the necessity for recombination between four plasmids (i.e., the packaging plasmid pMDLg/p encoding *gag-pol,* the pRSV-Rev plasmid encoding the *rev* accessory gene, the envelope plasmid pMD.G encoding VSV-G, and a lentiviral transfer vector plasmid that contains the lentiviral LTRs and packaging signal) for a replication-competent revertant virus to be generated. However, we have

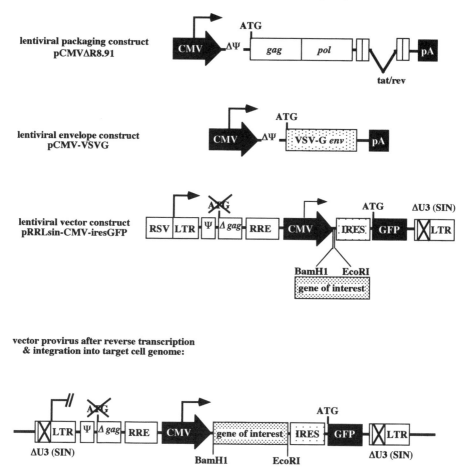

Fig. 4. Schematic maps of the third-generation lentivirus vector system.

generally observed a 0.5–1 log reduction in vector production titers with this third-generation split-genome system, presumably owing in part to lower efficiencies when cotransfecting four plasmids instead of three, and perhaps partly owing to the complete lack of the Tat *trans*-activator. Currently we have settled on a system, schematically illustrated in **Fig. 4**, that combines the most multiply attenuated second-generation packaging construct that still retains Tat and Rev (pCMVΔR8.91), with the self-inactivating transfer vector (pRRLsinCMVGFP) employed in third-generation systems, pseudotyped with VSV-G (pMD.G).

We have developed a number of vector constructs available to be packaged using the above system, based on the lentiviral SIN vector backbone *(33)*. The original vector construct pRRLsinCMVGFP (*see* **Fig. 4**) contains a 5' LTR in which the

HIV promoter sequence has been replaced with that of Rous sarcoma virus (RSV), a SIN 3' LTR containing a deletion in the U3 promoter region, the HIV packaging signal, and RRE sequences linked to a marker gene cassette consisting of GFP driven by the CMV promoter. As demonstrated above, the GFP marker gene allows easy quantitation of the transduction efficiency simply by UV fluorescence microscopy or flow cytometry *(15,16)*. Therefore, we have also constructed a version of pRRLsinCMVGFP that contains an internal ribosome entry site (IRES) just upstream of the GFP gene (pRRLsinCMViresGFP) with unique *Bam*H1 and *Eco*RI sites available to insert genes of interest. The IRES will result in reinitiation of translation from the same mRNA, thus linking expression of the gene of interest with GFP expression.

Furthermore, although the internal CMV promoter will work well in many cell types, in some cases the level of expression obtained is not adequate or silencing of the CMV promoter occurs over time. For these situations, we have developed transfer vectors that contain an alternative housekeeping promoter such as the phosphoglycerol kinase promoter in the vector construct pRRLsinPGKiresGFP, which should maintain high levels of constitutive activity. In addition, for the purposes of cardiac gene transfer, tissue-specific promoters can of course be used to drive cardiomyocyte-specific transgene expression.

References

1. Mulligan, R. C. (1993) The basic science of gene therapy. *Science* **260,** 926–932.
2. Crystal, R. G. (1995) Transfer of genes to humans: early lessons and obstacles to success. *Science* **270,** 404–410.
3. Leiden, J. M. (1995) Gene therapy-promise, pitfalls, and prognosis. *N. Engl. J. Med.* **333,** 871–873.
4. Verma, I. M. and Somia, N. (1997) Gene therapy—promises, problems and prospects. *Nature* **389,** 239–242.
5. Lafont, A., Guerot, C., and Lemarchand, P. (1996) Prospects for gene therapy in cardiovascular disease. *Eur. Heart J.* **17,** 1312–1317.
6. Partridge, T. A. and Davies, K. E. (1995) Myoblast-based gene therapies. *Br. Med. Bull.* **51,** 123–137.
7. Shi, Y., Ford, A., Vernami, P., and Zalewski, A. (1994) Transgene expression in the coronary circulation: transcatheter gene delivery. *Gene Ther.* **1,** 408–414.
8. Schulick, A. H., Newman, K. D., Virmani, R., and Dichek, D. A. (1995) In vivo gene transfer into injured carotid arteries. Optimization and evaluation of acute toxicity. *Circulation* **91,** 2407–2414.
9. Lewis, P. F. and Emerman, M. (1994) Passage through mitosis is required for oncoretroviruses but not for the human immunodeficiency virus. *J. Virol.* **68,** 510–516.
10. Naldini, L., Blomer, U., Gallay, P., et al., (1996) In vivo gene delivery and stable transduction of nondividing cells by a lentiviral vector. *Science* **272,** 263–267.
11. Burns, J. C., Friedmann, T., Driever, W., Burrascano, M., and Yec, J. K. (1993) Vesicular stomatitis virus G glycoprotein pseudotyped retroviral vectors: concen-

tration to very high titer and efficient gene transfer into mammalian and nonmammalian cells. *Proc. Natl. Acad. Sci. USA* **90,** 8033–8037.

12. Naldini, L., Blomer, U., Gage, F. H., Trono, D., and Verma, I. M. (1996) Efficient transfer, integration, and sustained long-term expression of the transgene in adult rat brains injected with a lentiviral vector. *Proc. Natl. Acad. Sci. USA* **93,** 11,382–11,388.

13. Miyake, K., Suzuki, N., Matsucka, H., Tohyama, T., and Shimada, T. (1998) Stable integration of human immunodeficiency virus-based retroviral vectors into the chromosomes of nondividing cells. *Hum. Gene Ther.* **9,** 467–475.

14. Blomer, U., Naldini, L., Verma, I. M., Trono, D., and Gage, F. H. (1996) Applications of gene therapy to the CNS. *Hum. Mol. Genet.* **5,** 1397–1404.

15. Kafri, T., Blomer, U., Peterson, D. A., Gage, F. H., and Verma, I. M. (1997) Sustained expression of genes delivered directly into liver and muscle by lentiviral vectors. *Nat. Genet.* **17,** 314–317.

16. Sakoda, T., Kasahara, N., Hammano, Y., and Kedes, L. (1999) A high-titer lentiviral production system mediates efficient transduction of differentiated cells including beating cardiac myocytes. *J. Mol. Cell Cardiol.* **31,** 2037–2047.

17. Page, K. A., Landau, N. R., and Littman, D. R. (1990) Construction and use of a human immunodeficiency virus vector for analysis of virus infectivity. *J. Virol.* **64,** 5270–5276.

18. Shimada, T., Fujii, H., Mitsuya, H., and Nienhuis, A. W. (1991) Targeted and highly efficient gene transfer into CD4+ cells by a recombinant human immunodeficiency virus retroviral vector. *J. Clin. Invest.* **88,** 1043–1047.

19. Buchschacher, G. L., Jr. and Panganiban, A. T. (1992) Human immunodeficiency virus vectors for inducible expression of foreign genes. *J. Virol.* **66,** 2731–2739.

20. Rebolledo, M. A., Krogstad, P., Chen, F., Shannon, K. M., and Klitzner, J. S. (1998) Infection of human fetal cardiac myocytes by a human immunodeficiency virus-1-derived vector. *Circ. Res.* **83,** 738–742.

21. Mochizuki, H., Schwartz, J. P., Tanaka, K., Brady, R. O., and Reiser, J. (1998) High-titer human immunodeficiency virus type 1-based vector systems for gene delivery into nondividing cells. *J. Virol.* **72,** 8873–8883.

22. Sussman, M. A., Hamm-Alvarez, S. F., Vilalta, P. M., Welch, S., and Kedes, L. (1997) Involvement of phosphorylation in doxorubicin-mediated myofibril degeneration. An immunofluorescence microscopy analysis. *Circ. Res.* **80,** 52–61.

23. Ueyama, T., Sakoda, T., Kauashima, S., et al. (1997) Activated RhoA stimulates c-fos gene expression in myocardial cells. *Circ. Res.* **81,** 672–678.

24. Price, J., Turner, D., and Cepko, C. (1987) Lineage analysis in the vertebrate nervous system by retrovirus- mediated gene transfer. *Proc. Natl. Acad. Sci. USA* **84,** 156–160.

25. Chen, C. and Okayama, H. (1987)High-efficiency transformation of mammalian cells by plasmid DNA. *Mol. Cell Biol.* **7,** 2745–2752.

26. Sakoda, T., Kaibuchi, K., Kishi, K., et al. (1992) smg/rap1/Krev-1 p21s inhibit the signal pathway to the c-fos promoter/enhancer from c-Ki-ras p21 but not from c-raf-1 kinase in NIH3T3 cells. *Oncogene* **7,** 1705–1711.

27. Sanes, J. R., Rubenstein, J. L., and Nicolas, J. F. (1986) Use of a recombinant retrovirus to study post-implantation cell lineage in mouse embryos. *EMBO J.* **5,** 3133–3142.

28. Radsak, K., Fuhrmann, R., Franke, R. P., et al., Induction by sodium butyrate of cytomegalovirus replication in human endothelial cells. *Arch . Virol.* **107,** 151–158.

29. Saemundsen, A. K., Kallin, B., and Klein, G. (1980) Effect of n-butyrate on cellular and viral DNA synthesis in cells latently infected with Epstein-Barr virus. *Virology* **107,** 557–561.

30. Ash, R. J. (1986) Butyrate-induced reversal of herpes simplex virus restriction in neuroblastoma cells. *Virology* **155,** 584–592.

31. Bohan, C., York, D., and Srinivasan, A. (1987) Sodium butyrate activates human immunodeficiency virus long terminal repeat-directed expression. *Biochem. Biophys. Res. Commun.* **148,** 899–905.

32. Zufferey, R., Nagy, D., Mandel, R. J., Naldini, L., and Trono, D. (1997) Multiply attenuated lentiviral vector achieves efficient gene delivery in vivo. *Nat. Biotechnol.* **15,** 871–875.

33. Dull, T., Zufferey, R., Kelly, M., et al. (1998) A third-generation lentivirus vector with a conditional packaging system. *J. Virol.* **72,** 8463–8471.

34. Zufferey, R., Dull, T., Mardel, R. J., et al. (1998) Self-inactivating lentivirus vector for safe and efficient in vivo gene delivery. *J. Virol.* **72,** 9873–9880.

II

CELL TRANSFER TO MYOCARDIUM

PROTOCOLS AND APPLICATIONS

5

Cell Therapy in the Heart

Cell Production, Transplantation, and Applications

Kevin S. Cahill, Catalin Toma, Mark F. Pittenger, Paul D. Kessler, and Barry J. Byrne

1. Introduction

Cardiac dysfunction resulting from various insults to the myocardium can ultimately lead to the development of heart failure. Owing to the limited regenerative capacity of adult cardiac tissue and the lack of a resident cardiac progenitor cell equivalent to the skeletal myoblast, the transplantation of myogenic cells into the myocardium has been investigated as a novel mechanism to repair damaged and dysfunctional myocardium. For maximal impact on cardiac function, the design of cellular therapies must carefully consider the identity of the transplanted cells as well as the method of cell delivery. This review details techniques for the purification of commonly investigated cell grafts, including skeletal myoblasts and mesenchymal stem cells, and the methods to deliver these grafts to the myocardium of laboratory animals.

Since the initial studies documenting the survival of atrial tumor-derived cell grafts in syngeneic myocardium (*1*) a variety of donor cell types have been evaluated (including fetal and adult cardiomyocytes, smooth muscle cells, skeletal muscle myoblasts, and mesenchymal stem cells) in an attempt to determine the most suitable cell type for cardiac repair (for review, *see* **ref. *2***). Skeletal myoblasts are a committed progenitor cell population found in close proximity to the mature skeletal myocytes. This cell population can be easily isolated from an adult muscle biopsy and propagated in tissue culture (*2,15*). Several reports have documented the ability of skeletal myoblasts to survive in healthy and damaged myocardium and ultimately improve systolic and diastolic function (*3–5*). Importantly, the ability of myoblasts to be utilized in

From: *Methods in Molecular Biology, vol. 219: Cardiac Cell and Gene Transfer*
Edited by: J. M. Metzger © Humana Press Inc., Totowa, NJ

autologous therapies obviates the need for life-long immunosuppression following transplantation.

Pluripotent stem cells capable of differentiation into mature cardiomyocytes have also been proposed for use in cellular therapies *(6)*. Mesenchymal stem cells (MSCs) are an adult bone marrow stem cell population with the potential for multilineage differentiation *(7,8)*. In culture, MSCs undergo rapid proliferation in an undifferentiated state and following exposure to appropriate induction conditions will differentiate into mesodermal lineages, including myocytes and cardiomyocytes *(8–10)*. Since MSCs are easily procured from bone marrow aspirates and readily undergo ex vivo expansion, they also have the potential to be useful in autologous cellular therapies. A functional improvement was demonstrated by Tomita and colleagues *(11)*, who reported that MSC-like cells isolated from rat bone marrow treated with 5-azacytidine could improve heart function in a cyroinjury model of cardiomyopathy.

To have the greatest positive impact on cardiac function, cell delivery strategies must be adapted to the type of myocardial damage that is present. One technique is direct injection of the cellular transplant into a specific region of the myocardium. This technique allows for the delivery of cells to a preselected area and holds promise for cell therapy for localized cardiac injury. For example, the fibrosis resulting from a transmural myocardial infarction can be visualized and then seeded with myogenic cells. This delivery strategy seems most amenable to situations in which a severe obstruction in arterial blood flow would preclude vascular delivery.

Alternatively, cell grafts can be delivered to the myocardium via the vasculature. It has been demonstrated that cell transplants will migrate across the capillary wall to engraft in the myocardium when arterially delivered *(12–14)*. In large animals and humans, this can be accomplished through the use of a catheter-mediated intracoronary infusion, whereas in rodents other techniques are needed to overcome the exceedingly small size of the vasculature. One technique for arterial cell delivery in rodents is an intraventricular cell injection. Of the cells delivered to the left ventricular cavity, a small percentage will enter the coronary circulation. Importantly, arterial delivery techniques allow the cells to engraft in all areas of the myocardium receiving coronary artery perfusion. This may allow for a maximal therapeutic effect when the myocardium is globally damaged, as is seen in muscular dystrophies with cardiac involvement or end-stage heart failure with global cardiomyopathy.

2. Materials

2.1. Myoblast Isolation and Culture Materials

1. 1X Dulbecco's modified Eagle's medium (DMEM) with L-glutamine, with 4.5 g/L glucose, without sodium pyruvate (Cellgro from Mediatech, Herndon, VA).
2. Phosphate-buffered saline (PBS), 1X solution without calcium and magnesium (Cellgro).

3. Fetal bovine serum (FBS) and horse serum (HS). Inactivate complement by incubation at 56°C for 30 min (Cellgro).
4. Penicillin and streptomycin stock solution (Cellgro), containing 10,000 IU per 100 mL penicillin and 10,000 µg/mL streptomycin.
5. Chick embryo extract (CEE, Gibco-BRL), for use in the myoblast culture media.
6. Myoblast culture media: DMEM with 20% FBS, 0.5% CEE, 5 mL of the penicillin/streptomycin stock solution. Sterilize the media by passage through a 0.22-µm filter.
7. Collagenase and trypsin-EDTA: trypsin-EDTA (Cellgro) 10X stock solution and 1% collagenase (Sigma St. Louis, MO).
8. Nylon mesh, 50-µm sterile.
9. Collagen-coated 60-mm tissue culture dishes.

2.2. Mesenchymal Stem Cell Isolation and Culture Materials

1. 1X DMEM with L-glutamine, with 1.0 g/L glucose, without sodium pyruvate (Cellgro).
2. FBS selected for MSC outgrowth (BioWhittaker, Walkersville, MD).
3. 100X MEM nonessential amino acid stock solution (Cellgro).
4. Mesenchymal stem cell culture media: DMEM (low glucose) with 10% selected FBS, 5 mL of the penicillin/streptomycin stock solution, and 5 mL of the nonessential amino acid solution. Sterilize the media by passage through a 0.22-µm filter.
5. 25-Gauge syringe, 3-mL needle, sterile nylon mesh.

2.3. Myoblast Delivery Materials

1. Standard surgical instruments and materials.
2. 29-Gauge insulin syringe.
3. Rodent ventilator (Harvard Apparatus, Holliston, MA).

3. Methods

3.1. Isolation of Myoblasts from Skeletal Muscle

3.1.1. Myoblast Harvest

The following procedure should be performed in a certified tissue culture hood, and all instruments and solutions should be properly sterilized.

1. Starting with 200–400 mg of freshly excised skeletal muscle, use scissors to cut the muscle into square pieces approx 2 mm in length.
2. Add the pieces to a 15-mL sterile conical tube containing 10 mL of PBS with 1X trypsin-EDTA and 1% collagenase. Incubate in a 37°C water bath for 15–30 min and gently vortex the tube once during the incubation. Stop the enzymatic digestion by transferring the supernatant into a 50-mL sterile conical tube containing 10 mL of DMEM supplemented with 10% FBS.
3. Triturate the neutralized solution by pipeting up and down several times with a 25-mL pipet. This should disperse the larger material present in the solution. Any

additional aggregates can be removed by passing the solution through a 30–60-μm nylon mesh.

4. Collect the cells by centrifugation at 200g for 5 min. Resuspend the cells in 1 mL of myoblast growth media and count the cells using a hemocytometer. Plate the cells at an approximate density of 1×10^5 cells/60-mm collagen-coated dish.
5. Culture cells in a 37°C incubator with 5% CO_2. One day after plating, perform two successive media changes to remove any nonadherent cell debris (*see* **Notes 1** and **2**).

3.1.2. Growth of Myoblast Cultures

The myoblasts will proliferate and become confluent in approx 2–3 d. Do not allow the cells to reach confluence, as they will begin to differentiate. Myoblasts should be trypsinized and replated at 1:4 dilutions when they become approx 80% confluent. Media should be changed every 2 d if the cells are not being split.

3.2. Isolation of Mesenchymal Stem Cells from Bone Marrow

The selection of MSCs from bone marrow is based on the phenomenon that MSCs readily adhere to tissue culture dishes, whereas hematopoietic and other contaminating cell types do not attach and/or do not readily expand in selected lots of serum. The purity and growth characteristics of MSC cultures may be variable and species-dependent. All MSC cultures should be characterized by flow cytometry and differentiation assays *(8)*. We have had the best results with rat and human MSC cultures, although certain strains of murine cultures are also useful.

3.2.1. MSC Harvest

This protocol will detail the harvest of MSCs from mice and should be performed in a tissue culture hood to minimize contamination of cultures. Isolation of MSCs from other species can be accomplished using this protocol with minor modifications.

1. Obtain 10 freshly dissected femurs. Dissect any remaining musculature from the femurs using forceps and scissors. Use an alcohol swab to clean the femurs and remove any remaining ligaments.
2. Using either scissors or a small bone cutter, carefully remove the proximal- and distalmost portions of the femur to provide access to the medullary cavity within the shaft.
3. Flush the bone marrow from the medullary cavity with PBS using a 3-mL syringe with a 25-gauge needle. This is accomplished by inserting the needle in the shaft and then rotating and moving the needle vertically while dispensing the PBS to completely dislodge the bone marrow from the medullary cavity. Collect the flow

through in a 15-mL conical tube.

4. Centrifuge the aspirate at 900*g* for 5 min and resuspend the cell pellet in 2-mL of MSC culture media. Pass the cellular solution through a 25-gauge needle several times to disrupt any cellular clumps and then pass the solution through nylon mesh to remove any contaminating bone fragments.

5. Plate the cells at an appropriate density so that after several days of growth MSC colonies are evenly spaced. This will vary with the strain of mouse used and the effectiveness of the harvest.

6. Change the medium daily for the first week to remove contaminating nonadherent cell types (*see* **Note 3**).

3.2.2. MSC Culture

1. Continue media changes every 2–3 d to ensure removal of hematopoietic cells. Colonies of MSCs should be seen 5–10 d after plating.

2. The rate of MSC proliferation will vary with the strain of mouse used. The MSCs should be trypsinized and replated at 1:4 dilutions when they become approx 80% confluent.

3.3. Delivery of Cellular Graft to Murine Myocardium

The following surgical techniques assume that the researcher has been trained in the basics of microsurgery in rodents. All surgeries are performed with the assistance of a dissecting microscope. Prior to in vivo myocardial delivery, the cells should be marked to allow for later identification in the myocardium. This can be accomplished through the use of membrane or DNA dyes such as CM-DiI or DAPI or through replication-defective recombinant viruses carrying marker genes. Our laboratory routinely utilizes recombinant adeno-associated virus vectors for the long-term transduction of MSCs and myoblasts.

3.3.1. Preparation of Cellular Grafts

1. Obtain the appropriate number of MSC- or myoblast-containing culture dishes. Remove the culture media and wash the cells twice with PBS prewarmed to 37°C.

2. Add 2–3 mL of PBS containing 1X trypsin-EDTA. Incubate at 37°C for 2–5 min. Monitor the reaction by microscopic examination of the culture for dissociated cells. Dislodge the cells by gently tapping the flask as necessary. MSC cultures may require an increased incubation time to remove all the cells completely. When all of the cells are in suspension, stop the enzymatic digestion by addition of 3 mL of DMEM with 10% FBS. Transfer the suspension to a 15-mL conical tube.

3. Pellet the cells by centrifugation at 1000*g* for 5 min. Resuspend the pellet in 1 mL of PBS and count the cells using a hematocytometer.

4. Again, pellet the cells by centrifugation at 1000*g* for 5 min. Resuspend the cell pellet in the appropriate volume of PBS to give a final concentration of 10^6 cells

per 25–50 µL. The cells should be injected as soon as possible following resuspension. Maintain the cells on ice until injection.

3.3.2. Direct Myocardial Injection of Cellular Grafts

The murine myocardial wall is exceeding thin, and care must be taken to ensure that the material is not injected into the ventricular cavity. The following protocol is designed to be performed in a mouse; however, most cardiac manipulations are technically easier to perform in a rat, and this protocol can easily be adapted to larger rodents. Sterile instruments and aseptic technique should be used at all times to decrease the chance of infection.

1. Appropriately anesthetize the animal. We routinely use ketamine and xylazine, although various other anesthetics are effective.
2. Using clippers first and then a razor, remove the hair from the thorax and the left axilla. Clean the shaved area with a 0.5% betadine solution and alcohol.
3. Place the animal on a positive pressure ventilator. This can be done by the passage of an 18-gauge angiocatheter through the oral cavity into the trachea (*see* **Note 4**). Connect the angiocatheter to the ventilator tubing. The ventilator settings depend on the weight of the animal. We routinely set the respiration rate to 115 breaths per minute and adjust the tidal volume to approximate normal respiratory activity visually. Secure the animal in the supine position with the upper limbs extended away from the thorax to a temperature-controlled operating surface. Monitor body temperature through the use of a rectal thermometer.
4. A lateral thoracotomy is performed to expose the heart. Make a 1–2-cm coronal incision through the skin approx 1 cm inferior to the left axilla. Use a fine-point high temperature cautery to ligate the superficial vessel running from the axilla inferiorly. Next use scissors to make an incision between two successive ribs. The intercostal musculature is only several millimeters thick, and care must be taken to ensure that the lung is not damaged. Cauterize any perforated vessels as needed. The thoracic wall can now be retracted as necessary to expose the myocardium adequately.
5. Once the area of interest in the heart is localized, use a 29-gauge needle to inject the cell suspension into the wall of the myocardium. Avoid advancing the needle into the ventricular cavity.
6. To close the incision, use 6-0 prolene to approximate the ribs and musculature. Care must be taken to ensure that the lungs are not inadvertently damaged and that the thoracic wall is secure and air-tight. Prior to completion of the closure, aspirate any air or fluid from the thorax by a 22-gauge angiocatheter connected to light suction. Finally, close the skin with 5-0 suture.
7. The animal can be weaned from the ventilator as the anesthetic begins to wear off. This process can be accelerated by the administration of a respiratory stimulant. Once the animal is spontaneously breathing, remove the tracheal tube.
8. The animal should be placed in a temperature-controlled recovery room and given antibiotics and pain medication following surgery.

3.3.3. Arterial Delivery of Myoblasts

Access to the left ventricular cavity can be obtained by a transdiaphragmatic injection. The murine heart is easily visible through the semitransparent diaphragm following a midline abdominal incision and retraction of the liver. Alternatively, several techniques can be utilized to increase coronary cell delivery involving dissection and occlusion of the great vessels. These techniques, however, require a highly trained microvascular surgeon and are beyond the scope of this review. The following procedure is designed for use in mice.

1. Anesthetize the animal by inhalation of isoflurane until the animal is unconscious. Monitor the breathing rate of the animal. Slow, labored breathing may indicate that too much anesthetic has been given.
2. Using clippers and then a razor, remove the hair from the abdomen. Clean the abdomen with a 0.5% betadine solution.
3. Use scissors to make a midline incision through the abdominal skin extending from the xyphoid process to about 2 cm inferiorly. Next, make an incision in the abdominal wall musculature along the linea alba.
4. Use a retractor to reflect the abdominal walls laterally. Locate the liver. Depress the liver with a cotton swab and use scissors to cut the falciform ligament. The diaphragm and inferior surface of the heart should be visible.
5. Using an insulin syringe containing the cells to be injected, advance the needle through the diaphragm and myocardial wall while pulling back gently on the plunger of the syringe. When the needle has entered the high-pressure left ventricle, a rush of bright red blood will enter the syringe. Retract the needle slightly and then inject the contents (*see* **Note 5**).
6. Following injection, remove the needle from the heart and apply immediate pressure to the injection site using a cotton swab. This step is essential to decrease the chance of pneumothorax. The injection site in the myocardial wall will seal spontaneously.
7. Close the abdominal wall incision with 6-0 prolene suture and then the skin with 5-0 suture.
8. The animal should be placed in a temperature-controlled recovery room and given antibiotics and pain medication following surgery.

4. Notes

1. The yield of myoblasts decreases with the age of the animal. Additionally, various techniques that injure the skeletal muscle 2–3 d before harvest can result in an increase in the yield of myoblasts.
2. Myoblast enrichment of the primary cultures can be accomplished based on the observation that myoblasts take longer to adhere to tissue culture dishes than fibroblasts. Thus, removing and replating the nonadherent myoblast suspension after 30–60 min of the initial plating will enrich for myoblasts. An increase in the cell yield can also be obtained by redigesting the muscle reminants following the initial enzymatic digestion of the muscle pieces.

3. The bone marrow aspirate can be centrifuged through a density gradient to remove contaminating cell types prior to plating. We centrifuge the aspirate at 1100g for 30 min in a 1.073 g/mL Percoll gradient. The nucleated cells collected at the interface and the upperlayer are then washed and plated.

4. Intubation can be accomplished in a mouse through the oral cavity or via a tracheotomy. To locate the laryngeal inlet, place the mouse supine on a platform inverted at approx 45 degrees. While using forceps to open the oral cavity, shine a bright light in the area of the mouse's neck. Look into the mouth and you will see a small circular light in the oral cavity. This is the laryngeal inlet and can be used as a guide to ensure that the esophagus is not inadvertently entered.

5. The maximum number of cells that can be delivered in a single intraventricular injection is approx 10^6. We routinely delivery this cell number in a volume of 100 µL. An increase in cell number may result in lethal cellular emboli. However, successive injections can be performed to increase the total number of cells that reach the myocardium. Prior to injection, it is useful to filter the cells through a 30-µm nylon mesh to avoid injection of large cell clumps that may produce lethal emboli. During injection it is helpful to have an assistant raise the xyphoid process with forceps and depress the liver with a cotton swab to increase visibility of the heart.

Acknowledgments

This research was supported by the National Institute of Standards and Technologies Advanced Technology Program (NIST/ATP), NHLBI, NIH (HL59412), and T32AI07110.

References

1. Koh, G. H., Soonpaa, M. H., Klug, M. G., and Field, L. J. (1993) Long-term survival of AT-1 cardiomyocyte grafts in syngeneic myocardium. *Am. J. Physiol.* **264,** H1727.

2. Kessler, P. D. and Byrne, B. J. (1999) Myoblast cell grafting into heart muscle: cellular biology and potential applications. *Annu. Rev. Physiol.* **61,** 219–242.

3. Taylor, D. A., Atkins, B. Z., Hungspreugs, P., et al. (1998) Regeneratng functional myocardium: improved performance after skeletal myoblast transplantation. *Nat. Med.* **4,** 929–933.

4. Rajnoch, C., Chachques, J. C., Berrebi, A., Bruneval, P., Benoit, M. O., and Carpentier, A. (2001) Cellular therapy reverses myocardial dysfunction. *J. Thorac. Cardiovasc. Surg.* **121,** 871–878.

5. Atkins, B. Z., Hueman, M. T., Meuchel, J., Hutcheson, K. A., Glower, D. D., and Taylor, D. A. (1998) Cellular cardiomyoplasty improves diastolic properties of injured heart. *J. Surg. Res.* **85,** 234–242.

6. Klug, M. G., Soonpaa, M. H., Koh, G. Y., and Field, L. J. (1996) Genetically selected cardiomyocytes from differentiating embryonic stem cells form stable intracardiac grafts. *J. Clin. Invest.* **98,** 216–224.

7. Haynesworth, S. E., Goshima, J., Goldberg, V. M., and Caplan, A. I. (1992) Characterization of cells with osteogenic potential from human bone marrow. *Bone* **13,** 81–88.
8. Pittenger, M. F., Mackay, A. M., Beck, S. C., et al. (1999) Multilineage potential of adult human mesenchymal stem cells. *Science* **284,** 143–147.
9. Saito, T., Dennis, J. E., Lennon, D. P., et al. (1995) Myogenic expresssion of mesenchymal stem cells within myotubes of mdx mice in vitro and in vivo. *Tissue Engin.* **1,** 327–343.
10. Makino, S., Fukuda, K., Miyoshi, S., et al. (1999) Cardiomyocytes can be generated from marrow stromal cells in vitro. *J. Clin. Invest.* **103,** 697–705.
11. Tomita, S., Li, R. K., Weisel, R. D., et al. (1999) Autologous transplantation of bone marrow cells improves damaged heart function. *Circulation* **100,** II247–II256.
12. Robinson, S. W., Cho, P. W., Levitsky, H. I., et al. (1996) Arterial delivery of genetically labeled skeletal myoblasts to the murine heart: long-term survival and phenotypic modification of implanted myoblasts. *Cell Transplant.* **5,** 77–91.
13. Taylor, D. A., Silvestry, S. C., Bishop, S. A., et al. (1997) Delivery of primary autologous skeletal myoblasts into rabbit heart by coronary infusion: a potential approach to myocardial repair. *Proc. Assoc. Am. Physicians* **109,** 245–253.
14. Toma, T., Pittenger, M. F., Cahill, K. S., Byrne, B. J., and Kessler, P. D. (2001) Human mesenchymal stem cells differentiate to a cardiomyocyte phenotype in the adult murine heart. *Circulation* **105,** 93–98.
15. Rando, T. A. and Blau, H. M. (1994) Primary mouse myoblast purification, characterization, and transplantation for cell-mediated gene therapy. *J. Cell Biol.* **125,** 1275–1287.
16. Yaffe, D. and Saxel, O. (1977) Serial passaging and differentiation of myogenic cells isolated from dystrophic mouse muscle. *Nature* **270,** 725–727.

6

Cardiac Cell Transplantation

Protocols and Applications

Steven M. White and William C. Claycomb

1. Introduction

Cellular transplantation into the heart is an emerging field with numerous applications for designing new therapeutic strategies for treating various types of heart disease. The two primary applications of cellular transplantation are to generate new functional myocardium and to deliver therapeutic agents such as growth factors into diseased hearts. Cardiac cellular transplantation experiments have been performed using different cell types, including cardiomyocyte cell lines *(1)*, primary cardiomyocytes *(2,3)*, skeletal myocytes *(4–6)*, and fibroblasts *(7)*. In performing cardiac cellular transplantation experiments, various animal models have been used to assess the efficacy of autologous *(8)*, syngeneic *(9)*, allogeneic, and xenogeneic *(1,10)* cellular transplants. Many investigators are currently focusing on using embryonic stem (ES) cells *(10,11)* and bone marrow-derived stem cells *(12,13)* for in vitro differentiation into cardiomyocytes for transplantation, or as direct sources for cardiac cellular transplantation. In order for cells to be useful for transplantation into injured myocardium, they must be able to survive in the recipient tissue, have limited capacity for replication, and become physically and electrically coupled to each other and the neighboring host myocardium so that they may all contract synchronously.

We have used the adult swine as a large animal model for studying the effects of cellular transplantation into injured myocardium *(1)*. Because the heart size and coronary anatomy closely resemble those of humans, the porcine animal model can provide valuable information regarding the efficacy of cellular

From: *Methods in Molecular Biology, vol. 219: Cardiac Cell and Gene Transfer*
Edited by: J. M. Metzger © Humana Press Inc., Totowa, NJ

transplantation as a therapy for heart disease. During the course of the experiments the animals undergo several procedures, depending on whether the cells are being transplanted into normal or infarcted myocardium. Cardiac catheterization is used to introduce an embolization coil into the left anterior descending (LAD) branch of the left coronary artery to induce a nonlethal myocardial infarction. The subsequent epicardial cellular injections are made using a median sternotomy to access the heart. There are several major issues related to performing cellular transplantation experiments including proper personnel and facilities, selection of cells to use for transplantation, and care for the animals used in the experiments. This chapter provides a detailed protocol for cardiac cellular transplantation in the porcine model and describes applications for this new and exciting therapy.

2. Materials

2.1. Personnel

For further information, *see* **Note 1**.

1. Cardiothoracic surgeon.
2. Cardiologist.
3. Anesthetist.
4. Cell culture technician (*see* **Note 2**).
5. Animal care providers (*see* **Note 3**).

2.2. Facilities

For further information, (*see* **Note 4**).

1. Animal care facility for large animals (adult swine).
2. Cardiac catheterization suite.
3. Surgical suite with anesthesia equipment.
4. Postoperative monitoring facility.

2.3. Cells

The following cell types have been used for transplantation into the heart:

1. Freshly isolated cardiomyocytes (fetal, neonatal, adult) *(1,7,14)*.
2. Cells from established cardiomyocyte cell lines (HL-1, AT-1) *(1)*.
3. Skeletal myocytes *(4–6)*.
4. ES cells (mouse) *(10,11)*.
5. Bone marrow-derived stem cells *(12,13)*.

2.4. Drugs, Media, and Reagents

2.4.1. Cell Transport for Transplantation Experiments

1. Cell culture medium specific for the cell type being used.
2. Ice for transporting cells.

2.4.2. Induction and Maintenance of General Anesthesia

1. Ketamine.
2. Acetylpromazine.
3. Pentobarbital.
4. Isoflurane.
5. Lidocaine.
6. Diltiazem.
7. Isotonic (normal) saline solution for intravenous administration.

2.4.3. Cardiac Catheterization

1. All drugs and solutions listed under **Subheading 2.4.2.**
2. Labetalol.
3. Lidocaine (*see* **Note 5**).
4. Diltiazem infusion bag (*see* **Note 6**).
5. Epinephrine.
6. Surgical soap
7. Iodine solution (Betadine).
8. Sterile water.
9. Renografin contrast solution.

2.4.4. Median Sternotomy Procedure

1. All drugs and solutions listed under **Subheading 2.4.2.**
2. Surgical soap.
3. Iodine solution (Betadine).
4. Sterile water.

2.4.5. Cellular Transplantation

1. Joklik's medium.
2. Ice.
3. Warm isotonic saline solution.

2.4.6. Postoperative Period

1. All drugs and solutions listed in **Subheadings 2.4.2.** and **2.4.3.** should be available.

2.4.7. Immunosuppression

1. FK-506.
2. Cyclosporine.
3. Prednisone.

2.4.8. Organ Harvesting

1. All drugs and solutions listed in **Subheadings 2.4.2.** and **2.4.3.**
2. Heparin.
3. Prednisone.

2.5. Equipment

2.5.1. Cell Transport for Transplantation

1. Sterile vial(s) (*see* **Note 7**).
2. Container for ice.

2.5.2. Induction and Maintenance of General Anesthesia

1. Sterile syringes (10 mL).
2. Sterile 22-gauge needles.
3. Sterile 18 gauge iv catheters.
4. Sterile iv connector tubing
5. Laryngoscope and blades.
6. Sterile endotracheal tubes (different sizes).
7. Pressure-controlled ventilator and anesthesia machine.
8. Arterial line kit.
9. Monitor capable of showing electrocardiogram (ECG), mean arterial blood pressure (MABP), and arterial O_2 saturation.
10. ECG electrodes.
11. Pulse oximetry electrode.

2.5.3. Cardiac Catheterization

1. All equipment listed in **Subheading 2.5.2.**
2. Functional cardiac catheterization suite with fluoroscopy.
3. Sterile drapes and towels.
4. Sterile 4 × 4-cm gauze sponges.
5. Sterile towel clips.
6. Sterile scalpel and scalpel blades.
7. Cordis introducer sheath (5–6-F; Cordis Co.).
8. Catheterization kit.
9. 5-F H1 embolization catheter.
10. Cooper embolization coil (0.5 × 10 mm; Cook Co.).
11. Guidewire.
12. Defibrillator (DC).

2.5.4. Median Sternotomy Procedure

1. All equipment listed in **Subheading 2.5.2.**
2. Sterile drapes and towels.
3. Sterile 4 × 4-cm gauze sponges.
4. Sterile towel clips.
5. Suction apparatus with sterile tips and tubing.
6. Sternal saw.
7. Sterile surgical instruments including the following:
   a. Scalpel blades.
   b. Scalpel handle.
   c. Traumatic and atraumatic forceps of different sizes.

    d. Curved and straight Metzenbaum scissors.
    e. Suture scissors.
    f. Needle holders of different sizes.
    g. Hand-held retractors.
    h. Sternal retractor.
8. Electrocautery apparatus
9. Sutures including the following types:
    a. 2-0 silk.
    b. 2-0 silk "pop-offs."
    c. 2-0 silk ties.
    d. 7-0 proline sutures.

2.5.5. Cellular Transplantation

1. Doppler thickening probes.
2. All surgical instruments listed in **Subheading 2.5.4.**, #7.
3. All sutures listed in **Subheading 2.5.4.**, #9.
4. Sterile 1-mL tuberculin syringes.
5. Sternal wires.
6. Sterile dressings and tape.

2.5.6. Postoperative Period

1. All equipment listed in **Subheading 2.5.2.** for anesthesia and monitoring.

2.5.7. Organ Harvesting

1. All equipment listed in **Subheading 2.5.2.** for anesthesia and monitoring.
2. All surgical equipment listed in **Subheading 2.5.4.**

3. Methods
3.1. Cell Transport for Transplantation

1. Prior to the transplantation experiments, the cells should be maintained according to the protocol for the specific cell type.
2. For transporting cells to the operating room for transplantation, cells should be suspended in sterile cell culture medium in a sterile vial and transported on ice (*see* **Note 8**).

3.2. Induction and Maintenance of General Anesthesia

1. Determine the weight (in kg) of the animal to be used (*see* **Note 9**).
2. Induce general anesthesia by administering 7 mg/kg ketamine im and 0.2 mg/kg acetylpromazine im followed by 25 mg/kg pentobarbital im.
3. Position the animal in the supine position on the procedure table and secure all limbs to the table.
4. Intubate the animal by using a laryngoscope to pass an endotracheal tube through the vocal cords into the main bronchus (*see* **Note 10**).
5. Connect the endotracheal tube to the pressure-controlled ventilator.

6. Ventilate the animal with 1–2% isoflurane.
7. Verify that the animal is under anesthesia and unresponsive to painful stimuli.
8. Obtain peripheral intravenous access (in any limb) by inserting a subcutaneous infusion catheter connected to intravenous tubing and a bag of normal saline solution.
9. Insert a peripheral arterial line for monitoring arterial blood pressure and blood gases during the cellular transplantation procedure.
10. Begin constant infusions of 3 mg/kg lidocaine iv and 2.5 mg/kg diltiazem iv to control ventricular rate and the onset of atrial arrhythmias.
11. Place ECG electrodes so that a 3-lead ECG may be used to monitor cardiac electrical activity during the procedure.

3.3. Cardiac Catheterization to Induce a Myocardial Infarction

1. Two days prior to the creation of the myocardial infarction, give the animals 200 mg labetalol (a β-adrenergic antagonist) each day in their feed to reduce the chance of mortality during the catheterization procedure.
2. Prepare each animal for the catheterization by following the protocol outlined in **Subheading 3.2.** *(1–11)* except for the placement of an arterial line (#9).
3. Give an iv infusion of normal saline supplemented with lidocaine (3 mg/kg over 20 min) and diltiazem (120 mg/h) during the procedure and for at least 2 h after the procedure to prevent ventricular arrhythmias (*see* **Note 11**).
4. Spread apart the rear legs and secure to the table.
5. Prepare the right groin for a surgical incision using sterile technique.
   a. Scrub the groin with surgical soap and sterile water using sterile gauze sponges.
   b. After scrubbing the area for at least 5 min, wipe the area clean with sterile towels to remove the soap lather.
   c. Apply iodine solution (Betadine) to the incision site using sterile gauze in a circular fashion starting from the site of the incision and spreading out to the periphery of the groin.
6. Locate the intended incision site by palpating the right femoral artery.
7. Create a sterile field around the intended incision site in the right groin by placing sterile towels and sheets around the incision site.
8. All subsequent steps should be performed in a sterile manner.
9. Make an approx 3-mm incision over the right common femoral artery using a sterile scalpel blade and create a small tunnel in the subcutaneous tissue with a hemostat.
10. Using the Seldinger technique, cannulate the femoral artery, insert the guidewire through the cannula, and advance the catheter over the guidewire.
11. Pass the catheter through the introducer sheath and advance the tip of the catheter to the aortic root under direct fluoroscopic guidance.
12. Perform coronary angiography by injecting Renografin contrast solution through the catheter so that the coronary anatomy may be studied (*see* **Note 12**).

13. Depending on the individual animal's coronary anatomy, either the terminal portion of the LAD or one of the obtuse marginal branches of the left circumflex artery may be chosen for the creation of the myocardial infarction (*see* **Note 13**).

14. Advance the 5-F H1 embolization catheter through the catheter already in place in the aortic root and maneuver it into the left main coronary artery and subsequently into either the middle to distal LAD artery or the proximal portion of a large obtuse marginal branch of the left circumflex artery.

15. With the embolization catheter in place and confirmed using angiography, deploy a Cooper embolization coil (0.5×10 mm) (Cook Co.) using a 0.035-in. guidewire.

16. ECG confirmation of myocardial infarction is demonstrated immediately by S-T segment elevation.

17. Symptomatic cardiac arrhythmias resulting from the deployment of the embolization coil should be treated according to the rhythm, and efforts should be made to resuscitate animals developing lethal arrhythmias using the following (*see* **Note 14**):
    a. DC cardioversion.
    b. 1 mg/kg epinephrine.
    c. 3 mg/kg lidocaine.

18. Perform repeat angiography to confirm that the vessel containing the embolization coil is occluded.

19. Remove the catheter apparatus from the animal.

20. Maintain pressure on the femoral artery for at least 10 min after the catheter is removed.

21. Monitor the animal and allow it to recover by following the protocol in **Subheading 3.6.**

22. Allow the animal to recover for 1 mo following the myocardial infarction, and prior to the cellular transplantation procedure.

3.4. Procedure for Performing a Median Sternotomy

1. Pepare each animal for the median sternotomy by following the protocol outlined in **Subheading 3.2.** *(1–11)*.

2. Begin preparing the chest for the incision by shaving any hair from the sternal and surrounding areas (*see* **Note 15**).

3. Using sterile water, surgical soap, and sterile gauze sponges, scrub the entire chest for at least 5 min (*see* **Note 16**).

4. Use sterile towels to dry the chest, removing all soap and water.

5. Apply iodine solution (Betadine) using sterile gauze sponges (*see* **Note 17**).

6. Create a sterile field by applying sterile towels and drapes around the intended incision site (*see* **Note 18**).

7. Perform all subsequent procedures using sterile technique by personnel properly scrubbed and dressed according to sterile technique (*see* **Note 19**).

8. Ensure the animal is under general anesthesia by applying a painful stimulus.

9. Ensure the sternal saw is working prior to making the incision.

10. Using a sterile scalpel blade, make a midline incision over the entire sternum.
11. Dissect down to the sternum using electrocautery to maintain hemostasis.
12. Ensure the entire sternum is accessible for splitting with the sternal saw.
13. Stop ventilation so that the lungs are deflated just long enough for the sternum to be split (*see* **Note 20**).
14. Position the sternal saw at the superior border of the sternum in the sternal notch and proceed inferiorly, splitting the sternum.
15. Continue ventilations once the sternum is completely split.
16. Insert a sternal retractor between the edges of the divided sternum and slowly open to provide an adequate working space.
17. After visualizing the heart, lift the anterior pericardium using atraumatic forceps with the help of the assistant, and cut longitudinally using Metzenbaum scissors.
18. Once an adequate view of the heart is obtained through the opening in the pericardium, suture the cut edges of the pericardium and tie to the sternal spreader using "pop-off" silk sutures.
19. Approximately three sutures on each edge of the cut pericardium are adequate to create a pericardial well in which the remainder of the procedure will take place.

3.5. Cellular Transplantation into the Myocardium

1. Transport the cells to be used for transplantation to the operating room on ice in small sterile vials at a concentration of 10^6 cells/20 µL culture medium (*see* **Note 21**).
2. The myocardial injection sites should be decided in advance depending on whether the heart is normal or if a myocardial infarction has been created (*see* **Note 22**).
3. For hearts with myocardial infarctions, the infarct zone is identified visually and confirmed using Doppler thickening probes placed on the surface of the myocardium (*see* **Note 23**).
4. Suture two probes (one over both normal and infarcted myocardium) to the epicardial surface with 7-0 proline sutures. These probes will be left in place for the duration of the animal's recovery until it is sacrificed 4–6 wk following the procedure.
5. For each injection, draw 100 µL of cells into a 1-mL tuberculin syringe with a 26-gauge needle.
6. Inject cells through the epicardium into the myocardium at various locations (*see* **Note 24**).
7. After each injection, place a 7-0 proline suture to mark each injection site for future gross and histologic examination.
8. Give each heart at least one sham injection of 100 µL culture medium without cells to serve as a control.
9. After the injections are made, fill the pericardium with warm saline solution and observe the heart for any bleeding.
10. Remove the saline with suction, and remove the sutures holdiı g the edges of the cut pericardium to the sternal retractor.
11. Leave the pericardium open (*see* **Note 25**).

12. Place drains within the pericardium and exit through the inferior portion of the incision.
13. Pass sternal wires (6) on needles through each half of the sternum at the same position on each side to accommodate approximation of the cut sternum.
14. Once all the sternal wires are in position, close the chest by grasping all the sternal wires and pulling the sternal borders together.
15. With the assistant holding the chest closed with the sternal wires, the surgeon takes each wire separately and twists it on itself so that it will hold its position and not slip.
16. After all the wires are twisted, cut each wire with surgical wire cutters, leaving an approx 0.5-cm tail of twisted wire.
17. Using a needle driver, fold the wire tails down toward the sternum so that they will not injure the overlying tissue.
18. After the ribcage is closed, place subcutaneous proline sutures followed by superficial sutures.
19. Dress the wounds by placing sterile gauze over the entire incision and securing the dressing with tape.

3.6. Postoperative Care of the Animal

1. Once the cellular transplantation procedure is complete, allow the animal to recover for 4 h under general anesthesia with the arterial line in place to monitor blood pressure.
2. During this recovery period, titrate bretylium and diltiazem to relative bradycardia or the presence of significant ventricular arrhythmias (*see* **Note 26**).
3. After 4 h, discontinue the anesthesia and allow the animal to regain consciousness.
4. Once the gag reflex begins to return, extubate the animal.
5. Leave ECG leads in place for a few hours to monitor cardiac electrical activity.
6. Return the animals to the animal care facility and maintain with an appropriate diet according to the institution's guidelines.
7. Allow animals to recover for 1 mo prior to harvesting the heart (*see* **Note 27**).

3.7. Immunosuppression Therapy

1. Immediately following the cellular transplantation procedure, start the animals on immunosuppressive therapy consisting of the following:
   a. 0.2 mg/kg FK-506 by oral gavage.
   b. 15 mg/kg cyclosporine by oral gavage.
   c. 0.35 mg/kg prednisone by oral gavage.
2. Maintain the animals on this immunosuppressive therapy from the time of cellular transplantation until they are sacrificed for harvesting of the heart (*see* **Note 28**).

3.8. Harvesting the Heart for Analysis

1. Prepare each animal for the median sternotomy to remove the heart by following the protocol outlined in **Subheading 3.2.** (*1–11*) with the exception of #9.
2. Open the chest through the same incision used for the previous sternotomy. Cut the wires holding the sternum together with wire-cutters, allowing the sternum to open.

3. Insert the sternal retractor to open the chest, exposing the heart in the cut pericardial sac.
4. Cut the heart free of any adhesions that may have developed since the last procedure.
5. Give the animal 1000 U/kg heparin iv to prevent blood clotting in the microvasculature of the heart.
6. Excise the heart by cutting the proximal aorta, pulmonary arterial trunk, and pulmonary veins, and allow the animal to exsanguinate.
7. The heart tissue is now ready to be processed according to the types of analyses desired (*see* **Note 29**).

3.9. Future Applications

Cardiac cellular transplantation is an exciting new therapy for the treatment of various types of heart disease. There have been many studies examining the efficacy of cellular transplantation as a means of generating functional myocardial tissue following an infarction. Although the data concerning the degree of functional improvement in ventricular function are not clear, it is clear that cellular transplantation into injured myocardium will play a major role as a therapeutic strategy in the near future. There are still many issues to be investigated with regard to the types of cells to be used for transplantation and the optimal method of delivery. Although this chapter has focused on the use of epicardial injections for cellular transplantation, other methods such as endocardial injections and intraarterial injections *(15)* have also been investigated. Instead of using direct injection as the method of delivery, it could be possible to deliver cells with altered cell surface protein expression into the systemic circulation and have them migrate to the heart. This could potentially make cellular transplantation minimally invasive.

An exciting area of cellular transplantation is the use of stem cells derived from various sources. The plasticity of stem cells makes them promising prospects for cardiac cellular transplantation with regard to their wide differentiation potential and ease of genetic manipulation. One application for genetically altering cells for transplantation is manipulating cells in vitro to reduce or alleviate their immunogenicity. Currently, there is controversy regarding appropriate sources of stem cells to be used in cellular transplantation. By genetically altering stem cells from different sources to render them nonimmunogenic, graft rejection could be alleviated and the donor pool for cells would be greatly increased, allowing for allogeneic and even xenogeneic transplantation.

Another potential application for cardiac cellular transplantation is in the treatment of certain congenital heart diseases. Most of the current studies in cardiac cellular transplantation focus on regenerating damaged myocardium as a result of an infarction. Although this is a promising use of cellular transplantation, the use of cellular therapy as a treatment for congenital heart malformations is also a potential therapeutic option. With the continuing development of early *in utero* diagnosis of cardiac malformations and growing experience with fetal surgery, it is possible that using cellular transplantation to reconstruct malformations or to deliver therapeutic agents that will alter cardiac morphogenesis directly to the heart will be a feasible therapy in the near future.

Cellular transplantation in the heart is a promising therapy not only for generating functional myocardial tissue but also for delivering growth factors and other therapeutic agents. It will be possible to alter cells genetically so that they constitutively or inducibly secrete therapeutic agents into the local tissue for purposes such as inducing angiogenesis, altering myocardial remodeling, or inhibiting local inflammation. These types of cellular therapies could play significant roles in many cardiovascular diseases, both acquired and congenital.

4. Notes

1. The personnel listed represent specialists in each area and are suggested, not required. For instance, the cardiologist or surgeon may be proficient in anesthesia, so that a separate person to deliver anesthesia may not be required. It is important that all of the personnel involved be experienced in dealing with the particular animal being used in the experiments.
2. The cell culture technician is the person responsible for providing the cells at the time of the transplantation experiments.
3. The type of animal care providers required will vary depending on the individual institution. We recommend that a licensed veterinarian be used as a consultant in the care of the animals, although veterinary technicians will be providing the daily care.
4. Although different institutions will vary in the facilities available for these types of experiments, all the facilities listed in **Subheading 2.2.** should be equipped similarly to those used for humans with respect to anesthesia and monitoring equipment.
5. Lidocaine (3 mg/kg) is given over 20 min.
6. 500 mg diltiazem (120 mg/h) is made in small infusion bags by the hospital pharmacy.
7. These can be any type of sterile vial (1–2 mL) routinely used in tissue culture.
8. For our experiments, we used cells suspended at a concentration of 10^6 cells/ 20 µL culture medium. Different numbers and concentrations of cells may be used depending on the goal of the experiment.
9. Animal weights are usually expressed in kilograms to facilitate drug dosing.
10. The person performing the intubation should be familiar with the unique upper airway anatomy of the adult swine.
11. Although the combination of lidocaine and diltiazem should be sufficient to control postoperative arrhythmias, additional agents such as β-receptor antagonists may also be useful.
12. Make sure enough images are obtained to ensure a complete and detailed view of the entire coronary anatomy.

13. Choosing a coronary branch that is too large could result in a lethal infarction. Also, if the goal of the experiment is to produce an animal with heart failure, choosing too small a vessel may not result in sufficient myocardial impairment to progress into clinical heart failure.
14. Prolonged resuscitation of animals with lethal arrhythmias is not advised.
15. Blot the chest with tape to remove any excess hair.
16. The animal should be scrubbed from the neck and shoulders down to the abdomen, and the entire chest should be cleaned from the most lateral regions (midaxillary lines in humans).
17. Apply the iodine solution by "painting" the chest, starting with the intended incision site and moving to the periphery of the region to be sterile. Take care not to reapply iodine solution to an area already covered.
18. Four sterile towels are typically placed first around the four sides of the incision site, creating a rectangle with the intended incision site in the middle. Adjacent towels are connected using sterile towel clips. Next, various large drapes are applied to cover exposed portions of the animal, table, and any neighboring equipment that could serve as a potential source of contamination.
19. Surgical personnel wearing caps and masks should scrub (at least 5 min) and wear sterile gowns and gloves as if this were a human surgical procedure.
20. This requires coordination between the surgeon and the person in charge of ventilations (and anesthesia).
21. The volume of cells in culture medium taken to the operating room depends on the number of injections intended for each cell type.
22. In experiments using hearts with infarcted myocardium, it is often desirable to make injections of cells into normal myocardium, in the middle of the infarct zone, and on the periphery of the infarct zone, close to normal myocardium.
23. Probes over normal myocardium should demonstrate ventricular thickening during systole (corresponding to the QRS complex on the ECG), whereas the probes over the infarcted myocardium will show thinning of the wall during ventricular systole owing to the presence of scar tissue. These probes measure ventricular wall thickness over time. The output of data from the ECG, Doppler thickening probes, and MABP can be measured simultaneously and viewed on the same video monitor.
24. When making injections, if localized cellular transplants are desired, it is important to pull back on the plunger of the syringe prior to injecting the cells to ensure that the tip of the needle is not in a vessel or the ventricular cavity. This is especially important when injecting cells into infarcted myocardium because of its thinner wall. If blood is seen when retracting the plunger, reposition the tip of the needle and reconfirm that the tip of the needle is in the myocardial interstitium.
25. Leaving the pericardium open allows the Doppler thickening probes and drains to exit through the incision site and remain attached to the animal postoperatively.
26. This requires close monitoring of the ECG to look for symptomatic arrhythmias.
27. This period is at least 4 wk to allow myocardial scar formation.
28. In this adult swine model, approx 60–70% of the animals survive the myocardial infarction and continue to recover for approx 1 mo.

29. Depending on the type of analyses desired, portions of the heart may be immediately processed for RNA isolation or fixed for histology or immunohistochemistry, depending on the particular experiment.

References

1. Watanabe, E., Smith, D. M., Jr, Delcarpio, J. B., et al. (1998) Cardiomyocyte transplantation in a porcine myocardial infarction model. *Cell Transplant* **7,** 239–246.
2. Koh, G. Y., Soonpaa, M. H., Klug, M. G., et al. (1995) Stable fetal cardiomyocyte grafts in the hearts of dystrophic mice and dogs. *J. Clin. Invest.* **96,** 2034–2042.
3. Reinecke, H., Zhang, M., Bartosek, T., and Murry, C. E. (1999) Survival, integration, and differentiation of cardiomyocyte grafts: a study in normal and injured rat hearts. *Circulation* 100:193–202.
4. Reinecke, H. and Murry, C. E. (2000) Transmural replacement of myocardium after skeletal myoblast grafting into the heart. Too much of a good thing? *Cardiovasc. Pathol.* **9,** 337–344.
5. Atkins, B. Z., Hueman, M. T., Meuchel, J. M., Cottman, M. J., Hutcheson, K. A., and Taylor, D. A. (1999) Myogenic cell transplantation improves in vivo regional performance in infarcted rabbit myocardium. *J. Heart Lung Transplant.* **18,** 1173–1180.
6. Kessler, P. D. and Byrne, B. J. (1999) Myoblast cell grafting into heart muscle: cellular biology and potential applications. *Annu. Rev. Physiol.* **61,** 219–242.
7. Sakai, T., Li, R. K., Weisel, R. D., et al. (1999) Fetal cell transplantation: a comparison of three cell types. *J. Thorac. Cardiovasc. Surg.* **118,** 715–724.
8. Li, R. K., Weisel, R. D., Mickle, D. A., et al. (2000) Autologous porcine heart cell transplantation improved heart function after a myocardial infarction. *J. Thorac. Cardiovasc. Surg.* **119,** 62–68.
9. Gojo, S., Kitamura, S., Hatano, O., et al. (1997) Transplantation of genetically marked cardiac muscle cells. *J. Thorac. Cardiovasc. Surg.* **113,** 10–18.
10. Dinsmore, J., Ratliff, J., Deacon, T., et al. (1996) Embryonic stem cells differentiated in vitro as a novel source of cells for transplantation. *Cell Transplant.* **5,** 131–143.
11. Klug, M. G., Soonpaa, M. H., Koh, G. Y., and Field, L. J. (1996) Genetically selected cardiomyocytes from differentiating embronic stem cells form stable intracardiac grafts. *J. Clin. Invest.* **98,** 216–224.
12. Orlic, D., Kajstura, J., Chimenti, S., et al. (2001) Bone marrow cells regenerate infarcted myocardium. *Nature* **410,** 701–705.
13. Tomita, S., Li, R. K., Weisel, R. D., et al. (1999) Autologous transplantation of bone marrow cells improves damaged heart function. *Circulation* **100,** II247–II256.
14. Li, R. K., Weisel, R. D., Mickle, D. A., et al. (2000) Autologous porcine heart cell transplantation improved heart function after a myocardial infarction. *J. Thorac. Cardiovasc. Surg.* **119,** 62–68.
15. Robinson, S. W., Cho, P. W., Levitsky, H. I., et al. (1996) Arterial delivery of genetically labelled skeletal myoblasts to the murine heart: long-term survival and phenotypic modification of implanted myoblasts. *Cell Transplant.* **5,** 77–91.

7

Cell Grafting for Cardiac Repair

Hans Reinecke and Charles E. Murry

1. Introduction

Despite impressive advances in the last decade in treating coronary athero-sclerosis, myocardial infarction remains the number one cause of death and disability in industrialized countries. A great deal of effort has been expended over the last 25 years toward identifying strategies to limit the amount of myocardium lost to infarction *(1,2)*. Although infarct size limitation remains a highly desirable goal, it has been extremely difficult to achieve clinically. A fundamental problem is the fact that ischemic myocardium dies quite rapidly, whereas most patients wait for more than 3 hours before seeking medical attention. Over the last 5 years, our group has become increasingly interested in working on strategies to enhance the repair phase of myocardial infarction *(3–7)*. Our long term goals are to induce muscular regeneration of the infarcted region. This chapter focuses on our work using skeletal muscle cell transplantation for cardiac regeneration.

Unlike many organs in the body, the heart cannot undergo regenerative healing after necrotizing injury. Two problems prevent regeneration. First, unlike smooth muscle, cardiomyocytes that survive the injury do not reenter the cell cycle to any significant extent *(8,9)*. Although very low rates of cardiomyocyte proliferation have been reported in injured hearts by some investigators, this clearly does not occur to a physiologically meaningful extent *(10)*. Second, unlike skeletal muscle, there are apparently no muscle stem cells in myocardium. Pluripotent somatic stem cells have recently been reported to exist in many tissues such as the brain *(11–13)*, bone marrow stroma *(14)*, and skeletal muscle *(15)*, but to date none have been described in the heart. There are recent

From: *Methods in Molecular Biology, vol. 219: Cardiac Cell and Gene Transfer*
Edited by: J. M. Metzger © Humana Press Inc., Totowa, NJ

reports that provide evidence for a circulating, bone marrow-derived cell capable of giving rise to cardiomyocytes in injured hearts *(16,17)*. If this is true, such cells might be one day manipulated to enhance cardiac repair; in any case, it is clear that their endogenous contribution cannot be physiologically significant.

1.1. Strategies For Cardiac Regeneration

The ideal way to repair a myocardial infarct would be to induce the heart to regenerate new muscle instead of forming a scar. In theory, this could be accomplished in at least three ways. First, the surviving cardiomyocytes could be induced to divide and migrate into the wound. The mechanism of cardiac myocyte withdrawal from the cell cycle is being studied in other labs *(18,19)*. Second, the fibroblasts of granulation tissue could be induced to differentiate into muscle cells. Our current understanding of cardiac differentiation does not permit transdifferentiation of wound fibroblasts to form cardiomyocytes. We have, however, previously induced cells in cardiac granulation tissue in vivo to form skeletal myofibers by adenoviral transfer of the myogenic determination gene, MyoD *(3)*. As molecular regulation of cardiac development becomes better understood, it may be possible to use a similar strategy to induce cardiomyocyte differentiation in healing infarcts. The final route toward muscle regeneration would be to graft cells into injured hearts to establish a new muscle tissue. In principal, these could be committed somatic cells such as cardiomyocytes or skeletal muscle cells, or they could be stem cells somehow programmed to differentiate into cardiomyocytes in vivo.

This chapter focuses on the grafting of adenovirally transduced skeletal myoblasts into the mouse heart, for purposes of cardiac repair. Relatively minor modifications of this protocol should permit one to use different cell types, different gene transfer vectors, or a different animal model customized to another experimental question.

2. Materials

2.1. Dissection of Skeletal Muscle

The microdissection should be carried out under aseptic conditions. Therefore, all tools should be sterilized, e.g., by autoclaving or ethylene oxide gas sterilization.

1. Dissecting microscope, e.g., Olympus SZ60.
2. Sterile underpads or similar.
3. Scalpel, blade (#10).
4. Small toothed tissue forceps (e.g., World Precision Instruments, Sarasota, FL).
5. Fine pointed jeweler's forceps (#4 or #5) (World Precision Instruments).

6. Dissecting scissors: straight blades with rounded tips (e.g., Codman, Raynham, MA; 46, #54-6526), curved iridectomy (e.g., Codman 63, #34-6503), and small spring loaded (Tiemann, Hauppauge, NY, #160-159).
7. Petri dishes (Falcon, Becton Dickinson Labware, Franklin Lakes, NJ).

2.2. Cardiac Surgery on Mice

All tools used for survival surgery on mice need to be sterilized by autoclaving, gas sterilization, or immersion in a germicidal solution according to manufacturer's specifications.

1. #3 scalpel handle (e.g., Codman, #11-5530) and #10 scalpel blade.
2. Small, toothed tissue forceps (e.g., Codman 89, #30-6530).
3. Fine hemostat (e.g., Jarit, Hawthorne, NY, #105-096).
4. Tissue scissors with straight, rounded blades (e.g., Codman 46, #54-6526).
5. Small, spring-loaded scissors (e.g., Tiemann, #160-161).
6. Spring loaded, Castro-Viejo-type needle holder (e.g., Storz, #E-3861).
7. Pediatric ophthalmic speculum for chest retractor (e.g., Cook eye speculum, infant; Miltex, Lake Success, NY).
8. 6-0 monofilament nylon suture (USSC).
9. 8-0 monofilament polypropylene suture (USSC).
10. Bipolar electrocautery device (e.g., Assi Polarmate).
11. 3-in. Cotton-tipped applicators.
12. 2×2-in. Gauze pads.
13. Small animal ventilator (e.g., Columbus Instruments CIV-101, Columbus, OH).
14. Avertin anesthetic (2,2,2-tribromoethanol, Aldrich). Concentrated stock dissolved in tertamyl alcohol (Aldrich) at 1 g/mL. Working stock diluted with normal saline to 25 µg/mL.
15. Isothermal pad (e.g., KAZ HP110, New York, NY).
16. Ophthalmic ointment.
17. Betadine.
18. Fiberoptic illumination (e.g., Zeiss KL 1500 LCD).
19. PE-90 endotracheal tube with beveled end, 2.5–3 cm total length.

2.3. Tissue Culture

1. Ham's F10 media (Gibco-BRL, Invitrogen, Carlsbad, CA).
2. Horse serum (ICN Flow, Costa Mesa, CA).
3. Antibiotic-antimycotic (100X, Gibco-BRL), contains 10,000 U of penicillin G, 10,000 (g streptomycin, and 25 µg of amphotericin B per mL, dilute 1:100 into media.
4. Gentamicin (50 mg/mL; Gibco-BRL), dilute 1:1000 into media (final conc. 50 µg/mL).
5. Enzyme solution: F10 plus 100 U/mL collagenase (purified collagenase CLSPANK; Worthington, Lakewood, NJ), 0.6 mg/mL pancreatin (Gibco-BRL),

antibiotics-antimycotics (1:100 diluted, final concentrations 100 U/mL penicillin G, 100 µg/mL streptomycin, 0.25 µg/mL amphotericin B), and 50 µg/mL gentamicin.

6. Recombinant human basic fibroblast growth factor (bFGF; a gift from Scios, Mountain View, CA). Basic FGF can be purchased from multiple commercial sources including R&D Systems (Minneapolis, MN), Gibco-BRL, or Sigma (St. Louis, MO).
7. F10 growth media: F10, 15% horse serum, 6 ng/mL bFGF, 100 U/mL penicillin G, 100 µg/mL streptomycin, 0.25 µg/mL amphotericin B, and 50 µg/mL gentamicin.
8. F10C differentiation media (referred to as F10C): F10, 10% horse serum, 6 µg/mL insulin (Sigma), 0.8 mM additional $CaCl_2$ (final calcium concentration 1.1 mM; add from a 1 M sterile $CaCl_2$ in ddH_2O stock solution).
9. Gelatin solution (2%) for coating of tissue culture plastic (Sigma, #G1393).
10. Trypan blue stain, ready to use (Gibco-BRL).
11. Hemocytometer.
12. Trypsin-EDTA (10X; Gibco-BRL), dilute 1:10 in Versene (Gibco-BRL).
13. Tissue culture plates, gelatin-coated, 150 mM(Falcon).
14. 6-well and 12-well plates, gelatin-coated, for staining and differentiation assays.

2.4. Borax Buffer for BrdU Staining

For 1 L borax buffer (sodium tetraborate, decahydrate, $Na_2B_4O_7 \cdot 10 \ H_2O$; Sigma, cat. no. B-9876):

1. Weigh out 38.14 g borax.
2. Add ~800 mL distilled H_2O.
3. pH to 8.5 with full-strength HCl (~12 N).
4. Stir until all the borax is dissolved (may have to do so overnight.)
5. Fill to 1000 mL with distilled H_2O.

3. Methods

3.1. Myoblast Cell Isolation

In our experiments, skeletal myoblasts were obtained from the hind limbs of 1–2-d-old Fischer 344 rats. If different species or different strains within a species are used as graft cell donor and graft cell recipient, the recipient's immune system should be suppressed or genetically compromised. Immune suppression can be achieved with cyclosporine A, whereas nude or severe combined immunodeficient animals are tolerant to a wide range of graft types.

1. To sterilize the skin, submerse the rat pups briefly in Betadine solution and place them onto a sterile underpad (*see* **Note 1**).
2. Quickly decapitate the pups with scissors and skin the carcasses.
3. Collect the hind limbs (20–40 per isolation) into a sterile Petri dish containing F10 media supplemented with antibiotics (100 U/mL penicillin G, 100 µg/mL

streptomycin, 0.25 µg/mL amphotericin B, and 50 µg/mL gentamicin), and keep them on ice.

4. Using a fresh Petri dish and cold F10 media, place the hind limbs one by one under a dissecting microscope.

5. Strip the muscles of surrounding adipose tissue and fascia, and bluntly dissect them from their tendons. The dissection process can be somewhat tedious and time-consuming (~2–3 h) but should be carried out carefully since it greatly determines the purity of the final myoblast preparation.

6. After the dissection under the microscope, transfer the preparation to a tissue culture laminar flow hood. Mince the muscles with iridectomy scissors until a fine slurry is formed.

7. Digest the slurry in 8 mL F10 supplemented with 100 U/mL collagenase, 0.6 mg/mL pancreatin, and antibiotics (100 U/mL penicillin G, 100 µg/mL streptomycin, 0.25 µg/mL amphotericin B, and 50 µg/mL gentamicin). Continue each round of digestion for ~20 min at 37°C (in water bath or incubator) with constant agitation to assist dispersal. If continuous agitation is not available, occasional manual agitation is recommended. After each round, triturate the preparation vigorously with a 10-mL pipet to assist breakdown of the tissue structure and thus force the release of myoblasts.

8. Allow the tissue pieces to settle by gravity and collect the supernatant. The first round is generally discarded since it contains mostly erythrocytes (although this should be independently verified by each investigator by phase contrast microscopy).

9. Collect the supernatants from each other round and mix the supernatant 1:1 with F10 growth media. In our experience 5–6 rounds resulted in complete digestion; thus a total volume of 50 mL enzyme solution (for muscle tissue from 20–40 hind limbs and ~8 mL fresh enzyme solution per round) should be sufficient.

10. After the final round, pool all supernatants, and filter the cell suspension through sterile gauze to remove undispersed tissue fragments and mature myofibrils.

11. At the final step, resuspend the cells in F10 growth media and count them using Trypan blue dye exclusion to determine cell number and viability.

3.1.1. Variation: Satellite Cell Isolation

1. The following procedure has been used successfully to isolate satellite cells from both rat and mouse skeletal muscle. Remember that the number of satellite cells in mice and rats declines with age (*20,21*).

2. Excise the tibialis anterior (TA), extensor digitorum longus (EDL), soleus, gastrocnemius, quadriceps, and hamstrings, and place them into a tissue culture dish containing 10 mL Dulbecco's modified Eagle's medium (DMEM) plus antibiotics (100 U/mL penicillin G, 100 µg/mL streptomycin, 0.25 µg/mL amphotericin B, and 50 µg/mL gentamicin).

3. Carefully discard tendons, all bone, and fat, and thoroughly mince the muscle tissue with a scalpel.

4. Digested the muscle tissue at 37°C with 0.1% pronase (Calbiochem, La Jolla, CA) for 1 h in a water bath or incubator with constant agitation to assist dispersal.

If continuous agitation is not available, occasional manual agitation is recommended.

5. Triturate the tissue vigorously and pass it through a 10-μm filter (Millipore, Bedford, MA).
6. Collect the cells by centrifugation.
7. Plate the cells on gelatin-coated plates in DMEM containing 20% fetal bovine serum, 15% horse serum, and 6 ng/mL recombinant human bFGF, plus antibiotics.

The primary satellite cell isolates typically contain ~50–60% desmin-positive satellite cells; the other cells are presumably fibroblasts.

3.2. Myoblast Cell Culture

1. After cell counting, plate the cells on gelatin-coated dishes at a density of 5 × $10^3/cm^2$. Add bFGF twice daily (6 ng/mL), and replace the complete medium once per day. It is important to keep a ~12 h rhythm between the bFGF feedings to avoid depletion of this growth factor, which would cause terminal differentiation of myoblasts. The adherent cells typically grow with a doubling time of ~18 h and contain ~60% desmin-positive myoblasts as determined with an anti-human desmin antibody (D33) *(22)*; the other cells are presumably fibroblasts. To avoid myogenic differentiation, which inevitably occurs at higher densities, it is very important to keep proliferating myoblast cultures subconfluent at all times.
2. Passage the cultures every ~3–4 d (1:5 split).
3. To identify the grafts, tag the proliferating myoblast cultures with (bromodeoxyuridine (BrdU; 10 μ*M*) overnight prior to grafting.
4. Evaluate the quality of the myoblast preparation in a differentiation assay.
5. Grow the test cultures to near confluency and then switch to F10 supplemented with 10% horse serum, 6 μg/mL insulin (Sigma), 0.8 m*M* $CaCl_2$, and no bFGF (referred to as F10C). Under these media conditions, myoblasts undergo cell fusion in 24–48 h to form multinucleated myotubes, which often contract (twitch) more or less regularly.

See **Fig. 1A** for a myoblast culture and **Fig. 1B** for a differentiated culture showing myotubes stained with anti-desmin antibody *(22)*.

Fig. 1. (**A**) Fischer rat myoblasts in culture. Myoblasts appear spindle-, oval-, or round-shaped and mononucleated under growth conditions. Phase contrast. Original magnification ×400. (**B**) Desmin immunostaining of differentiated Fischer rat skeletal muscle cells. The culture shown was differentiated for 3 d, fixed with methanol, and stained with an anti-desmin monoclonal antibody *(22)*. Desmin is the major intermediate filament of all muscle cells (skeletal, cardiac, and smooth muscle cells). The diaminobenzidine precipitate gives rise to the dark cytoplasm. The nuclei are counterstained with hematoxylin. By day 3 of differentiation, most of the myoblasts have

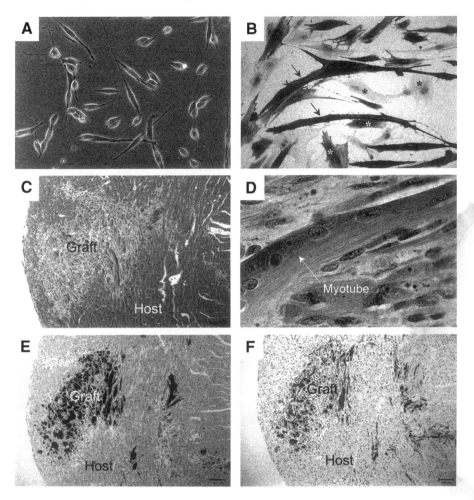

Fig. 1. (*contintued*) fused to form multinucleated myotubes (arrows). Some desmin-positive cells are mononucleated (white asterisks) and may represent not yet fused myoblasts. Unstained cells (black asterisks) probably represent fibroblasts. Original magnification ×1000. (**C**) Fischer rat myoblast graft at 1 wk after grafting into a normal nude mouse heart. The area of the graft appears in lighter gray. One million myoblasts transduced with an adenovirus encoding the gap junction protein connexin43 were injected into the left ventricle. Hematoxylin and eosin staining. Scale bar-100 μm. (**D**) One week after grafting, the myoblasts had fused to form multinucleated myotubes often showing cross-striations. Hematoxylin and eosin staining. Original magnification ×400. (**E**) Fast skeletal myosin heavy chain immunostaining of serial section. The dark color of immunoreactive cells is caused by the diaminobenzidine precipitate. Scale bar 100-μm. (**F**) Connexin43 immunostaining of serial section. The diaminobenzidine precipitate (dark gray) reveals expression of the adenovirus-encoded transgene (connexin43) in the graft cells. Scale bar 100-μm.

3.2.1. Variation: Satellite Cell Differentiation

1. Induce myogenic differentiation of satellite cell cultures by switching the cells to DMEM supplemented with 10% horse serum, 6 µg/mL insulin, and antibiotics.

3.3. The AdEasy System

Recombinant adenoviruses provide a versatile system for gene expression studies and therapeutic applications. The AdEasy system used in our laboratory was developed by He et al. *(23)* and, as of this writing, the required plasmids can be obtained at no charge from this lab. Packaging cells (human embryonic kidney 293 cells) are available at a minimal charge from the American Type Culture Collection. In addition, commercial kits are available for the generation of adenoviruses from Stratagene or Qbiogene (former Quantum Biotechnologies, Carlsbad, CA). The AdEasy system simplifies the generation and production of adenoviruses. A recombinant adenoviral plasmid is generated with a minimum of enzymatic manipulations, employing homologous recombination in bacteria rather than in eukaryotic cells. Following transfections of such plasmids into a mammalian packaging cell line, viral production can be conveniently followed with the aid of green fluorescent protein (GFP), encoded by a gene incorporated into the viral backbone. Other constructs lacking GFP or mammalian promoters are available as well. Clonal viral stocks can be obtained from this procedure without plaque purification *(23)*. The authors provide such excellent and updated protocols for the construction of adenoviruses using the AdEasy system on the world wide web (http://www.coloncancer.org/adeasy.htm) that we could do no better in describing the method here. The concentration of the adenovirus is determined with a spectrophotometer at 260 nm. An OD_{260nm} of 1 is equivalent to 10^{12} virus particles per mL. Readers interested in the generation and propagation of adenoviruses and gutted vectors are referred to Chapters 1 and 2.

3.4. Infection of Myoblast Cultures with Adenovirus

Note that working with adenoviruses is biohazardous. Proper sterile techniques should be used, and decontamination of all tools (pipets, tips, vacuum tubing, and so on) and surfaces with bleach is necessary.

1. Grow myoblasts for 5–6 d, and carry out the infection the day before grafting. The optimal multiplicity of infection (MOI) varies widely and hence needs to be determined for a given cell type (e.g., test MOI range 1–1000 particles/cell).
2. Infect the myoblasts with 1000 MOI for 2 h under constant agitation in a dry incubator (37°C, 5% CO_2). The dry air in the incubator only protects the shaker from corrosion; it will not affect the infection itself or the efficiency of infection. Also, if a shaker is not available, occasional (every 10 min) manual agitation is sufficient.

3. After 2 h of infection, aspirate the adenovirus containing media, rinse the plates twice with warm phosphate-buffered saline (PBS), and add fresh F10 growth media supplemented with BrdU (*see* **Subheading 3.5.**).

3.5. Cell Labeling with BrdU

To provide a marker for cells after grafting, supplement the F10 growth media with 10 µ*M* BrdU the night before harvest (Roche-Boehringer, Indianapolis, IN; 1:1000 dilution of 10 m*M* BrdU stock solution in PBS; filter-sterilize [0.2-µm pore size] and freeze aliquots at –80°C; do not freeze-thaw more than twice). BrdU is a thymidine analog that is incorporated during DNA synthesis. Thus, for high labeling efficiency, cell replication is necessary (e.g., adult heart muscle cells that are mitotically quiescent represent a poor target for BrdU labeling). For alternative cell labeling methods, *see* **Notes 2 and 3**.

3.6. Preparation of Myoblast Cell Suspensions for Grafting

For further information, *see* **Note 4**.

1. Immediately prior to grafting, aspirate the medium.
2. Rinse the plates once with Versene, and incubate them with 0.05% (1X) Trypsin-Versene (Gibco-BRL) (just enough to cover the plate, ~5 mL per 150-mm plate).
3. Pellet the cells by centrifugation, and wash them twice in a large volume (~10–15 mL) of the respective medium without supplements such as serum, antibiotics, or growth factors.
4. Count the cells before the final centrifugation step. Trypan blue (Gibco-BRL) dye exclusion should be used to determine cell viability before grafting.
5. Resuspend the final pellet in the desired volume of supplement-free medium by gentle up and down pipeting. Limit the injection volume for the rat heart to 70 µL, and for the mouse heart to 7 µL.

When grafting cells with high metabolic activity, such as cardiomyocytes, keep the cells on ice no longer than ~30 min prior to grafting. Skeletal muscle cells are less sensitive and can be kept on ice for 2 h without a noticeable decrease in viability. It is recommended to check the cell viability by Trypan blue after grafting; moreover, some cells should be replated to determine viability. (Enough cells for these assays always remain in the tube.)

3.7. Mouse Surgery

1. Obtain male nude mice from Taconic Farms (NCR-nu/nu homozygotes) or from Charles River (CD-1 [ICR]-nu/nu homozygotes). Surgery is easiest with adults weighing 20 g or more, but we have successfully used animals weighing as little as 16 g.
2. Anesthetize the mice with an intraperitoneal injection of avertin (0.018–0.022 mL/g body weight), using the working solution described above.

3. Cover the eyes with sterile ophthalmic ointment to prevent corneal drying.
4. Place the mouse supine on an isothermal pad, its paws taped to the surface, and its incisors hooked over a 00 silk thread taped to the pad. For injections into the normal heart, the mouse is positioned in a supine position and all four paws are taped to the pad on their respective sides. For inducing myocardial infarctions, however, the left coronary artery is better visualized if the left and right hind limbs are taped to the right side.
5. Position the surgical board nearly upright, and transilluminate the mouse's throat with a fiber optic light source.
6. Gently retract the tongue, and advance a cotton-tipped applicator to the level of the glottis to absorb secretions. With a properly positioned light source, the tracheal opening is readily visualized by the bright light emanating from it.
7. Gently advance the PE-90 endotracheal tube into the tracheal opening, taking care not to damage the surrounding soft tissues.
8. Confirm proper intubation by connecting the endotracheal tube to the respirator and checking for synchrony between the chest expansion and ventilator cycle.
9. Accomplish ventilation with room air supplemented with a low flow of oxygen, using a tidal volume of 0.5–0.7 mL and a respiratory rate of 100 breaths/min. The endotracheal tube will not form a tight seal with the tracheal wall: the ventilator volume setting therefore does not reflect the animal's actual tidal volume. It is useful to compare chest excursions before and after connection to the ventilator to approximate the correct volume setting for the ventilator. It is easy to overventilate a mouse inadvertently, resulting in pulmonary barotrauma and post-operative respiratory failure.
10. Sterilize the mouse's left chest with Betadine, and swing a surgical microscope into place for the remainder of the operation.
11. Make a 2–2.5-cm incision in the skin, parallel to and ~5 mM lateral to the sternum.
12. Using blunt dissection, separate the pectoralis and serratus muscles from one another to expose the chest wall.
13. Using a small, spring-loaded scissors, enter the pleural cavity through an intercostal space at the cephalad end of the incision.
14. Taking care not to damage the left lung, cut three ribs caudal to the incision. Inspect the wound and control sources of bleeding by electrocautery.
15. Place the rib spreader into the wound and retract to expose the heart and lungs. Identify the left phrenic nerve as the white, cord-like structure coursing along the lateral surface of the pericardium.
16. Open the thin, membranous pericardium using a fine hemostat while avoiding damage to the phrenic nerve.

3.8. Mouse Coronary Occlusion

Before attempting coronary occlusion in the mouse, the reader is referred to the detailed publications by Michael et al. *(24)* and Guo et al. *(25)* outlining their techniques. Guo et al. also have an excellent web site describing the mouse myocardial infarct model, <http://www.usouthal.edu/ishr/help/mouseinfarct/>. Michael et al. *(24)* performed vascular casting studies to determine the mouse coronary anatomy and described several common anatomic variations. The principal challenge to performing coronary occlusion is properly identifying the coronary arteries. Dark vessels present on the heart's surface are coronary veins. The coronary arteries are pale, almost ghostly vessels, best seen under bright illumination with a fiberoptic light source.

1. Occlude the left coronary artery by passing an 8-0 suture with a tapered needle under the artery and through the superficial myocardium. The site of occlusion depends on the experimenter's objectives. Proximal occlusions lead to large infarcts, a greater incidence of heart failure, and, correspondingly, higher mortality. As one progresses distally, less and less myocardium is placed at risk. For this study, occlude the artery approximately midway between the left atrial appendage and the left ventricular apex.
2. Perform a brief test occlusion by crossing the sutures before they are tied. When the suture is properly placed, myocardium distal to the suture should blanch, giving a sharp interface with the normal red-brown color of perfused myocardium.
3. For permanent coronary occlusions, tie the suture 3 times. Michael et al. *(24)* and Guo et al. *(25)* have described techniques for inducing coronary occlusion followed by reperfusion.

We have performed coronary occlusions in over 1000 mice, and our long-term survival rate is 85–90%.

3.9. Cell Injection

Use a Hamilton syringe and a 30-gauge needle for cell injections. A Hamilton syringe is used because of the low void volume.

1. Resuspend the cells just prior to aspiration by gently flicking their tube.
2. Draw the suspension into the syringe and extrude bubbles. We typically use a volume of 7 μL for mouse heart injections after we found that volumes >10 μL cause myocardial failure and death.
3. Advance the syringe in a cranial-to-caudal approach until the needle contacts the epicardial surface of the anterior left ventricle. Take care to avoid major coronary arteries or veins.
4. Using a shallow angle, manually advance the needle such that the tip can still be visualized in the superficial myocardium, while still having the needle's bevel far enough within the wall to minimize backflow.
5. Inject the cell suspension manually over a 5-s period. A successful injection produces a blanch in the surrounding myocardium, presumably owing to transient compression of the coronary microvasculature. The blanch fades over a several-minute period.

3.10. Surgical Closure

1. After checking for hemostasis, close the chest wall in layers (ribs, muscle, and skin separately) using 6-0 monofilament nylon suture.
2. Disconnect the endotracheal tube from the respirator, and observe the mouse for spontaneous respiration.
3. Once regular respirations occur, remove the endotracheal tube.
4. Give the mouse a 0.5-mL subcutaneous injection of normal saline to replace fluid losses.
5. Transfer the animals to a warmed box, and monitor them regularly until they have recovered fully from anesthesia, typically ~60 min. Then return them to their cages.

3.11. Tissue Handling

1. At defined time points, harvest hearts and briefly rinse them in 0.9% NaCl solution.
2. Depending on the antigens to be studied, fix hearts either by immersion in 4% phosphate-buffered paraformaldehyde or methyl Carnoy's solution (60% methanol, 30% chloroform, 10% glacial acetic acid).
3. After overnight fixation, transversely section the hearts, and embed them in paraffin by routine methods. *See* **Fig. 1C** for an example of a successful graft (hematoxylin and eosin [H&E] staining). **Figure 1D** shows a differentiated myotubes within the graft (H&E staining). In **Fig. 1E**, the graft is identified by immunostaining for fast skeletal myosin heavy chain with the antibody MY-32 *(26)*. **Figure 1F** demonstrates expression of the adenovirus-encoded transgene in the grafted cells (in this case the gap junction protein connexin43, identified by a polyclonal anti-connexin43 antibody *(27)*.

4. Notes

1. Myoblast cell isolation. In general, all primary cell isolations carry a high risk of microbial contamination owing to the involvement of an animal (in addition to the investigator!). Furthermore, in most laboratories it is not possible to dedicate a laminar flow hood to just animal/ tissue dissection work, which may help to reduce contamination sources. However, even if primary cell isolations are carried out in a regular laboratory, one can easily avoid common contamination sources (e.g., human skin, room air) by wearing professional sterile gloves (or spray-sterilize nonsterile gloves with 70% ethanol) and a face mask. We also found it useful to include gentamicin (spectrum: gram-positive and gram-negative bacteria) in the antibiotic-antimycotic mix.
2. Identification of graft cells. In our grafting studies, unambiguous identification of the grafted cells was desired. In some cases the graft and host had such a different morphology that distinguishing the two was not a problem. In addition, owing to the transplantation grafting technique (single injection of a concentrated cell suspension into the left ventricular wall), the graft cells usually appeared as a distinguishable island surrounded by host myocardium. However, if only few

cells are grafted, if cells are grafted intravascularly, or if only a few cells engraft into the target organ in a nonlocalized fashion, a label of some kind is required to identify the grafted cells.

Furthermore, a label is absolutely required if "transdifferentiation" of the graft cell phenotype into the host cell phenotype is investigated. If long-term stability of the cell tag is desired, a genetic label is recommended. For example, one can isolate the graft cells from male donors and graft into female recipients. The graft cell-associated Y-chromosome can be detected via Southern blotting *(28)* or, better still, by a combination of *in situ* hybridization to mark lineage and antibody staining to identify phenotype *(29)*. Other genetic labels include the use of transgenic mice for the isolation of the graft cell population. For example, the ROSA26 mouse is transgenic for the enzyme β-galactosidase (lacZ), which is expressed ubiquitously, and the detection assay (X-Gal assay) gives rise to blue cells *(30)*. Another elegant variant is the green fluorescent protein (GFP) transgenic mouse, in which all cells exhibit green fluorescence owing to the ubiquitous activity of the chicken β-actin promoter *(31)*. Both the lacZ and the GFP label also can be detected by antibody staining. The investigator should keep in mind that detection of the genetic label might require specific fixation protocols (e.g., native GFP can only be detected in frozen tissue sections). An alternative strategy is the transduction of graft cells with adenoviral or retroviral vectors encoding a reporter gene prior to grafting. Cells infected with adenovirus, however, inflict a strong immune response in the host, and, therefore, experiments require the use of immune-compromised animals (e.g., nude mice or rats), which are more cost- and logistics-intensive (e.g., specified pathogen-free animal facilities).

A setback to the use of retroviruses is their relatively poor infection efficiency in primary cells. A protocol yielding a higher efficiency retroviral infection of primary myoblasts, however, was developed by Springer and Blau *(32)*. This protocol combines multiple rounds of infection with centrifugation, and, in our hands, it also yields significantly increased infection efficiencies in fetal cardiomyocytes.

3. Identification of BrdU-labeled graft cells. The detection of BrdU-labeled graft cells in the tissue sections requires some extra steps in addition to a generic immunostaining protocol.
   a. Deparafinize and dehydrate paraffin slides as usual.
   b. If diaminobenzidine is used as a chromagen, quench the slides in methanol (0.3% H_2O_2 for 30 min at room temperature), and rinse them twice in PBS (2×5 min). Then transfer them into 1.5 N hydrochloric acid (HCl) at 37°C for 15 min. The HCl treatment denatures the DNA, thereby exposing the BrdU epitope for antibody recognition.
   c. Briefly rinse the slides in distilled water, and incubate them in 0.1 M borax buffer 2×5 min. Borax (hydrated sodium borate) stabilizes the open DNA strands.
   d. Wash the slides (2×5 min) in PBS. Nonspecific binding of antibodies is blocked by incubation with serum. (We use 1.5% serum of the secondary antibody host species.)

e. Proceed with the anti-BrdU antibody incubation per conventional immunocytochemistry.
4. Preparation of cell suspensions for grafting. As a general rule, the graft cells should be prepared immediately before the injection. One should keep in mind that the metabolic demands of different cell types vary dramatically. For example, cardiomyocytes are very demanding cells with low ischemic tolerance, whereas skeletal myoblasts are much less demanding and have a relatively high ischemic tolerance. These cell type-specific characteristics become even more important when cells are kept at high concentrations in a very low media volume ($\sim$1–2 $\times$ 10^5/μL), as may be necessary for the injection of a high number of cells (1–10 $\times$ 10^6/injection into the heart). It is recommended to check the viability (Trypan blue stain) of a given cell type after forcing the high-density cell suspension through the small size needle (27–30-gauge for cardiac injections in rats and mice).

Acknowledgments

This work was supported in part by grants from the National Heart, Lung, and Blood Institutes.

References

1. Braunwald, E. (1974) Editorial: reduction of myocardial-infarct size. *N. Engl. J. Med.* **291,** 525–526.
2. Braunwald, E. and Maroko, P. R. (1974) The reduction of infarct size—an idea whose time (for testing) has come. *Circulation* **50,** 206–209.
3. Murry, C. E., Kay, M. A., Bartosek, T., Hauschka, S. D., and Schwartz, S. M. (1996) Muscle differentiation during repair of myocardial necrosis in rats via gene transfer with MyoD. *J. Clin. Invest* **98,** 2209–2217.
4. Murry, C. E., Wiseman, R. W., Schwartz, S. M., and Hauschka, S. D. (1996). Skeletal myoblast transplantation for repair of myocardial necrosis. *J. Clin. Invest.* **98,** 2512–2523.
5. Reinecke, H., Zhang, M., Bartosek, T., and Murry, C. E. (1999) Survival, integration, and differentiation of cardiomyocyte grafts: a study in normal and injured rat hearts. *Circulation* **100,** 193–202.
6. Reinecke, H., MacDonald, G. H. Hauschka, S. D., and Murry, C. E. (2000) Electromechanical coupling between skeletal and cardiac muscle: implications for infarct repair. *J. Cell Biol.* **149,** 731–740.
7. Reinecke, H. and Murry, C. E. (2000) Transmural replacement of myocardium after skeletal myoblast grafting into the heart. Too much of a good thing? *Cardiovasc. Pathol.* **9,** 337–344.
8. Soonpaa, M. H. and Field, L. J. (1997). Assessment of cardiomyocyte DNA synthesis in normal and injured adult mouse hearts. *Am. J. Physiol* **272,** H220–H226.
9. Soonpaa, M. H. and Field, L. J. (1998). Survey of studies examining mammalian cardiomyocyte DNA synthesis. *Circ. Res.* **83,** 15–26.

10. Anversa, P. and Kajstura, J. (1998) Ventricular myocytes are not terminally differentiated in the adult mammalian heart. *Circ. Res.* **83,** 1–14.

11. Vescovi, A. L. and Snyder, E. Y. (1999) Establishment and properties of neural stem cell clones: plasticity in vitro and in vivo. *Brain Pathol.* **9,** 569–598.

12. Bjornson, C. R., Rietze, R. L., Reynolds, B. A., Magli, M. C., and Vescovi, A. L. (1999) Turning brain into blood: a hematopoietic fate adopted by adult neural stem cells in vivo. *Science* **283,** 534–537.

13. Jiang, Y., Vaessen, B., Lenvik, T., Blackstad, M., Reyes, M., and Verfaillie, C. M. (2002) Multipotent progenitor cells can be isolated from postnatal murine bone marrow, muscle, and brain. *Exp. Hematol.* **30,** 896–904.

14. Pittenger, M. F., Mackay, A. M., Beck, S. C., et al. (1999) Multilineage potential of adult human mesenchymal stem cells. *Science* **284,** 143–147.

15. Jackson, K. A., Mi, T., and Goodell, M. A. (1999) Hematopoietic potential of stem cells isolated from murine skeletal muscle [see comments]. *Proc. Natl. Acad. Sci. USA* **96,** 14,482–14,486.

16. Jackson, K. A., Majka, S. M., Wang, H., et al. (2001) Regeneration of ischemic cardiac muscle and vascular endothelium by adult stem cells. *J Clin. Invest.* **107,** 1395–1402.

17. Bittner, R. E., Schofer, C., Weipoltshammer, K., et al. (1999) Recruitment of bone-marrow-derived cells by skeletal and cardiac muscle in adult dystrophic mdx mice. *Anat. Embryol. (Berl.)* **199,** 391–396.

18. MacLellan, W. R. and Schneider, M. D. (2000). Genetic dissection of cardiac growth control pathways. *Annu. Rev. Physiol* **62,** 289–319.

19. Pasumarthi, K. B., Tsai, S. C., and Field, L. J. (2001) Coexpression of mutant p53 and p193 renders embryonic stem cell-derived cardiomyocytes responsive to the growth-promoting activities of adenoviral E1A. *Circ. Res.* **88,** 1004–1011.

20. Snow, M. H. (1977) The effects of aging on satellite cells in skeletal muscles of mice and rats. *Cell Tissue Res.* **185,** 399–408.

21. Gibson, M. C. and Schultz, E. (1983). Age-related differences in absolute numbers of skeletal muscle satellite cells. *Muscle Nerve* **6,** 574–580.

22. Van Muijen, G. N., Ruiter, D. J., and Warnaar, S. O. (1987) Coexpression of intermediate filament polypeptides in human fetal and adult tissues. *Lab. Invest.* **57,** 359–369.

23. He, T. C., Zhou, S., da Costa, L. T., Yu, J., Kinzler, K. W., and Vogelstein, B. (1998) A simplified system for generating recombinant adenoviruses. *Proc. Natl. Acad. Sci. USA* **95,** 2509–2514.

24. Michael, L. H., Entman, M. L., Hartley, C. J., et al. (1995) Myocardial ischemia and reperfusion: a murine model. *Am.J Physiol* **269,** H2147–H2154.

25. Guo, Y., Wu, W. J., Qiu, Y., Tang, X. L., Yang, Z., and Bolli, R. (1998) Demonstration of an early and a late phase of ischemic preconditioning in mice. *Am. J. Physiol* **275,** H1375–H1387.

26. Havenith, M. G., Visser, R., Schrijvers-van Schendel, J. M., and Bosman, F. T. (1990) Muscle fiber typing in routinely processed skeletal muscle with monoclonal antibodies. *Histochemistry* **93,** 497–499.

27. Nagy, J. I., Li, W. E., Roy, C., et al. (1997) Selective monoclonal antibody recognition and cellular localization of an unphosphorylated form of connexin43. *Exp. Cell Res.* **236,** 127–136.

28. Beauchamp, J. R., Pagel, C. N., and Partridge, T. A. (1997) A dual-marker system for quantitative studies of myoblast transplantation in the mouse. *Transplantation* **63,** 1794–1797.

29. Mezey, E., Chandross, K. J., Harta, G., Maki, R. A., and McKercher, S. R. (2000) Turning blood into brain: cells bearing neuronal antigens generated in vivo from bone marrow. *Science* **290,** 1779–1782.

30. Zambrowicz, B. P., Imamoto, A., Fiering, S., Herzenberg, L. A., Kerr, W. G., and Soriano, P. (1997) Disruption of overlapping transcripts in the ROSA beta geo 26 gene trap strain leads to widespread expression of beta-galactosidase in mouse embryos and hematopoietic cells. *Proc. Natl. Acad. Sci. USA* **94,** 3789–3794.

31. Okabe, M., Ikawa, M., Kominami, K., Nakanishi, T., and Nishimune, Y. (1997) 'Green mice' as a source of ubiquitous green cells. *FEBS Lett.* **407,** 313–319.

32. Springer, M. L. and Blau, H. M. (1997). High-efficiency retroviral infection of primary myoblasts. *Somat. Cell Mol. Genet.* **23,** 203–209.

III

VECTORS FOR CARDIAC GENE TRANSFER

IN VITRO AND IN VIVO ASSAYS AND APPROACHES

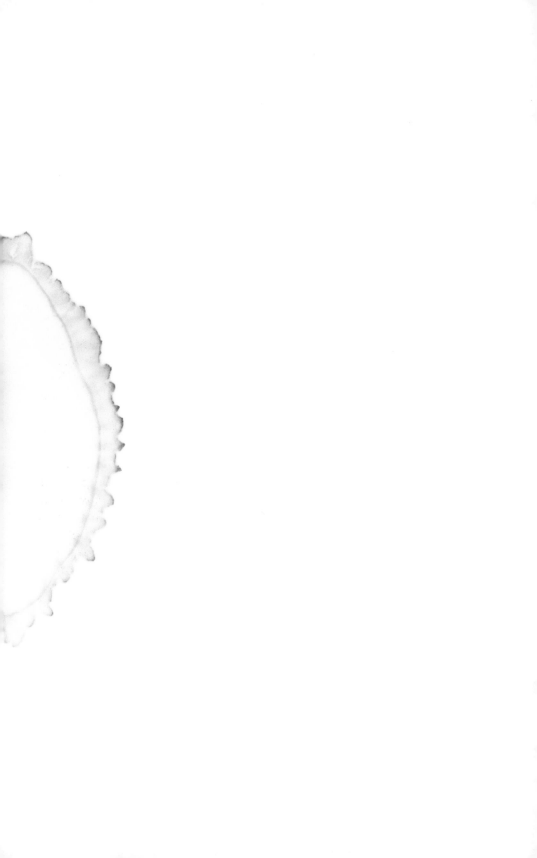

8

Suppressor tRNAs

Protocols and Applications for Cardiac Gene Transfer

Massimo Buvoli, Ada Buvoli, and Leslie A. Leinwand

1. Introduction

Although tRNA-mediated suppression has been mainly used to study chain-terminating mutations in bacteria and yeast *(1,2)*, suppressor tRNAs have also been employed for a variety of other purposes. For example, by introducing a nonsense mutation into the diphtheria toxin-coding sequence, its expression in vivo can be regulated by the presence or absence of a suppressor tRNA. This technique has provided new approaches to cancer therapy *(3)* as well as to the study of visual system development in *Drosophila melanogaster (4)*.

In addition, since nonsense mutations result in a large number of human genetic diseases *(5)*, suppressor tRNAs have been studied as possible therapeutic tools for somatic gene therapy. Ideally, suppression therapy should eliminate the translation block caused by a nonsense mutation without interfering with the termination process at the natural stop codons. Both the ability to suppress a nonsense mutation in the β-globin mRNA (β° thalassaemia) and a partial restoration of DNA repair activity were successfully achieved in vitro *(6,7)*.

Recently we have extended these last studies in vivo by testing the ability of multimerized suppressor tRNAs to rescue a reporter gene with an ochre mutation expressed in the heart of a transgenic mouse *(8)*. The advantage of our system resides in the possibility of achieving a controlled level of suppression activity by choosing the number of suppressor tRNA genes that can be multimerized on a single plasmid. Consequently, potential toxic effects on cell metabolism *(9)* should be minimized.

From: *Methods in Molecular Biology, vol. 219: Cardiac Cell and Gene Transfer*
Edited by: J. M. Metzger © Humana Press Inc., Totowa, NJ

This chapter describes the procedure to assembly tandem multimerized suppressor tRNA genes (*see* **Subheading 3.1.**), the assay to determine suppression activity in cultured cells (*see* **Subheading 3.3.**), and the surgical procedure for injecting plasmids that carry suppressor tRNA genes into the mouse heart (*see* **Subheading 3.4.**).

2. Materials

2.1. Construction and Cloning of Multimerized tRNA Genes

1. Restriction and modifying enzymes (New England Biolabs, Beverly, MA).
2. Plasmid: pUC 18 (Gibco-BRL, Rockville, MD).
3. Polymerase chain reaction (PCR) reagents: BIOTAQ DNA Polymerase and BIO-X-ACT DNA Polymerase (Bioline, Springfield, NJ); nucleotides (Gibco-BRL); synthetic oligonucleotides (Integrated DNA Technologies, Coralville, IA).
4. Purification of PCR products: PCR reactions were purified using QIAquick gel extraction kit (QIAGEN, Valencia, CA).
5. TAE electrophoresis buffer (50X): combine 242.2 g of Tris base, 57.1 mL of glacial acetic acid, and 100 mL of 0.5 M EDTA, pH 8.0. Adjust to 1 L with H_2O. Store at room temperature.
6. Agarose gel loading buffer (6X): Mix 25 mg of bromophenol blue, 25 mg of xylene cyanol, 7 mL of H_2O, 3 mL of glycerol, 100 µL of 1 M Tris-HCl, pH 7.5, and 20 µL of 0.5 M EDTA, pH 7.5.
7. Molecular size and weight standards: Hyper Ladder I (ISC BioExpress, Kaysville, UT).

2.2. Escherichia Coli Transformation

1. DH5α competent cells (Gibco-BRL).
2. Selective growing media: LB and LB agar (Gibco-BRL) supplemented with 100 µg/mL ampicillin. To prepare plates for chromogenic selection spread 20 µL of 5-bromo-4-chloro-3-indolyl-β-D-galactoside (X-Gal) stock solution and 40 µL of isopropyl-β-D-thiogalactose (IPTG) stock solution over the entire surface of an LB agar plate with a sterile spreader.
3. Ampicillin stock solution (1000X): dissolve the ampicillin sodium salt, (Sigma, St. Louis, MO) in H_2O at a concentration of 100 mg/mL. Sterilize by filtration and store at –20°C.
4. X-Gal stock solution: dissolve X-Gal (Sigma) in dimethylformamide to make a 40 mg/mL solution. Wrap it in aluminum foil and store at –20°C.
5. IPTG stock solution: dissolve IPTG in H_2O to make a 20 mg/mL solution. Sterilize by filtration and store at –20°C.

2.3. Analysis of Recombinant DNA Clones

1. Small-scale isolation of plasmid DNA: DNA was purified using PERFECTprep plasmid DNA preparation kit (5 Prime → 3 Prime, Boulder, CO).
2. Primers for sequencing: 24-mer Reverse Sequencing Primer (-48) and 17-mer Sequencing Primer (-40) (New England Biolabs).

3. Solutions for large-scale isolation of plasmid DNA: *STE solution*: combine 1 mL of 1 M Tris-HCl, pH 8.0, 2 mL of 5 M NaCl, and 0.2 mL of 0.5 M EDTA, pH 8.0. Adjust the volume to 100 mL with H_2O. Sterilize by filtration. *Solution 1:* Dissolve 9 g of glucose, 25 mL of 1 M Tris-HCl, pH 8.0, and 20 mL of 0.5 M EDTA, pH 8.0, in H_2O. Adjust the volume to 1 L. Autoclave for 15 min at 10 lb/sq. in. and store at 4°C. *Solution 2* (made fresh every time): combine 4 mL of 5 M NaOH, 86 mL of H_2O and 10 mL of 10% sodium dodecyl sulfate (SDS). *Solution 3:* dissolve 294.4 g of potassium acetate and 115 mL of glacial acetic acid in H_2O. Adjust the volume to 1 L. Store at room temperature.

2.4. Analysis of Suppressor tRNA Activity

2.4.1. COS-7 Transfection

1. Cell culture medium for COS-7 cells: Dulbecco's modified Eagle's medium (DMEM; Gibco-BRL), supplemented with 10% fetal bovine serum (Hyclone, Logan, UT), 2 mM L-glutamine and containing 100 U/mL penicillin G sodium and 100 μg/mL streptomycin sulfate.
2. L-glutamine 100X stock solution (Gibco-BRL).
3. Penicillin and streptomycin 100X stock solution (Gibco-BRL).
4. Trypsin-EDTA 10X stock solution: (Gibco-BRL).
5. PBS: dissolve 5 g of NaCl, 0.25 g of KCl, 0.85 g of anhydrous Na_2HPO_4, and 1.25 g of KH_2PO_4 in a final volume of 1 L H_2O . Sterilize by autoclaving for 20 min at 10 lb/sq. in. on liquid cycle. Store at room temperature.
6. FuGENE (Roche, Indianapolis, IN).
7. Buffers for cell and tissue extractions: *Buffer C:* 0.25 M Tris-HCl, pH 7.8; *Buffer H:* combine 25 μL of 1 M glycylglycine pH 7.8, 15 μL of 1 M $MgSO_4$, 8 μL of 0.5 M EGTA, pH 7.8, and 2 μL of 0.5 M dithiothreitol. Adjust the volume to 1 mL with H_2O.
8. Homogenizer: IKA-Turrax T 25 homogenizer (IKA Labortechnik Staufen, Germany).

2.4.2. Reporter Gene Assay (CAT Assay)

1. Bio-Rad protein assay (Bio-Rad, Hercules, CA).
2. [^{14}C]chloramphenicol 50–60 mCi/mmol (NEN, Boston, MA).
3. Acetyl-CoA: dissolve 10 mg of acetyl-CoA (Roche) in 3 mL of H_2O to make a 4 mM solution. Aliquot and store at –20°C.
4. *Buffer E:* for each sample prepare 47 μL of a cocktail containing 23 μL of 2 M Tris-HCl pH 7.4, 4 μL of [^{14}C]chloramphenicol, and 20 μL of acetyl-CoA. Prepare a master mix according to the number of samples.
5. Thin-layer chromatography (TLC) plates: Baker-flex silica gel IB 20 × 20 cm (J.T. Baker, Phillipsburg, NJ).

2.5. Direct DNA Injection into the Mouse Heart

1. Avertin 100% stock solution for anesthesia: dissolve 10 g of 2,2,2-tribromoethanol (Aldrich, Milwaukee, WI) in 10 mL of tert-Amyl alcohol (Aldrich) by

vortexing for several minutes. Be sure to completely dissolve the small crystals formed after combining the two reagents. Dilute to 2.5% working solution in sterile phosphate-buffered-saline (PBS). Store both solutions protected by light at 4°C.

2. Surgical instruments: microdissecting straight forceps (RS-5130), small curved hemostatic forceps (RS-7111), straight scissors (RS-5882), cautery unit, clip applier, and clipper (Roboz, Rockville, MD); hot bead sterilizer (Fine Science Tools, Foster City, CA); Chromic Gut 4-0 (Ethicon, Somerville, NJ); permabond 910, cyanoacrylate adhesive (Permabond International, Englewood, NJ); syringes: 50- or 100-μL Hamilton syringes (Reno, NE); 26G$^{1/2}$ and 30G$^{1/2}$ needles (Becton Dickinson, Franklin Lakes, NJ).

3. Methods

3.1. Construction of Plasmids Carrying Multimerized Suppressor tRNA Genes

Plasmids containing 2–16 copies of the ochre suppressor tRNA gene (tRNAsu$^+$ gene) were generated following the scheme shown in **Fig. 1**. Since 16 copies of tRNAsu$^+$ span only about 3040 nucleotides, the cloning of multimerized suppressor tRNA genes in a more efficient viral delivery system should also be considered.

The original plasmids containing the tRNAsu$^+$ gene (pSV1GT-ser ochre), the CAT ochre (pRSVcat[oc27]), and the CAT wt (pRSV*cat*) reporter genes were obtained from Uttam RajBhandary (Department of Biology, Massachusetts Institute of Technology, Cambridge, MA). Since the same laboratory has also generated the human serine-derived amber and opal suppressor tRNA genes *(10)*, plasmids carrying a combination of different suppressor tRNAs can also be generated.

1. Amplify the tRNAsu$^+$ gene from pSV1GT-ser ochre plasmid with the primers 50 UP (complementary to nucleotides 63–83 upstream of the suppressor tRNA gene) and TERM (complementary to nucleotides 16–36 downstream of the suppressor tRNA gene) carrying appropriate restriction sites (**Fig. 1** and *see* **Note 1**). For the PCR reaction (100 μL), mix 10 ng of plasmid, 1X BIO-X-ACT OptiBuffer, 1.5 mM MgCl$_2$, 0.5 μM each primer, 0.2 mM each dNTP, and 4 U of BIO-X-ACT. Use the following PCR cycling parameters: 25 PCR cycles at 94°C for 20 s, 56°C for 20 s, and 72°C for 35 s.

2. Purify the PCR product on agarose gel. Mix 1.2 g of agarose, 2 mL of 50X TAE, and H$_2$O to a final volume of 100 mL. Dissolve the agarose in a microwave, cool the solution to 50°C, add 5 μL of a 10 mg/mL ethidium bromide stock solution, and pour in a gel tray with a large well comb. Mix the sample with loading buffer (1X final) and run the gel in 1X TAE containing 0.5 μg/mL of ethidium bromide. Purify the PCR fragment using a QIAquick gel extraction kit according to the

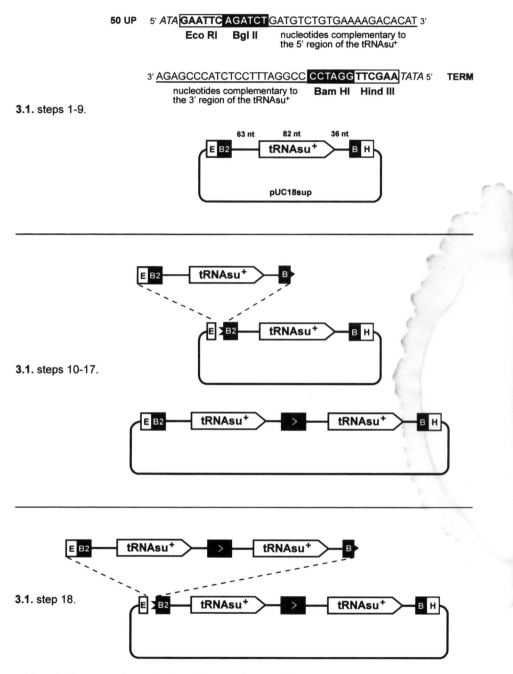

50 UP   5′ *ATA* GAATTC AGATCT *GATGTCTGTGAAAAGACACAT* 3′

Eco RI   **Bgl II**   nucleotides complementary to
the 5′ region of the tRNAsu⁺

3′ AGAGCCCATCTCCTTTAGGCC CCTAGG TTCGAA *TATA* 5′   **TERM**

nucleotides complementary to   **Bam HI**   **Hind III**
the 3′ region of the tRNAsu⁺

3.1. steps 1-9.

3.1. steps 10-17.

3.1. step 18.

Fig. 1. Construction of plasmids carrying multimerized suppressor tRNA genes. Illustration of the steps outlined in **Subheading 3.1.**

manufacturer's protocol. Quantify the amount of DNA recovered on an agarose gel, by comparison with a known amount of the same size DNA marker.

3. Digest 5 μg of plasmid pUC 18 (since this vector carries the β-galactosidase gene, it generates blue colonies in the presence of the chromtogenic substrate X-Gal) and 1 μg of PCR product with the restriction endonucleases *Eco*RI and *Hin*dIII in NEBuffer 2 at 37°C for 2 h. Use 60 U of each enzyme in a 100 μL reaction.

4. Purify and quantify the samples from the previous step, on a 1.2% agarose gel as previously described (*see* **step 2**).

5. Ligate 20 ng of digested and purified pUC18 and 10 ng of digested and purified PCR insert with 400 U of T4-Ligase in a 20 μL reaction (*see* **Note 2**). Incubate the reaction for 2 h at room temperature and then overnight at 14°C.

6. Transform *E. coli* DH5α competent cells with 3 μL of ligation mixture according to the manufacturer's instructions. After the heat shock, put the sample on ice and add 0.9 mL of LB. Incubate the cells for 1 h at 37°C with agitation.

7. Transfer cells in an Eppendorf tube, pellet for 20 s in a microfuge at 12,000*g*, and resuspend in 100 μL of LB. Plate cells on an LB ampicillin (100 μg/mL) agar plate containing X-Gal and IPTG. (Inactivation of the plasmid's β-galactosidase by insertion of the tRNA fragment results in recombinant white colonies.) Incubate at 37°C overnight.

8. Inoculate 3 mL of LB (containg 100 μg/mL ampicillin) with a single white colony. Inoculate several clones.

9. Extract the DNA using PERFECTprep plasmid DNA preparation kit according to the manufacturer's protocol. Elute the DNA in 50 μL of H_2O and digest 5 μL at 37°C for 1 h in the presence of NEBuffer 2 and the restriction endonucleases *Eco*RI and *Hin*dIII (10 U each) in a 20 μL reaction. Analyze the products of the digestion on a 1.2% agarose gel. Select a clone releasing a 200-nt-long insert containing the suppressor tRNA gene. Sequence the tRNAsu[+] gene to be sure that no mutations were introduced during the PCR amplification step.

10. Multimerize the suppressor tRNA gene as follows:

11. Digest 2.5 μg of pUC 18 containing the tRNAsu[+] gene (pUC18sup) with 60 U of both *Eco*RI and *Bam*HI in 80 μL reaction containing NEBuffer 2. Incubate the reaction at 37°C for 2 h. Purify and quantify the 200-nt-long fragment containing the tRNAsu[+] gene as described in **step 2**.

12. Digest 0.5 μg of pUC18sup with 30 U of *Bgl*II in a 50 μL reaction containing NE Buffer 3. After 1 h at 37°C add 20 U of *Eco*RI and incubate the reaction for 1 additional hour (*see* **Note 3**). Purify and quantify the ~2800-nt-long fragment, corresponding to the pUC18sup as described in **step 2**.

13. Ligate 20 ng of the digested pUC18sup and 12.5 ng of the 200-bp fragment with 400 U of T4-Ligase in a 20 μL reaction. Incubate the reaction for 2 h at room temperature and then overnight at 14°C.

14. Transform the DH5α *E. coli* competent cells as previously described (**step 6**). Plate on LB containing ampicillin (100 μg/mL) without chromogenic selection.

15. Analyze the recombinant clones carrying two copies of the tRNAsu[+] by PCR using the 17-mer Sequencing Primer and the 24-mer Reverse Sequencing Primer

located on the pUC 18 backbone. Aliquot a master PCR solution (500 µL) containin 1X BIOTAQ buffer, 1.5 mM MgCl$_2$, 0.15 mM each primer, 0.2 mM each dNTP, and 2 U of BIOTAQ DNA Polymerase in 10 PCR tubes. Using a sterile micropipet tip, pick a white colony and streak it first on a new LB agar plate (record plate) containing ampicillin (100 µg/mL). Resuspend the bacteria left in the tip directly in one PCR reaction mix by pipeting the solution a few times through the tip. Use the following PCR cycling parameters: 28 cycles at 94°C for 30 s, 58°C for 40 s, and 72°C for 1 min.

16. Analyze the PCR products on a 1.2% agarose gel. Choose a clone carrying a 400-nt insert containing two copies of the tRNAsu$^+$ gene.
17. Recover the corresponding clone from the record plate and inoculate it in 3 mL LB containing ampicillin (100 µg/mL). Extract the DNA as previously described (**step 9**).
18. Multimerize the tRNAsu$^+$ genes by repeating **steps 11–18**. When the desired number of tRNAsu$^+$ copies has been obtained (*see* **Note 4**), purify large amounts of the multimerized plasmids as described in the next section.

3.2. Large-Scale Isolation of Plasmid DNA

1. In a 15-mL Falcon tube, inoculate a single colony into a starter culture of 3 mL LB containing ampicillin (100 µg/mL). Incubate at 37°C for 5–8 h with shaking.
2. In a 4-L flask inoculate 750 mL LB containing ampicillin (100 µg/mL) with 2 mL of the starter culture. Incubate overnight with vigorous shaking.
3. The following morning harvest the cells by centrifigation at 5000g for 10 min at 4°C.
4. Wash the pellet in 50 mL of ice-cold STE solution and recentrifuge as in **step 3**.
5. Resuspend the bacterial pellet in 24 mL of solution 1. Add 48 mL of solution 2, mix by inverting the tube a few times, and incubate at room temperature for 5 min. Add 36 mL of chilled solution 3, mix by inverting the tube a few times, and incubate on ice for 20 min. Centrifuge at 20,000g for 40 min. Decant the supernatant containing the plasmid into a new tube through cheesecloth. Precipitate the DNA by adding 0.6 vol of room temperature isopropanol. Mix and let stand at room temperature for 10 min.
6. Recover the DNA by centrifugation at 15,000g. Carefully remove the supernatant, wash the pellet with 5 mL of 70% ethanol at room temperature, and centrifuge at 15,000g for 10 min. Carefully remove the supernatant, dry the DNA pellet briefly under vacuum, and resuspend it in 6 mL of TE (10 mM Tris-HCl, pH 7.5, 1 mM EDTA, pH 7.5). Store 3 mL at –20°C for future plasmid preparations.
7. In a 15-mL falcon tube mix the remaining 3 mL of DNA solution and 5.1 g of solid cesium chloride; adjust the volume to 5.6 mL with TE. Mix and warm the solution to 37°C to facilitate the dissolution of the cesium chloride. Add 200 µL of ethidium bromide (10mg/mL). Centrifuge the solution at 9000g for 10 min at room temperature. Transfer 5.3 mL of clear solution above the pellet to a Quick-seal Beckman centrifuge tube (13 × 51 mm). For optimal plasmid banding, the total weight of the tube should be 9.8–10 g. Seal the tube and centrifuge at 361,267g for 15 h at 20°C in a 65VTI Beckman rotor.

8. At the end of the centrifugation, carefully remove the tube, place it in a rack, and insert a needle on the top of it to allow air to enter when the DNA band is recovered. Use a 5-mL hypodermic syringe equipped with an $18G^{1/2}$ needle to withdraw the plasmid DNA gently (lower band) without disturbing the chromosomal and nicked circular DNA (upper band).

9. Reband the plasmid by transferring the solution to a new Quick-seal tube. Fill the tube with a solution prepared by dissolving 4.7 g of cesium chloride in 4.1 mL of TE and 100 µL of ethidium bromide (10 mg/mL). Seal the tube, repeat the centrifugation as before (**step 7**), and recover the plasmid DNA as previously described.

10. Bring the DNA solution to 3 mL with TE in a 15-mL Falcon tube. To remove the ethidium bromide from the DNA, add an equal volume of iso-amyl alcohol. Mix the organic and aqueous solutions by vigorously shaking the tube. Centrifuge at 450g for 5 min at room temperature. Discard the upper organic phase and repeat the extraction until the lower aqueous phase becomes clear.

11. Dialyze the DNA overnight at 4°C against two changes of 3000X volume excess of 10 mM Tris-HCl, pH 7.5 (*see* **Note 5**). After dialysis, precipitate the DNA by adding 0.3 M Na-acetate, pH 5.4, and 2 vol of ethanol. Resuspend DNA in sterile USP (0.145 M NaCl) or water.

12. Determine the DNA concentration spectrophotometrically by adsorption at 260 and 280 nm.

3.3. Determination of Suppressor tRNA Activity in Cultured Cells

Plasmids carrying multiple copies of suppressor tRNA genes should be tested in cultured cells before injection into the heart. This assay is carried out by comparing the CAT activity produced by extracts from cells transfected with the plasmid expressing the wild-type CAT gene and that produced by extracts from cells cotransfected with the plasmid expressing the CAT gene carrying a nonsense mutation and a multimerized construct *(8)*. Constructs have to show a proportional relationship between the number of suppressor tRNA genes and the rescued CAT activity.

Multimer constructs can also be tested in vivo, by injection into the mouse heart (*see* **Subheading 3.4.**) following the same principle described above.

3.3.1. Transient COS-7 Cell Transfection

1. The day before transfection, wash a confluent 100-mm dish of COS-7 twice with 10 mL of PBS, remove PBS, and add 1 mL of trypsin 1X. Incubate at 37°C for 2 min, shake the plate to detach the cells completely, recover the suspension, and dilute the cells 1:3 in DMEM. Cells should be 60–80% confluent on the day of transfection.

2. For each transfection, use 4 µg of plasmid expressing the CAT (ochre, amber, opal) reporter gene and 8 µg of a multimerized suppressor tRNA plasmid. To determine the level of suppression, transfect the cells with 4 µg of wild-type

CAT plasmid mixed with 8 μg of DNA carrier (i.e., pUC 18) to maintain the total DNA mass. Transfect the cells using FuGENE according to the manufacturer's instructions.

3. After 48 h, remove the media and wash the cells 3 times with PBS, drain, add back 1 mL of PBS, and scrape the cells with a sterile cell scraper. Transfer the cells to an Eppendorf tube and collect them by centrifugation at 12,000*g* for 10 s. Wash the cell pellet with 1 mL of ice-cold PBS and once more recover the cells by centrifugation. Resuspend the cell pellet in 150–200 μL of buffer C.
4. Disrupt the cells by three cycles of freezing in dry ice and thawing at 37°C. Centrifuge at 12,000*g* for 5 min at 4°C to pellet the cellular debris. Transfer the supernatant to a fresh tube.
5. Determine the protein concentration using the Bio-Rad Protein assay. Incubate the extract at 65°C for 10 min to inactivate endogenous deacetylases. Centrifuge at 12,000*g* for 2 min at 4°C. Save the supernatant and store it at –80°C.

3.3.2. CAT Assay

1. Assay 10–60 μL of cell/tissue extract (*see* **Note 6**). Adjust the volume of each sample to 103 μL with buffer H and then add 47 μL of buffer E. Incubate for 2 h at room temperature.
2. Add 1 mL of ethyl acetate and vortex each sample for 20 s. Centrifuge at 12,000*g* for 5 min at room temperature.
3. Transfer each upper phase to a new tube and dry the mixtures under vacuum.
4. Redissolve the samples in 15 μL of ethyl acetate and apply them, a few microliters at a time, on a TLC plate (be sure to spot the samples above the level of the solvent used for chromatography; *see* next steps).
5. Prepare a TLC chamber containing 95% chloroform, 5% methanol.
6. Put the plate in the chamber, close the lid, and run the chromatography for 1 h and 45 min.
7. Air-dry the plate at room temperature, wrap it in Saran wrap, and expose it in a phosphorimager cassette (*see* **Note 7**).

3.4. Direct DNA Injection into the Mouse Heart

Direct DNA transfer into cardiac muscle is performed by injection of purified naked DNA with a hypodermic needle. Transgene expression is maximal at 2–3 wk post injection and it is stable for few months. Although the major limitation of this procedure is represented by the relatively small number of cardiocytes that are transduced *(11)*, it can be employed to study cardiac gene regulation in both physiologic and pathologic conditions. Direct injection of suppressor tRNA genes into the heart can be used to control the expression of specific cardiac genes (as previously discussed for the diphtheria toxin) as well as for therapeutic purposes.

1. Immobilize the mouse on its back by holding the tail and the skin behind the ears with the fingers of the left hand.

2. Anesthetize the mouse with 12–15 µL of 2.5% avertin solution injected intraperitoneally through a 26G$^{1/2}$ needle (*see* **Note 8**). Avoid damage to the abdominal organs by inserting the needle for ~5 mm to the left of the mouse midline, around one-third of the distance from the umbilicus to the pubis.

3. After withdrawal to painful stimulation (tail pinch) is obtained, place the mouse in the supine position, with the upper limbs extended and taped to the surgical table. Surgical anesthesia occurs in 5–10 min, lasts ~30 min, and is followed by 1–2 h of partial anesthesia.

4. Before the heart surgery, fill a 50-µL Hamilton syringe with 20–40 µg of plasmid in a volume of 15–25 µL of saline solution.

5. Shave the hair around the sternum and disinfect the area with iodophor swabs.

6. Make a superficial 1–1.5-cm-long incision in the skin along the side of the sternum.

7. To expose the ribs, dissect the chest muscles with the microdissecting straight forceps. Gently insert the forceps under the transverse pectoral muscle and then under the deep pectoral muscle (*see* **Note 9**).

8. To save critical time at the end of the procedure, insert a chromic gut through the transverse pectoral and the deep pectoral muscle.

9. Locate the space between the ribs where the heartbeat is clearly seen; cut the rib just below it with straight scissors (*see* **Note 10**).

10. Open the chest with small curved hemostatic forceps; avoid injuring the heart and the lungs. Widen the incision by turning and opening the forceps. Since at this stage the respiration is abolished (owing to equalization of the external and intrapleural pressures), the procedure should be completed as fast as possible (15–20 s).

11. To push the heart out of the thoracic cavity, position the index and the middle finger of the left hand on the mouse shoulders, and then press the right upper quadrant of the abdomen with the left thumb (*see* **Note 11**).

12. Remove the hemostatic forceps. Inject the DNA solution through a 30-gauge needle. Administer the injection within few seconds. Deliver the DNA into the myocardium of the left ventricle, avoiding the ventricular cavity.

13. Return the heart back to the chest by gently pushing it with the right index finger. Immediately suture the muscles with the preinserted gut.

14. Squeeze the mouse's chest to expel the trapped air before applying a thin layer of cyanoacrylate adhesive (*see* **Note 12**).

15. Squeeze the chest a second time before the glue dries.

16. Close the skin with one staple.

17. Place the mouse under a heat lamp until it begins to move spontaneously (*see* **Note 13**).

3.5. Harvesting the Heart

If multimerized constructs are also tested in vivo, harvest the hearts according to the following procedure.

1. Sacrifice the mouse by cervical dislocation. Cut the anterior ribs on each side of the sternum. Expose the heart and separate it from the atria using small scissors.
2. Wash the heart in ice-cold PBS by squeezing the ventricles a few times with the forceps. Cut the heart into small pieces and transfer them in a 5-mL polypropylene Falcon tube.
3. Homogenize the sample on ice for 20–25 s at maximum power in 600–800 µL of cold buffer H.
4. Centrifuge the homogenate at 5000g for 30 min at 4°C. Transfer the supernatant to a new tube and determine its protein concentration using the Bio-Rad protein assay. Store the extract at –80°C.
5. Determine the CAT activity as described in **Subheading 3.3.2.**

4. Notes

1. The multimerization procedure is based on the observation that, although two different restriction endonucleases can often generate compatible ends, the new chimeric site is no longer cleavable by the original enzymes used. A list of enzymes generating compatible ends can be easily found in any enzyme catalog (i.e., NEB). Choose cloning/multimerization sites that don't cleave the gene of interest.
2. In general, we found that a concentration of vector equivalent to 1 µg/mL and a molar ratio vector/insert of 1:5–10 represent the optimal conditions to obtain a high number of recombinant colonies.
3. The activity of some restriction endonucleases may be critically affected by the number of bases flanking their recognition sites. Thus, for an efficient double digestion, cut the plasmid with *Bgl*II first and then with *Eco*RI (*see* the NEB catalog—Cleavage close to the end of a DNA fragment paragraph—for information about the major restriction endonuclases).
4. The optimal number of tRNAsu$^+$ genes has to be determined experimentally. Although plasmids carrying up to 16 copies of the gene are stable in both bacterial and mammalian cells, we do not know whether more copies will result in plasmid rearrangements.
5. It is important to dialyze the DNA in a large volume of Tris-HCl in order to completely remove traces of cesium chloride and other metal ions that have very toxic effects. For the same reason do not include EDTA in the dialysis buffer.
6. If different samples are compared, normalize their volumes according to their protein concentration.
7. In general, three radioactive spots are detectable. The slowest migrating spot corresponds to nonacetylated chloramphenicol, whereas the two faster migrating spots correspond to the two monoacetylated chloramphenicol forms. The presence of an additional spot, corresponding to the diacetylated chloramphenicol, indicates that the assay is out of linear range (conversion >40–50% with % acetylated = counts in acetylated forms/counts in acetylated forms + counts in nonacetylated chloramphenicol). If this happens, dilute the extract in 1% bovine serum albumin and repeat the assay.

8. Anesthesia represents one of the most critical parameters of the procedure since each mouse strain reacts differently to small overdoses of avertin. To avoid critical depression of respiration, use suboptimal doses of avertin when a new mouse strain is employed. If withdrawal to painful stimulation is not achieved, administer a booster (corresponding to ~10% of the initial dose) until an adequate anesthesia is obtained. If necessary, repeat the booster dose during the procedure.

9. Avoid any damage to the chest muscles since their integrity is essential to reduce the formation of pneumothorax after the chest wall is repaired.

10. Cut the rib approximately in the middle, without damaging the internal mammary artery running along the inside surface of the chest wall. If the corresponding intercostal artery is visualized, cauterize it before the incision.

11. This represents the most critical step of the procedure. Care should be taken to avoid exteriorization of the lungs, injuries to the great vessels, and laceration of the intercostal muscles around the incision. If the exteriorization of the heart does not occur in few seconds, the survival rate will decrease substantially.

12. Treatment with cyanoacrylate adhesive prevents additional air from becoming trapped in the thorax before the chest repair. This reduces the formation of persistent pneumothorax, and greatly increases the number of survivors.

13. If respiration does not restart regularly, a few tail pinches can help to restore the normal respiratory rhythm. Repeat the stimulation if necessary. Injection of 0.1–0.2 mg of dexametazone intraperitoneally can sometimes facilitate the recovery of sensitive mouse strains more prone to develop respiratory complications. In general, mortality ranges between 10–40% depending on the mouse strain employed.

References

1. Steege, D. A. and Soll, D. G. (1979) Suppression, in *Biological Regulation and Development*, (Goldberger R. F., ed.), Plenum, New York, pp. 433–475.
2. Hinnebusch, A. G. and Liebman, S. W. (1991) Protein synthesis and translational control in *Saccharomyces cerevisiae*, in *The Molecular and Cellular Biology of the Yeast Saccharomyces: Genome Dynamics, Protein synthesis, and Energetics* (Broach, J. R., Pringle, J. R., and Jones, E. W., eds.), Cold Spring Harbor Laboratory Press, Cold Spring Harbor, NY, pp. 672–686.
3. Robinson, D. F. and Maxwell, I. H. (1995) Suppression of single and double nonsense mutations introduced into diphtheria toxin A-chain gene: a potential binary system for toxin gene therapy. *Hum. Gene Ther.* **6,** 137–143.
4. Kunes, S. and Steller H. (1991) Ablation of *Drosophila* photoreceptor cells by conditional expression of a toxin gene. *Genes Dev.* **5,** 970–983.
5. Atkinson, J. and Martin, R. (1994). Mutations to nonsense codons in human genetic disease: implications for gene therapy by nonsense suppressor tRNAs. *Nucleic Acids Res.* **22,** 1327–1334.
6. Temple, G. F., Dozy, A. M., Roy, K. L., and Kan, Y. W. (1982) Construction of a functional human suppressor tRNA gene: an approach to gene therapy for β-thalassaemia. *Nature* **296,** 537–540.

7. Panchal, R. G., Wang, S., McDermott, J., and Link, C. J., Jr. (1999) Partial functional correction of xeroderma pigmentosum group A cells by suppressor tRNA. *Hum. Gene Ther.* **10,** 2209–2219.

8. Buvoli, M., Buvoli, A., and Leinwand, L.A. (2000) Suppression of nonsense mutations in cell culture and mice by multimerized suppressor tRNA genes. *Mol. Cell. Biol.* **20,** 3116–3124.

9. Hudziak, R. M., Laski, U. L., RajBhandary, U. L., Sharp P. A., and Capecchi, M. R. (1982). Establishment of mammalian cell line containing multiple nonsense mutations and functional suppressor tRNA genes. *Cell* **31,** 137–146.

10. Capone, J. P., Sharp, P. A., and RajBhandary, U. L. (1985) Amber, ochre and opal suppressor tRNA genes derived from a human serine tRNA gene. *EMBO J.* **4,** 213–221.

11. Li, K., Welikson, R. E., Vikstrom, K. L., and Leinwand, L. A. (1997) Direct gene transfer into the mouse heart. *J. Mol. Cell. Cardiol.* **29,** 1499–1504.

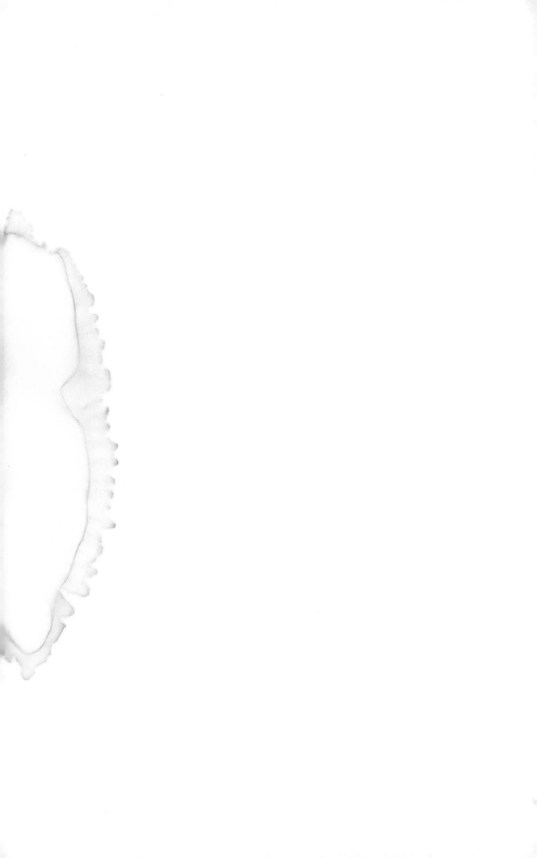

9

Antisense Oligonucleotides

Design, Construction, and Applications to Cardiac Allograft Transfer

Leora B. Balsam, Douglas N. Miniati, and Robert C. Robbins

1. Introduction

Antisense oligonucleotide technology has emerged as an important technique for manipulating gene expression. The theory behind this technique derives from an understanding of transcription and translation. Synthetic oligodeoxyribonucleotide chains are engineered complementary to a given messenger RNA (mRNA). By binding to the mRNA, the oligonucleotide prevents protein translation. This blockade may be mediated by RNAase-H degradation of the RNA-oligonucleotide complex. In addition to negative effects on protein translation, oligonucleotides may inhibit mRNA transcription through triple helix formation with complementary DNA regions *(1–3)*.

Several challenges have been met in the application of antisense oligonucleotide technology to in vivo systems. First, oligonucleotides are unstable in the intracellular milieu; they are susceptible to breakdown by numerous nucleases *(4)*. This problem has been overcome by the chemical engineering of phosphorothioate oligonucleotides. By replacing one of the nonbridging oxygen atoms at the internucleoside phosphate linkage with a sulfur atom, these constructs become more resistant to nuclease digestion. Second, adequate delivery of oligonucleotides to target tissue can be difficult. Intravenous routes result in systemic effects that may prove toxic and nonspecific. Local application to tissue may not result in adequate uptake. Various modalities of gene transfer, including virus- and lipid-mediated transfection, have been described, but these bear potential toxicities as well as limited efficiency. We have refined a technique for pressure-mediated delivery of oligonucleotides to ex vivo cardiac allografts that is safe and efficacious *(5–8)*. This technique has been used

From: *Methods in Molecular Biology, vol. 219: Cardiac Cell and Gene Transfer*
Edited by: J. M. Metzger © Humana Press Inc., Totowa, NJ

in other vascular tissue, including human vein grafts; a recent randomized controlled trial demonstrated the utility of ex vivo gene therapy in preventing neointimal hyperplasia in human vascular bypass grafts *(9)*. Although the technique is still evolving, it is clear that it may hold important clinical applications in the field of cardiovascular surgery and transplantation.

In the discussion that follows, we describe our method for pressure-mediated oligonucleotide transfection of cardiac allografts. It has been used successfully for the transfection of single-stranded antisense molecules as well as double-stranded transcription factor enhancer sequences.

2. Materials

2.1. Oligonucleotide Preparations

Commercially available antisense oligonucleotides with a phosphorothiate backbone are dissolved in phosphate-buffered saline (PBS) to 80 μM concentration. This construct can be fluorescein-conjugated and used to measure transfection efficiency. Oligodeoxynucleotides can be stored at –20°C.

2.2. Animals and Heart Procurement Procedure

1. Adult male PVG rats weighing 200–300 g (Harlan Sprague-Dawley, Indianapolis, IN).
2. Isofluorane inhalational anesthesia.
3. Sodium pentobarbital (50 mg/mL stock).
4. Heparin (1000 U/mL).
5. Stanford cardioplegia: sodium bicarbonate 25 mEq/L, potassium chloride 30 mEq/L, 5% dextrose, 1.3% mannitol.

2.3. Pressure Chamber

A commercially designed 8 × 24-in. steel chamber (Travaglio Consulting Engineers, Kensington, CA) is employed that uses compressed air to establish pressurization and can be manually pressurized and depressurized at a slow rate.

2.4. Determination of Transfection Efficiency: Tissue Processing and Fluorescence Microscopy

1. Cryostat cooled to –20°C and capable of making 5-μm sections.
2. OCT embedding compound.
3. Fluorescence microscope (Leica DMRB).
4. Hoechst 33342 dye (Sigma).

3. Methods

3.1. Design of Antisense Oligonucleotides

We have used both single-stranded antisense oligonucleotides as well as double-stranded sequences corresponding to promoter or enhancer sequences for transcription factors. The latter exert their effect through competitive binding of transcription factors. However, we will limit the discussion below to the design of single-stranded antisense oligonucleotides.

In the literature, oligonucleotides with successful antisense effects have been engineered to 5' translation initiation sites, 3' untranslated areas, and internal sequences of mRNA. The success of each molecule in exerting its antisense effect may be limited by a complex mRNA tertiary structure that may "hide" the complementary sense sequence. Thus, designing a successful antisense molecule may require some trial and error. In general, these molecules should be approx 14–20 nt in length; this confers adequate sequence specificity and affords reproducible pressure-mediated transfection (*see* **Notes 1–3**). Longer oligonucleotides and plasmids exhibit poor transfection with this technique.

1. Synthesize oligonucleotides of appropriate length (we recommend 14–20 nt) on a phosphorothiate backbone. The sequence should be complementary to a selected mRNA region. Such oligonucleotides are commercially made to order (Sigma-Genosys). For determining transfection efficiency, fluorescein-conjugated oligonucleotides are also needed (*see* **Note 4**).
2. Suspend the oligonucleotides in ice-cold PBS to a final concentration of 80–160 μ*M*. They can be stored at –20°C, although we tend to prepare them fresh with each experiment. Fluorescein-conjugated oligonucleotides should be stored away from light.

3.2. Procurement of Cardiac Allograft and Local Delivery of Oligonucleotides

The following technique of heart procurement is well described in the literature and is based on the model of Ono and Lindsey *(10)*. Most of our experiments are performed with PVG male donor rat hearts as described below.

1. Anesthetize PVG male donor rats (weight 200–300 g) with 2–3% isofluorane and 50 mg/kg intraperitoneal sodium pentobarbital.
2. When adequate anesthesia is achieved, perform a midline laparotomy. Identify the inferior vena cava, and inject heparin at a dose of 300–500 U.
3. Perform a sternotomy and crossclamp the thoracic aorta. Transect the distal pulmonary artery.
4. Deliver 3 mL of cold Stanford cardioplegia antegrade proximal to the aortic crossclamp using a 25-gauge needle.
5. Following arrest of cardiac contractions, deliver 1.2 mL of cold antisense oligonucleotide solution proximal to the aortic crossclamp at a rate of 1 mL/min. We have tried various concentrations of oligonucleotide and find that 80–160 μ*M* works best *(8)*.
6. A single 5-0 Tevdek tie is used to ligate the vena cavae and pulmonary veins *en masse*.
7. Explant the heart and place it in a vial containing 2 mL of ice-cold antisense oligonucleotide solution, on ice.

3.3. Pressure-Mediated Delivery of Oligonucleotides

1. Place the vial and surrounding ice bath in the pressure chamber.
2. Pressurize the chamber at a rate of 4 atm/min. We find transfection of over 40% at pressures of 3–9 atm.
3. Incubate the sample in the chamber for 45 min. This includes the time for pressurization and depressurization.
4. Depressurize at 0.4 atm/min.
5. To measure transfection efficiency, proceed with the next section. If effective transfection is already established, remove the heart from the vial and perform the heterotopic transplantation.

3.4. Assessment of Transfection Efficiency in Rat Myocardium

To assess transfection efficiency, fluorescein-conjugated oligonucleotides should be used for the above steps.

1. Remove heart from pressure chamber and rinse with PBS.
2. Embed transverse sections in OCT compound and snap-freeze in liquid nitrogen.
3. Allow the tissue to equilibrate to –20°C and cut to 5-μm sections with a cryostat.
4. Place the sections on polylysine-coated glass slides.
5. Air-dry the slides at room temperature away from light for 30 min.
6. Place a drop of Hoechst 33342 dye (5–20 μg/mL) over the tissue. This dye intercalates DNA and should stain all nuclei.
7. Coverslip the slide.
8. Following a 10-min incubation period at room temperature, examine the slides at 400× under a fluorescence microscope with the fluorescein isothiocyanate (FITC) filter followed by the appropriate Hoechst filter. The total number of FITC-staining nuclei is divided by the total number of Hoechst-staining nuclei to determine transfection efficiency.

3.5. Summary

We have described a highly efficient technique for ex vivo gene delivery to cardiac allografts. Unlike virus- or lipid-mediated transfection techniques, which may trigger inflammatory responses, this method appears to be relatively nontoxic. However, despite the success of this method, the mechanism underlying it is poorly understood. This will provide a substrate for many interesting future studies.

4. Notes

1. Oligonucleotide length will determine specificity. Hence, we caution against using short constructs. We have found that delivery of larger constructs, including plasmids, to the cell is less efficacious; hence we use 14–20-mers.
2. Certain oligonucleotide sequences have been shown to have nonspecific effects including immune stimulation and growth factor binding. These include CG

sequences and G quartets (GGGG) *(11)*; these should be avoided in designing antisense molecules.

3. Each experiment should include a series of control "scrambled oligonucleotides" to ensure that the effect seen is secondary to an antisense mechanism rather than other nonspecific effects.

4. FITC-labeled oligonucleotides are appropriate for determining transfection efficiency, but they may mitigate antisense inhibition of transcription/translation. Once efficient transfection is established, we have used non-fluorescein-conjugated oligonucleotides for further studies.

References

1. Crooke, S. T. (1997) Advances in understanding the pharmacological properties of antisense oligonucleotides. *Adv. Pharmacol.* **40,** 1–49.
2. Stein, C. A. and Cheng, Y. C. (1993) Antisense oligonucleotides as therapeutic agents—is the bullet really magical. *Science* **261,** 1004–1012.
3. Jen. K. Y. and Gewirtz, A. M. (2000) Suppression of gene expression by targeted disruption of messenger RNA: available options and current strategies. *Stem Cells* **18,** 307–319.
4. Akhtar, S., Kole R., and Juliano, R. L. (1991) Stability of antisense DNA oligodeoxynucleotide analogs in cellular extracts and sera. *Life Sci.* **49,** 1793–1801.
5. Mann, M. J., Gibbons, G. H., Hutchinson, H., Poston R. S., Hoyt, E. G., Robbins, R. C., and Dzau, V. J. (1999) Pressure-mediated oligonucleotide transfection of rat and human cardiovascular tissues. *Proc. Natl. Acad. Sci.* **96,** 6411–6416.
6. Poston, R. S., Mann, M. J., Hoyt, E. G., Ennen, M., Dzau, V. J., and Robbins, R. C. (1999) Antisense oligodeoxynucleotides prevent acute cardiac allograft rejection via a novel, nontoxic, highly efficient transfection method. *Transplantation* **68,** 825–832.
7. Feeley, B. T., Miniati, D. N., Park, A. K., Hoyt, E. G., and Robbins, R. C. (2000) Nuclear factor [kappa]B transcription factor decoy treatment inhibits graft coronary artery disease after cardiac transplantation in rodents. *Transplantation* **70,** 1560–1568.
8. Feeley, B. T., Poston, R. S., Park, A. K., et al. (2000) Optimization of ex vivo pressure mediated delivery of antisense oligodeoxynucleotides to ICAM-1 reduces reperfusion injury in rat cardiac allografts. *Transplantation* **69,** 1067–1074.
9. Mann, M. J., Whittemore, A. D., Donaldson, M. C., et al. (1999) Ex-vivo gene therapy of human vascular bypass grafts with E2F decoy: the PREVENT single-centre, randomised, controlled trial. *Lancet* **354,** 1493–1498.
10. Ono, K. and Lindsey, E. S. (1969) Improved technique of heart transplantation in rats. *J. Thorac. Cardiovasc. Surg.* **57,** 225–229.
11. Stein, C. A. (1995) Does antisense exist? *Nat. Med.* **1,** 1119–1121.

10

Theoretical and Technical Considerations for Gene Transfer into Vascularized Cardiac Transplants

Guanyi Lu and D. Keith Bishop

1. Introduction

The transfer of genes encoding immunomodulatory agents into allografts holds promise as an inductive therapy in transplantation (reviewed in **refs. 1–3**). This approach is clinically applicable, since vascularized transplants are routinely perfused at the time of organ harvest and therefore may be transfected by perfusion. However, many fundamental aspects of this technology must be addressed before it may be optimally applied to clinical transplantation. For example, it has been suggested that immunosuppressive gene therapy may provide advantages over conventional immunosuppression *(1–3)*. Notably, gene transfer should allow for the persistent, local release of the agent within the microenvironment of the graft, thereby negating the deleterious side effects of systemic immunosuppression. Although this feature of immunosuppressive gene transfer is attractive, it has not been validated. Indeed, adenovirus mediated transfer of CTLA4Ig in liver allografts results in readily detectable levels of the transgene product in the sera *(4)*. Hence, local secretion of the transgene product may result in systemic immunosuppression and increased susceptibility to infections and neoplasia. This fundamental aspect of immunosuppressive gene therapy has not been fully addressed and should be rigorously investigated.

Questions regarding the duration of immunosuppressive gene expression in transfected allografts have not been adequately addressed. Observations made in other gene transfer systems *(5–13)* suggest that transgene expression might be transient in transfected allografts. Although this would limit the use of gene transfer as a gene replacement therapy or in the treatment of chronic diseases,

From: *Methods in Molecular Biology, vol. 219: Cardiac Cell and Gene Transfer*
Edited by: J. M. Metzger © Humana Press Inc., Totowa, NJ

transient gene expression may be beneficial in the context of transplantation. For example, transient production of an immunosuppressive agent may provide an inductive therapy aimed at inhibiting alloreactive T-cell priming, altering the function of graft-reactive cells, and/or inducing regulatory cells. In addition, transient expression may avoid complications associated with prolonged exposure to the immunosuppressive agent. However, the silencing of transgene expression reported in other systems is generally associated with the development of an immune response to the transgene product and/or the DNA delivery vector *(5–13)*. The transfer of an immunosuppressive gene would probably mute the vector-induced immune response *(14–18)*, thereby allowing transgene expression to persist within the graft. Indeed, we have reported that adenovirus-mediated transfection of cardiac allografts with transforming growth factor-β1 (TGF-β1) results in transgene expression for at least 60 d *(19)*. Clearly, a better understanding of the mechanisms that regulate the duration of immunosuppressive gene expression is warranted, and systems that allow controlled transgene expression must be developed.

Finally, the choice of vectors for gene delivery into solid organs is currently limited. For example, *retroviral vectors* represent an attractive vehicle for gene delivery since they integrate into the host genome, thereby ensuring sustained gene expression (reviewed in **ref. 20**). The major disadvantage of retroviral vectors is that they only transfect dividing cells and therefore are of limited use in adult solid organ transplantation. *Lentiviral vectors* are appealing in that, unlike current retroviral vectors, they capable of transfecting nondividing cells in vivo (reviewed in **ref. 21**). Since lentiviral vectors have been developed relatively recently, very little is known about the immune response to these vectors. Furthermore, current lentiviral vectors have restricted tissue and species specificities, thereby posing additional limitations for their use in organ transplantation. Much attention has been recently given to *adeno-associated virus* (AAV) (reviewed in **ref. 22**). AAV has been reported to have decreased immunogenicity, which allows for prolonged transgene expression in vivo. However, AAV-delivered transgene expression is markedly delayed in vivo, requiring several weeks to reach peak levels (reviewed in **ref. 23**). Hence, delayed transgene expression may be inappropriate in the context of organ transplantation, in which the need for the immunosuppressive transgene product may be immediate.

Adenoviral vectors are capable of transfecting a wide variety of cell types, and they may be produced inexpensively at high titers (reviewed in **refs. 20** and **24**). These features make adenoviral vectors attractive for in vivo gene transfer strategies aimed at transfecting quiescent cells, including the parenchymal cells of solid organ transplants. However, in vivo administration of adenoviral vectors induces an immune response in naive animals, and the use of these vectors in humans is further complicated by the fact that most individuals have preexisting immunity to adenovirus. Indeed, the antiadenoviral immune response has been implicated in inflammation and loss of transgene expression in a variety of transfected tissues including the lung *(11)*, liver *(12)*, and muscle *(13)*. Despite the numerous reports emphasizing the limitations of adenoviral vectors, we have found that the degree of inflammation and tissue damage and the duration of transgene expression is dependent on which tissue is transfected with adenovirus. Specifically, adenoviral-mediated gene transfer of β-galactosidase into cardiac isografts does not result in overt inflammation within the graft, even though a vigorous antiadenoviral immune response is induced *(25)*. This contrasts to the inflammatory response that occurs in the liver when adenovirus is administered intravenously. These observations *(25)* indicate that, although adenoviral vectors may be used to deliver transgenes effectively in the context of cardiac transplantation, they may not be suitable for transfection of all solid organ transplants.

Cationic liposomes provide a nonimmunogenic DNA delivery vehicle for in vivo gene transfer (reviewed in **refs. *26–28***). Cationic lipids bind and condense plasmid DNA spontaneously to form complexes that have a high affinity for cell membranes. These DNA-liposome complexes are readily endocytosed, and the endosomal membrane is subsequently disrupted, releasing the plasmid into the cytoplasm. However, the transfection efficiency of DNA-liposome complexes is relatively low compared with that of adenoviral vectors, and it is estimated that only 1 in 1000 plasmids reach the nucleus and are expressed *(27)*. Nonetheless, several reports have documented the ability of DNA-liposome complexes to transfect vascularized cardiac transplants *(19,29–32)*. With improvements in lipid formulations, it is now possible to increase transfection efficiency without lipid toxicity *(33)*. Indeed, we have used the experimental lipid GAP DLRIE/DOPE to transfect vascularized cardiac allografts effectively with either TGFβ1 *(19)* or viral interleukin-10 (IL-10) *(32)* and have demonstrated the suppressive effects of the transgene product in vivo.

In summary, although immunosuppressive gene therapy holds promise as a modality for solid organ transplantation, many issues must be addressed to optimize this technology for clinical use. We have adapted the mouse vascularized cardiac transplant model *(34)* as an experimental system in which to test the efficacy and mechanisms of action of immunosuppressive gene therapy in the setting of transplantation. The immunobiology of transplant rejection has been well studied in this experimental model *(35–40)*. Hence, details of immunologic analyses are not discussed here, rather, details of the transfection and transplantation procedure are emphasized.

2. Materials

2.1. Equipment

1. Operating microscope: Wild-M690 (Wild Heerbrugg, Switzerland).

2.2. Instruments

Surgical instruments may be obtained from Roboz.

1. Dumont tweezer (fine forceps, curved), #7, 115 mm, two.
2. Dumont tweezer (fine forceps), straight, #5, 110 mm, two.
3. Castro-Viejo microdissecting scissors, straight, 3 1/2 in.
4. Vannas microdissecting scissors, straight, 3 in.
5. Castro-Viejo scissors, angular, blunt, 3 1/2 in.
6. Microsuturing needle holder, curved.
7. Forceps, straight, toothed, 12 mm.
8. Scissors, straight, 12 mm.
9. Needle holder, straight.

2.3. Self-Made Instruments

1. Paper clip retractor, two.
2. Mouse restrainer, four.
3. Mouse surgical pad.

2.4. Suture

1. 4-0 white twisted cotton suture (Deknatel DSP).
2. 7-0 silk tie.
3. 10-0 Dermalon suture with TE-70 4-mm needle (Sherwood Davis & Geck).
4. 4-0 Sofsilk suture with 3/8-in. cutting needle (USSC).

2.5. Cautery

1. Fine-tip, low-temperature cautery (Solan Surgical Products).

3. Methods

3.1. Donor and Recipient Preparation

1. Anesthetize the mice with 4% chloral hydrate in phosphate-buffered saline (PBS) intraperitoneally with approx 0.01 mL/g of body weight.
2. Shave the hair from the operating area and disinfect the area with 75% ethanol.

3.2. Organ Perfusion and Harvest

1. Open the abdominal cavity and inject 0.1 mL of heparin into the inferior vena cava using a 30-gauge needle and a tuberculin syringe.
2. Enter the thoracic cavity via a butterfly incision.
3. Invert the entire thoracic wall over the animal's head and secure the thoracic wall in place with a hemostat.

4. Ligate and divide the inferior vena cava (IVC) and right superior vena cava (SVC) with 7-0 silk ties. The left SVC is also ligated but does not need to be divided.
5. Carefully separate the thymus from the aorta.
6. Ligate the distal portion of the descending aorta and all bifurcations above it.
7. Using a tuberculin syringe with a 30-gauge needle, perfuse the heart *in situ* with 200 µL Ringer's lactate solution containing the DNA delivery vector. We routinely perfuse cardiac grafts with 5×10^8–1×10^9 adenoviral vectors *(19,25)* or DNA-liposome complexes containing 375 µg of plasmid DNA and 125 µg of the cationic lipid GAP-DLRIE/DOPE (Vical, San Diego, CA) *(19,32)*. This DNA-lipid ratio is critical to ensure optimal DNA-liposome mediated transfection of cardiac grafts *(32)*. Vials containing 2 mg GAP-DLRIE/DOPE are reconstituted with 1 mL Ringer's lactate solution and may be used for at least 1 wk when stored at 4°C. DNA-liposome complexes are formed immediately prior to use by admixing plasmid DNA, reconstituted lipid, and Ringer's solution and are allowed to form at room temperature for 10 min prior to perfusion.
8. Successful perfusion is indicated by the absence of fluid spillover from the aorta. During the perfusion, the heart will slowly turn pale in color and will continue to beat weakly.
9. Following perfusion, gently ligate the ascending aorta.
10. Slip the lower blade of the angular scissors under both the aorta and pulmonary artery, and push the blade slightly away from the heart.
11. Cut the aorta and pulmonary artery at the same length.
12. Lay a mass ligature around the heart, and retract the heart to the right side over the mass ligature.
13. Carefully ligate the tissue under the heart. Care should be taken to ensure that this tie is placed under the ligature of the IVC and the right SVC and to collect all pulmonary veins and the left SVC.
14. Separate the heart from the body under the mass ligation with scissors.
15. Place the perfused heart into iced Ringer's lactate solution for 30 min prior to transplantation.

3.3. Cardiac Transplantation

This procedure was adapted from the technique described by Corry et al. *(34)*.

1. Make a long midline abdominal incision and retract the skin and muscle with paper clip retractors.
2. Place the intestine to the upper-left side and cover with PBS wetted gauze.
3. Mobilize a small segment of the aorta and vena cava under the renal bifurcation.
4. Then cut the lumber artery and vein behind the aorta and the IVC with a fine-tip cautery.
5. Place two 4-0 cotton ties under the aorta and IVC. Tie half-hitch knots, beginning with the proximal ligature first.
6. According to the diameters of donor's aorta and pulmonary artery, make longitudinal incisions in the recipient's aorta and IVC with a pair of microscissors.
7. Anastomose aorta and pulmonary artery end to side to the recipient's aorta and IVC, respectively, using 10-0 suture.

8. Slowly remove the distal 4-0 cotton tie first, followed by removal of the proximal cotton tie. The heart will be filled with the recipient's blood and will resume contraction spontaneously.
9. Monitor graft function by daily abdominal palpation.

3.4. Permutations: Retransplantation of Transfected Cardiac Transplants

3.4.1. Applications

At least two experimental questions prompted us to develop a technique for retransplanting transfected cardiac allografts into naive, secondary recipients. The first addresses the question of what is the duration of "therapeutic" transgene expression following the initial transfection of the cardiac transplant. We have shown that transgene expression persists within the cardiac transplant for at least 8 weeks following adenoviral *(19,25)* or DNA-liposome complex *(19)* mediated transfection. Our retransplantation technique allows one to determine the duration for which an immunosuppressive transgene product is produced at levels required to subvert the immune system and prevent rejection. The second application addresses the question of whether gene transfer strategies may be employed to restrict the progression of chronic allograft rejection and whether they may be applicable in the setting of other cardiovascular diseases. Chronic allograft rejection is initiated by transient depletion of CD4+ T cells as described *(39)*. Approximately 30 d post transplant, the allograft is harvested, transfected with the transgene of interest, and retransplanted into SCID mice that have been reconstituted with T-cells obtained from mice bearing chronically rejected allografts *(39)*.

3.4.2. Cardiac Transplant Perfusion and Harvest

1. Make a longitudinal midline incision extending from the xiphoid process to the symphysis pubis.
2. Expose the entire abdominal cavity using the paper clip retractors.
3. Invert the gut onto the upper-left side and cover it with PBS wetted gauze. The transplanted heart should also be covered with a small PBS-wetted gauze.
4. Gently retract the heart to a different position, exposing the adhesions around the heart.
5. Using a fine-tip cautery, separate the transplanted heart form the surrounding adhesions. This process may be extremely difficult because of extensive adhesions and revascularization. It is critical to stop even minor bleeding with cautery to prevent fatal hemorrhage following retransplantation.
6. Mobilize the proximal and distal portions of the aorta and vena cava near the transplanted heart as far as possible.
7. Cut all lumbar bifurcations under the aorta and vena cava.

8. Gently separate the mobilized proximal aorta from the vena cava.
9. Place a 4-0 cotton tie around the proximal aorta as far from the transplanted heart as possible.
10. Place two 7-0 silk ties under the mobilized distal aorta and vena cava and inject 0.1 mL of heparin through the IVC.
11. Tighten the cotton tie around the proximal aorta and one of the silk ties around the distal aorta and vena cava.
12. If transfection of the transplant is to be performed, perfuse the heart with either adenoviral vectors or DNA-liposome complexes at this time. The perfusate volume and the concentration of adenovirus or DNA-liposome complexes are the same as those described above for primary transfection.
13. Using a tuberculin syringe with a 30-gauge needle, perfuse the transplant *in situ* through the distal aorta. After perfusion, the transplanted heart will become pale, making pathologic changes in the transplant more obvious by gross examination.
14. Ligate the second 7-0 silk tie around the distal aorta and vena cava between the transplanted heart and the needle track through which the heart was perfused.
15. Cut the distal aorta and vena cava between two silk ties.
16. Divide the transplanted heart from the body by cutting the proximal aorta and vena cava below the cotton tie around the aorta.
17. Place the heart in iced Ringer's lactate solution.

3.4.3. Retransplantation

The initial steps of recipient preparation for retransplantation are identical to those performed for primary transplantation. However, the lengths of the incisions for the anastomoses on the recipient's aorta and vena cava are different, because of differences in the diameters of the transplant-associated vessels that are anastomosed during primary transplantation and retransplantation. The ascending aorta, which is used during primary transplantation, is much larger than the descending aorta that is used for retransplantation. Similarly, the pulmonary artery used in primary transplantation is much smaller than the IVC used in retransplantation. Hence, the incision in the recipient's descending aorta and vena cava must be adjusted accordingly.

1. Anastomose the transplant-associated aorta and vena cava end to side to the recipient's aorta and vena cava, respectively, with 10-0 suture.
2. Slowly remove the 4-0 cotton ties at both ends of the mobilized aorta and vena cava. The retransplanted heart will be perfused with the recipient's blood and will resume contraction spontaneously.
3. Since the blood vessel stem of the retransplanted heart is much longer than that of the primary transplanted heart, the vessels must be properly secured following the anastomoses. This is accomplished by using the intestine and other tissues to temporarily hold the stem temporarily in an upright position.

References

1. Knechtle, S. J. (1996) Gene therapy and transplantation—a brief review. *Transplant. Proc.* **28(suppl 1),** 19–23.
2. Bromberg, J. S., DeBruyne, L. A., Sung, R. S., and Qin, L. (2000) Gene transfer to facilitate transplantation, in *Gene Therapy in Inflammatory Diseases* (Evans, C. H. and Robbins, P. D., eds.), Birkhauser Verlag, Basel, pp. 163–204.
3. Giannoukakis, N., Thomson, A. W., and Robbins , P. D. (1999) Gene therapy in transplantation. *Gene Ther.* **6,** 1499–1511.
4. Olthoff, K. M., Judge, T. A., Gelman, A. E., et al. (1998) Adenovirus-mediated gene transfer into cold-preserved liver allografts: Survival pattern and unresponsiveness following transduction with CTLA4Ig. *Nat. Med.* **4,** 194–200.
5. Blaese, R. M., Culver, K. W., Miller, A. D., et al. (1995) T lymphocyte-directed gene therapy for ADA-SCID: initial trial results after 4 years. *Science* **270,** 475–480.
6. Riddell, S. R., Elliot, M., Lewinsohn, D. A., et al. (1996) T-cell mediated rejection of gene-modified HIV-specific cytotoxic T lymphocytes in HIV-infected patients. *Nat. Med.* **2,** 216–223.
7. Tripathy, S. K., Black, H. B., Goldwasser, E., and Leiden J. M. (1996) Immune responses to transgene-encoded proteins limit the stability of gene expression after injection of replication-defective adenovirus vectors. *Nat. Med.* **2,** 545–550.
8. Kay, M. A., Landen, C. N., Rothenberg, S. R., et al. (1994) In vivo hepatic gene therapy: complete albeit transient correction of factor IX deficiency in hemophilia B dogs. *Proc. Natl. Acad. Sci. USA* **91,** 2353–2357.
9. Connelly, S., Mount, J., Mauser, A., et al. (1996) Complete short-term correction of canine hemophilia A by *in vivo* gene therapy. *Blood* **88,** 3846–3853.
10. Kozarsky, K. F., McKinley, D. R., Austin, L. L., Raper, S. E., Raper, Stratford-Perricaudet, L. D., and Wilson, J. M. (1994) *In vivo* correction of low density lipoprotein receptor deficiency in the Watanabe heritable hyperlipidemic rabbit with recombinant adenoviruses. *J. Biol. Chem.* **269,** 13,695–13,702.
11. Yang, Y., Li, Q., Ertl, H. C. J., and Wilson, J. M. (1995) Cellular and humoral immune responses to viral antigens create barriers to lung-directed gene therapy with recombinant adenoviruses. *J. Virol.* **69,** 2004–2015.
12. Yang, Y., Jooss, K. U., Su, Q., Ertl, H. C. J., and Wilson, J. M. (1996) Immune responses to viral antigens versus transgene product in the elimination of recombinant adenovirus-infected hepatocytes *in vivo. Gene Ther.* **3,** 137–44.
13. Vilquin, J.-T., Guerette, B., Kinoshita, I., et al. (1995) FK506 immunosuppression to control the immune reactions triggered by first-generation adenovirus-mediated gene transfer. *Hum. Gene Ther.* **6,** 1391–1401.
14. Lee, M. G., Abina, M. A., Haddada, H., and Perricaudet, M. (1995) The constitutive expression of the immunomodulatory gp 19k protein in E1-, E3- adenoviral vectors strongly reduces the host cytotoxic T cell response against the vector. *Gene Ther.* **2,** 256–262.
15. Ilan, Y., Droguett, G., Chowdhury, N. R., et al. (1997) Insertion of the adenoviral E3 region into a recombinant viral vector prevents antiviral humoral and cellular

immune responses and permits long-term gene expression. *Proc. Natl. Acad. Sci. USA* **94**, 2587–2592.

16. McCoy, R. D., Davidson, B. L., Roessler, B. J., Huffnagle, B. B., and Simon, R. H. (1995) Expression of human interleukin-1 receptor antagonist in mouse lungs using a recombinant adenovirus: effects on vector-induced inflammation. *Gene Ther.* **2**, 437–442.
17. Qin, L., Ding, Y., Pahud, D. R., Robson, N. D., Shaked, A., and Bromberg, J. S. (1997) Adenovirus-mediated gene transfer of viral IL-10 inhibits the immune response to both alloantigen and adenoviral antigen. *Hum. Gene Ther.* **8**, 1365–1374.
18. Chan, S. Y., Louie, M. C., Piccotti, J. R., et al. (1998) Genetic vaccination-induced immune responsiveness to the HIV protein Rev: emergence of the IL-2 producing helper T lymphocyte. *Hum. Gene Ther.* **9**, 2187–2196.
19. Chan, S. Y., Goodman, R. E., Szmuszkovicz, J. R., et al. (2000) DNA-liposome versus adenoviral mediated gene transfer of TGFβ1 in vascularized cardiac allografts: Differential sensitivity of CD4$^+$ and CD8$^+$ T cells to TGFβ1. *Transplantion* **70**, 1292–1301.
20. Kay, M. A., Glorioso, J. C., and Naldini, L. (2001) Viral vectors for gene therapy: the art of turning infectious agents into vehicles of therapeutics. *Nat. Med.* **7**, 33–39.
21. Trono, D. (2000) Lentiviral vectors: turning a deadly foe into a therapeutic agent. *Gene Ther.* **7**, 20–23.
22. Monahan, P. E. and Samulski, R. J. (2000) AAV vectors: is clinical success on the horizon? *Gene Ther.* **7**, 24–30.
23. Russell, D. W. and Kay, M. K. (1999) Adeno-associated virus vectors and hematology. *Blood* **94**, 864–874.
24. Wilson, J. M. (1996) Adenoviruses as gene-delivery vehicles. *N. Engl. J. Med.* **334**, 1185–1187.
25. Chan, S. Y., Li, K., Piccotti, J. R., et al. (1999) Tissue specific consequences of the anti-adenoviral immune response: Implications for cardiac transplants. *Nat. Med.* **5**, 1143–1149.
26. Gao, X. and Huang, L. (1995) Cationic liposome-mediated gene transfer. *Gene Ther.* **2**, 710–722.
27. Crystal, R. G. (1995) The gene as the drug. *Nat. Med.* **1**, 15–17.
28. Li, S. and Huang, L. (2000) Nonviral gene therapy: promises and challenges. *Gene Ther.* **7**, 31–34.
29. Ardehali, A., Fyfe, A., Laks, H., Drinkwater, D. C., Qiao, J.-H., and Lusis, A. (1995) Direct gene transfer into donor hearts at the time of harvest. *J. Thorac. Cardiovasc, Surg.* **109**, 716–720.
30. Fyfe, A. I., Ardehali, A., Laks, H., Drinkwater, D. C., and Lusis, A. J. (1995) Biologic modification of the immune response in mouse cardiac isografts using gene transfer. *J. Heart Lung Transplant.* **14**, S165–S170.
31. Dalesandro, J., Akimoto, H., Gorman, C. M., et al. (1996) Gene therapy for donor hearts: ex vivo liposome-mediated transfection. *J. Thorac. Cardiovasc. Surg.* **111**, 416–422.

32. DeBruyne, L. A., Li, K., Chan, S. Y., Qin, L., Bishop, D. K., and Bromberg, J. S. (1998) Cationic lipid-mediated gene transfer of viral IL-10 prolongs graft survival in a vascularized cardiac allograft model. *Gene Ther.* **5,** 1079–1087.

33. Stephan, D. J., Yang, A.-Y., San, H, et al. (1996) A new cationic liposome DNA complex enhances efficiency of arterial gene transfer in vivo. *Human Gene Ther.* **7,** 1803–1812.

34. Corry, R. J., Winn, H. J., and Russell, P. S. (1973) Primarily vascularized allografts of hearts in mice: the role of H-2D, H-2K, and Non-H-2 antigens in rejection. *Transplantation* **16,** 343.

35. Bishop, D. K., Shelby, J., and Eichwald, E. J. (1992) Mobilization of T lymphocytes following cardiac transplantation: evidence that CD4 positive cells are required for cytotoxic T lymphocyte activation, inflammatory endothelial development, graft infiltration, and acute allograft rejection. *Transplantation* **53,** 849–857.

36. Chan, S. Y., DeBruyne, L. A., Goodman, R. E., Eichwald, E. J., and Bishop, D. K. (1995) In vivo depletion of CD8 positive T cells results in Th2 cytokine production and alternate mechanisms of allograft rejection. *Transplantation* **59,** 1155–1161.

37. Piccotti, J. R., Chan, S. Y., Goodman, R. E., Magram, J., Eichwald, E. J., and Bishop, D. K. (1996) IL-12 antagonism induces Th2 responses, yet exacerbates mouse cardiac allograft rejection: evidence against a dominant protective role for Th2 cytokines in alloimmunity. *J. Immunol.* **157,** 1951–1157.

38. Piccotti, J. R., Li, K., Chan, S. Y. et al. (1998) Alloantigen-reactive Th1 helper development in IL-12 deficient mice. *J. Immunol.* **160,** 1132–1138.

39. Piccotti, J. R., Li, K., Chan, S. Y., Eichwald E. J., and D.K., Bishop. (1999) Cytokine regulation of chronic cardiac allograft rejection: evidence against a role for Th1 in the disease process. *Transplantation* **67,** 1548–1555.

40. Bishop, D. K., Chan, S. Y., Eichwald, E. J., and Orosz, C. G. (2001) Immunobiology of allograft rejection in the absence of interferon-gamma: CD8+ effector cells develop independent of CD4+ cells and CD40 – CD40L interactions. *J. Immunol.* **166,** 3248–3255.

11

Isolation, Culture, and Gene Transfer of Adult Canine Cardiac Myocytes

Jennifer C. Hirsch, Andrea R. Borton, and Joseph M. Metzger

1. Introduction

The ability to isolate individual canine cardiac myocytes that maintain normal rod-shaped morphology and contractility with stimulation is integral to the study of cardiac myocyte function and response to intervention in vitro. The literature is replete with the use of isolated murine and rat myocytes for the investigation of cardiac physiology. Methods include morselization or perfusion of the myocardium with various enzymatic solutions to disperse cells. Similar methods have been translated to larger species with variable yield and viability.

The method outlined has been used extensively in our laboratory with reproducible high yield and viability. Cells obtained can be maintained in culture for up to 7 days with maintenance of normal rod-shaped morphology and contractility with field stimulation.

This technology is a powerful tool for analysis of cardiac physiology on a cellular level. Through gene transfer, it is possible to alter different components of the myocyte such as myofilament expression or ion channel content to elucidate further important mechanisms involved in contractile function. Various pharmaceutical manipulations can also be employed to determine cellular responses in normal and genetically altered myocytes. The ability to maintain adult myocytes in culture for an extended period allows for a longer therapeutic window for pharmaceutical and gene manipulation. These myocytes retain the ability to undergo electrical stimulation, allowing for analysis of calcium transients and sarcomere shortening at various time intervals following genetic and pharmacologic interventions. In addition, unlike rat myocytes,

From: *Methods in Molecular Biology, vol. 219: Cardiac Cell and Gene Transfer*
Edited by: J. M. Metzger © Humana Press Inc., Totowa, NJ

canine myocytes do not become refractory to stimulation if not exposed to early phasic stimulation.

2. Materials

2.1. Stock Solutions, Perfusion Solutions, and Cell Culture Media

1. Stock solutions are maintained for the production of fresh perfusion solutions prior to each preparation. Stock solutions consist of 1 *M* NaCl, 0.5 *M* KCl, 0.5 *M* KH_2PO_4, 100 m*M* $MgSO_4$, and 100 m*M* $CaCl_2$ (**Table 1**). Solutions are all made with dH_2O in 1-L quantities. Solutions are membrane-sterilized by filtration through a 0.22-µm filter (Millipore, Bedford, MA) into autoclave-sterilized bottles. These solutions can be maintained for 6 mo at room temperature. Sterile technique should be employed whenever the solutions are accessed.

2. Prepare the solutions used for myocardial perfusion and cell isolation 1–5 d prior to the scheduled experiment. Keep the solutions at 4°C for up to 2 wk. Adjust the pH to 7.4 for all solutions with 1 *M* HCl or 1 *M* NaOH. After pH adjustment, measure solutions to the desired volume using a volumetric flask and then filter through a 0.22-µm filter (Millipore) into autoclave-sterilized bottles.

   a. Krebs-Hensleit buffer (KHB) with calcium is used for washing and preparation of the myocardium and initial myocardial perfusion. KHB is comprised of 118 m*M* NaCl, 4.8 m*M* KCl, 1.2 m*M* KH_2PO_4, 1.2 m*M* $MgSO_4$, 1.0 m*M* $CaCl_2$, 25 m*M* HEPES, and 11 m*M* glucose. Two liters of KHB with calcium are required for one canine experiment (**Table 1**).

   b. Calcium-free modified Tyrode's (MT) solution is used for the second myocardial perfusion. It is comprised of 118 m*M* NaCl, 4.8 m*M* KCl, 1.2 m*M* KH_2PO_4, 1.2 m*M* $MgSO_4$, 25 m*M* HEPES, 11 m*M* glucose, 0.68 m*M* glutamine, 5 m*M* sodium pyruvate, 2 m*M* mannitol, and 10 m*M* taurine. One liter of MT is required for one canine experiment (**Table 1**). Enzymes (*see* **Subheading 2.1.4.**) are added to MT immediately before using.

   c. Use the incubation solution to resuspend the cells after initial isolation. It is produced by aliquoting 100 mL of MT that has been pH adjusted and adding 2% (2 g) bovine serum albumin (BSA, fraction V, Boehringer-Mannheim, Indianapolis, IN). Then sterile filter the solution as for the above solutions.

3. Dulbecco's modified Eagle's medium (DMEM): DMEM (with high glucose, with L-glutamine, with phenol red, without sodium pyruvate; Gibco-BRL, Grand Island, NY) with 10% fetal bovine serum (FBS; Gibco-BRL), and 1% penicillin/streptomycin (use 5 mL/500 mL media of stock). Use 5000 U/mL penicillin, 5000 µg/mL streptomycin; Gibco-BRL, and serum-free DMEM with 1% penicillin/streptomycin for cell resuspension and culture.

4. Enzymes: hyaluronidase 0.15 mg/mL (Type I-S, Sigma, St. Louis, MO) and collagenase 0.4 mg/mL (Type 2, Worthington, Lakewood, NJ) are used for tissue digestion.

5. Solutions for apparatus maintenance: 70% ethanol, sterile-filtered dH_2O, and sterile-filtered dH_2O with 1% penicillin/streptomycin.

Table 1
Stock and Perfusion Solutions

Final concentrations	MW	Stock	g in 1 L stock	2 L KHB	1 L MT
118 mM NaCl	58.44	1 M	58.44 g	236 mL	118 mL
4.8 mM KCl	74.53	0.5 M	37.27 g	19.2 mL	9.6 mL
1.2 mM MgSO$_4$ · 7 H$_2$O	246.47	100 mM	24.65 g	24 mL	12 mL
1.2 mM KH$_2$PO$_4$	136.1	0.5 M	68.05 g	4.8 mL	2.4 mL
1.0 mM CaCl$_2$ · 2 H$_2$O	147	100 mM	14.70 g	20 mL	—
0.68 mM glutamine	146.1	Add fresh	—	—	0.1 g
11 mM glucose	180.2	Add fresh	—	3.96 g	1.98 g
25 mM HEPES	260.3	Add fresh	—	13 g	6.5 g
5 mM sodium pyruvate	110.0	Add fresh	—	—	0.55 g
2 mM mannitol	182.2	Add fresh	—	—	0.364 g
10 mM taurine	125.1	Add fresh	—	—	1.25 g

2.2. Surgical Instruments

1. Stainless steel surgical instruments required for explantation and preparation of the myocardium: #10 Bard-Parker surgical blade, scalpel handle, rib spreader, two Debakey forceps, Castro-Viejo vascular needle driver, Metzenbaum scissors, iris scissors, and small hemostat.
2. Autoclave the surgical instruments prior to each preparation. Store instruments to be reused during the myocyte isolation (one Debakey forceps and iris scissors) in a sterile beaker containing 70% ethanol during the experiment.

2.3. Glassware

1. Use standard laboratory grade Pyrex glassware. Autoclave the necessary glassware prior to each preparation, including: 500-mL beaker (two), 250-mL beaker (two), 150-mL beaker (two), 100-mL beaker (two), and 50-mL beaker (one), and 8 × 8-in. Pyrex baking dish (one).
2. Either reusable autoclaved Pyrex 1-L bottles or 1-L sterile disposable bottles may be used for the storage of solutions.

2.4. Perfusion Apparatus, Cellectors, and Triturators

1. The perfusion apparatus used for myocyte isolation consists of two solution reservoirs positioned above and connected to a double-barreled warming coil with a changeover stopcock (Baker perfusion set, #50-8382, Harvard, Holliston, MA) (**Fig. 1**). Polyethylene tubing is used to connect the solution reservoirs to the Baker apparatus as well as to create the bubble traps and drain lines. The height of the reservoirs should be ~65 cm with the bubble traps set to the same level.

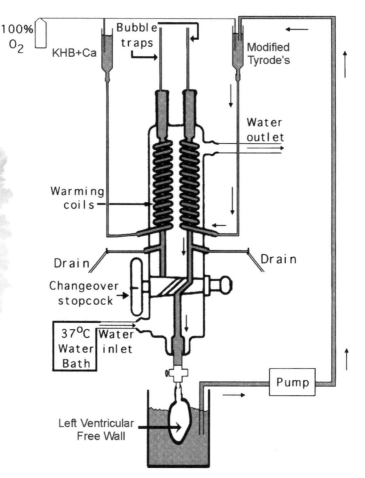

Fig. 1. Heart perfusion apparatus.

Three-way stopcocks are placed at the end of each drain line and at the outlet of the "Baker" apparatus. A gas dispenser (Fisher Scientific, Pittsburgh, PA) is used to bubble 100% oxygen into the solution reservoirs.

2. The tissue is triturated with a sterile, silanized Pasteur pipet that has been fire-polished after the tapered end is removed.
3. Pass isolated cells through a sterile 230-μm mesh sieve (Cellector, Bellco, Vineland, NJ).

2.5. Cell Plating

1. Place 18-mm square glass coverslips (No. 1, Corning Cover Glass, Fisher Scientific, Pittsburgh, PA) into each well of a 6-well tissue culture plate treated by vacuum gas plasma (Becton-Dickinson, Franklin Lakes, NJ).

2. Each coverslip is coated with 100-μL of mouse laminin (Gibco-BRL). Laminin is diluted to a final concentration of 40 μg/mL with phosphate-buffered saline, aliquoted into 1-mL quantities, and stored at –80°C. After an aliquot has been thawed, it should be disposed of rather than reused.

3. Methods

3.1. Setup

1. Prepare solutions as shown in **Table 1**:
   a. KHB-Ca^{2+} (2 L), Ca^{2+}-free MT (1 L), incubation solution with 2% BSA (100 mL), DMEM + P/S, DMEM + P/S + 10% FBS.
   b. Autoclave the necessary glassware.
2. Wash out the perfusion apparatus with serial rinses of the following solutions:
   a. Approximately 100 mL of EtOH + sterile filtered dH$_2$O in each syringe and tubing.
   b. Approximately 100 mL of sterile filtered dH$_2$O in each syringe and tubing, repeat.
   c. Approximately 100 mL of sterile filtered dH$_2$O + P/S in each syringe and tubing.
   d. Clean out the water bath with EtOH and Lysol, and then fill it with dH$_2$O and turn on.
3. Place KHB-Ca^{2+} in the left syringe and Ca^{2+}-free MT in the right syringe. Flush system to make sure no bubbles remain and oxygenate left syringe for 10–15 min prior to experiment. Turn on the water bath to warm the perfusion solutions.

3.2. Animal Surgery

3.2.1. Preparation

1. Set up dissecting area:
   a. Four blue pads, roll of tape, and opaque trash bag.
   b. Full bucket of ice X 3; into each bucket place one of the following:
      i. 500-mL beaker filled with KHB-Ca^{2+}; this is used for the initial cooling and rinsing of the heart.
      ii. 8 × 8-in. baking dish half filled with cold KHB-Ca^{2+}. This will be used to dissect the left ventricular free wall away from the remainder of the heart followed by the ligation of major perforating vessels.
      iii. One sterile 150-mm Petri dish. Half of the Petri dish should be filled with KHB-Ca^{2+}.
         (1) For the cannulation dish, mount a 10-mL syringe containing KHB-Ca^{2+} with the tip of the syringe resting at the surface of the Petri dish.
   c. One 250-mL beaker with 70% EtOH (~50–100 mL) for sterilizing and storing instruments during the experiment.
   d. Prepare collagenase solution in a sterile 50-mL beaker: Add 12 mg hyaluronidase, 32 mg collagenase, and 40 mg BSA to 25 mL of Ca^{2+}-free MT. Ultimately this will be diluted up to 80 mL when it is added to the preprimed perfusion apparatus.

i. Prepare extra enzyme solution in sterile 250-mL beaker: Add 30 mg hyaluronidase, 80 mg collagenase, and 100 mg BSA to 200 mL of Ca^{2+}-freeMT. Keep in a 37°C incubator until needed.

2. Sedate the dog with 0.07 mL/kg intramuscular injection of BAG (butorphanol,

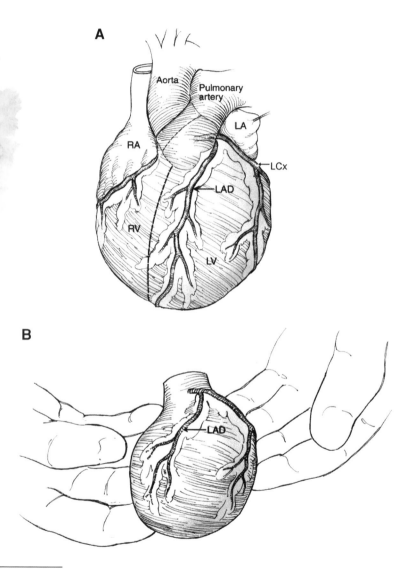

Fig. 2. (**A**) Anterior view of the explanted heart. The dashed line represents the line of dissection for the left ventricular free wall and aortic cuff. RA, right atrium; LA, left atrium; RV, right ventricle; LV, left ventricle; LAD, left anterior descending coronary artery; LCx, left circumflex coronary artery. (**B**) Excised portion of the left ventricular free wall with the aortic cuff as seen from the epicardial surface. Note the LAD, which

100 mg), acepromazine (25 mg), glycopyryolate (5 mg)/50 mL saline—may be stored at 4°C for 1 mo) in housing kennel. Bring the animal to the lab, inject with 500 U/kg intravenous heparin (the cephalic vein is the easiest for access) to prevent clotting of blood in the coronaries, and wait for 5 min.

3.2.2. Heart Explantation and Preparation

1. Euthanize the dog with pentobarbital iv (390 mg/mL) 1 mL/5 kg (*see* **Note 1**), place in a right lateral decubitus position, prep the left chest with 95% EtOH, perform a left thoracotomy, and remove the heart with a several centimeter cuff of aortic root (*see* **Note 2**).
2. Rinse the heart in ice-cold KHB-Ca^{2+}, making sure as much blood as possible is gently squeezed from the heart. Then transfer the heart to the 8 × 8-in. baking dish containing ice-cold KHB-Ca^{2+}.
3. Excise the left ventricular free wall perfused by the left anterior descending (LAD) coronary (**Fig. 2A** and **B**). Start at the apex of the heart, enter the right ventricle, and excise the right ventricular free wall along with the pulmonary

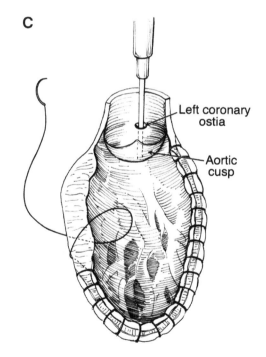

C

Left coronary ostia

Aortic cusp

Fig. 2. (*continued*) is the perfusion vessel for the excised myocardium and the left circumflex coronary artery along the superior margin. (**C**) Endocardial view of the excised left ventricular free wall with suture approximation of the endocardial and epicardial surfaces. The angiocatheter is seen in the left coronary ostia and is advanced into the proximal LAD, just distal to the takeoff of the left circumflex. A pursestring suture is placed around the coronary ostia to secure the angiocatheter.

artery and then the right and left atria. The left ventricle with the aortic root should remain. Enter the left ventricular cavity through the mitral valve orifice. Transect the left ventricular free wall approx 2–3 cm lateral to the LAD all the way to the apex. Complete the excision by transecting the septum approx 1 cm medial to the LAD up to the aortic root. Cut the aorta to leave a small cuff of arterial wall around the left coronary ostia.

4. Loosely approximate the epicardium and endocardium with a running 6-0 Prolene suture. Carefully ligate major perforating vessels and the left circumflex artery at the transected end. Place a pursestring suture around the left coronary ostia with a 4-0 silk suture (**Fig. 2C**), (*see* **Note 3**).

5. Cannulate the left coronary ostia with a 14-gauge angiocatheter. Advance into the proximal LAD. Secure in place with the silk pursestring. Wrap extra suture around the catheter and retain the long ends to secure further to the perfusion apparatus. Mount the catheter on the 10-mL syringe containing KHB-Ca^{2+} in the mounting Petri dish. Gently perfuse the heart to assess flow and identify any major leaks. Adjust the catheter as needed. Ligate any persistent leaks. There should not be significant resistance when one is pushing on the syringe plunger.

3.3. Myocardial Perfusion

1. Start slow drip of Ca^{2+}-KHB on the perfusion apparatus, and check for bubbles. Transfer cannula with the heart to the perfusion apparatus, wrap the ends of the pursestring suture around the stopcock, and turn on flow completely.

2. Perfuse with Ca^{2+}-KHB for 10 min (*see* **Note 4**). Wipe off oxygenator, and transfer to Ca^{2+}-free MT after ~5 min. Check to make sure effluent from the myocardium is clear. The heart will begin to contract after 3–5 min. This is an indication of adequate perfusion and warming of the tissue.

3. Perfuse with Ca^{2+}-free MT.
   a. After 1 min, collect fluid for 1 min to determine flow rate (~20 mL/min is desired; *see* **Note 5**).
   b. After 3 min, add the 25 mL collagenase/hyaluronidase solution to the Ca^{2+}-free MT syringe. The final volume should be 80 mL. It is necessary to determine the volume of solution that is contained within the tubing of your perfusion apparatus prior to the initial experiment. The volume in the syringe can be adjusted so that the total volume in the system is 55 mL prior to the addition of the 25 mL of enzyme solution, which will bring the final volume to 80 mL.
   c. After 15 min, change the enzyme solution if the original is cloudy.
   d. Total perfusion time with collagenase solution should be 30 min (*see* **Note 6**).

3.4. Cell Isolation

1. Remove the heart and cannula from the perfusion apparatus.

2. Remove the cannula and suture. Transfer the heart to a sterile 150-mm Petri dish. Lift the endocardial flap by incising the endocardium circumferentially with the iris scissors that had been set aside in EtOH (*see* **Note 7**). Remove the digested

myocardium from between the epicardium and endocardium by dissecting at the myocardial epicardial plane with iris scissors. The digested myocardium should be removable as essentially one large piece. Mince any partially digested pieces with the iris scissors. Transfer entire digested portion of the myocardium (usually 80–90% of the original tissue mass) to two 150-mL beakers. Add 25 mL of fresh collagenase/hyaluronidase solution to each beaker.

3. Swirl gently for 3 min in water bath. Remove supernatant with a pipet and discard. Resuspend tissue in 25 mL of collagenase/hyaluronidase solution and repeat. The first and second digests are discarded.

4. Do the remaining digests for 3–5 min (*see* **Note 8**). For digest 3 and beyond, remove the supernatant with a 10-mL pipet and place it in sterile 15-mL conical tubes (one to three tubes will be needed). Avoid any undigested clumps of tissue. Then centrifuge the conical tubes at $45g$ for 10 s. Remove the supernatant and resuspend the cell pellet in a total of 5 mL incubation solution (5 mL is the total combined volume for all conical tubes for a given digest). Place the resuspended cells in a 15-mL conical tube that is stored in a 37°C incubator while the remaining digests are performed. When placing each additional conical tube into the incubator, gentle invert the prior tubes to prevent hypoxia.

5. Place a drop of cell suspension on a cover slip and view on a light microscope to check viability. Steps 4 and 5 should be repeated with each digest.

6. Starting with the fourth digest, gently triturate the minced tissue with a wide-bore silanized Pasteur pipet, and then swirl in the water bath. Repeat trituration at the end of the digests prior to removal of the supernatant.

7. For the sixth and subsequent digests, repeat step 6. Then pass the supernatant through the cellector (*see* **Note 9**), which is placed in a 150 mM petri dish with the top of the dish used to keep the dish at an angle. Transfer the filtered supernatant to 2×15-mL tubes and then continue as described in **step 4**. Approximately 8–12 digests will be needed (*see* **Note 10**).

8. When all the digests are complete, spin each tube for 10 s at $45g$ and resuspend the cell pellets using a 10-mL Pasteur pipet and combine into two to three (depending on cell density) conical tubes containing 10 mL of incubation solution each. Cell pellets should have a pale salmon color. If the pellet is white or gray, then most of the cells are dead and that pellet should be disposed of rather than combined with the other digests (this is often the case with digest 3).

9. The final phase is to bring the calcium concentration up to the level in DMEM. The canine cardiac myocytes are highly sensitive to calcium and will die if this is done too quickly. Therefore, add back 14.6 µL of 100 mM CaCl$_2$ every 5 min to each tube (10 mL) for 1 h. This will bring the final [Ca^{2+}] to 1.8 mM. After adding back calcium, centrifuge each tube at $45g$ for 6–10 s. This time will vary based on projected cell number and viability. Viability can be increased by decreasing the spin time, but yield will increase (*see* **Note 11**).

10. Carefully resu pend the pellet in serum-free DMEM + P/S (volume will depend on projected m yocyte yield [10–30 mL]; this volume is referred to as the dilution factor).

3.5. Cell Plating

3.5.1. Preparation

1. Warm up DMEM + P/S and DMEM + P/S + 10% FBS in a 37°C water bath.
2. In preparation for plating cells, you will need to do the following in the hood during the digests. This usually requires the assistance of an additional person.
   a. Determine the number of 6-well plates that will be needed for your desired experiment (a poor prep [yield $<2 \times 10^6$] usually provides enough cells for 15 plates; a good prep [yield $>7 \times 10^6$] will provide cells for over 60 plates).
   b. Place the 6-well plates in the hood with the covers off. Place 1–18-mm^2 cover slips into each well. UV the plates for 10 min. The covers can then be replaced.
   c. When you begin the calcium addback, the cover slips can be laminin-coated. Thaw the necessary amount of laminin on ice (0.6 mL per plate). Aliquot 100 μL (40 μg/mL) of laminin per cover slip. This is done by first touching each edge of the cover slip with the pipet tip to allow a small amount of laminin to seep under the cover slip by capillary action. This will help to keep the cover slips from floating in the media. Then draw a large circle with the laminin on the cover slip to form ultimately a large single bubble of laminin on the center of the cover slip (*see* **Note 12**). UV with the covers off for 10 min. Replace the covers and leave in the hood until ready to use. The plates should be used in 30–45 min so that the laminin does not dry on the cover slips.
3. Clean and dry off the hemocytometer.

3.5.2. Cell Counting and Resuspension

1. To resuspend the cells in DMEM + P/S, carefully mix by pipeting several times with a 5-mL pipet followed by a Pasteur pipet. It is important to avoid the creation of air bubbles during this phase, as this will lower cell viability.
2. Transfer a small aliquot of resuspended cells with a sterile Pasteur pipet to a hemocytometer. Count nine fields: live (rod-shaped) cells *vs* dead (non-rod-shaped) cells. Viability is the percentage of rod-shaped cells to the total (rod- and non-shaped). Expected viability is 40–60 %.

$$\text{number of rod-shaped cells in nine fields} = \text{total live cells}$$

$$\text{total live cells} \div 9 = \text{number of cells} \times 10^4$$

$$\text{number of cells multiplied by the dilution factor} = \text{total number of cells isolated}$$

3. Dilute cells so that the concentration is 1×10^5 rod-shaped cells/mL. Cells are plated in DMEM + P/S + 5% FBS. This is accomplished by using 50% DMEM + P/S and 50% DMEM + P/S +10% FBS; therefore the final FBS concentration is 5%.

Example: Isolate **4.2** $\times 10^6$ cells. The volume for resuspension is **42** mL (1×10^5 cells/mL). Therefore, use 21 mL of DMEM + P/S + 10% FBS and 21 mL of DMEM + P/S (**Note**: this is a total of 21 mL including initial dilution factor,

so if the cells were initially suspended in 15 mL of DMEM + P/S,
then an additional 6 mL needs to be added).

4. Remove excess laminin from coverslips with a sterile Pasteur pipet connected to a vacuum (*see* **Note 13**).
5. Resuspend the cells using a Pasteur pipet prior to each set of plates. Then aliquot 200 μL/cover slip (= 2×10^4 cells/cover slip) and place in the center of the cover slip where the laminin was located. It is important to keep the cells in a bubble of media to allow attachment. Therefore take care when transferring to the incubator and when opening and closing the incubator door. If the cells "splash off" the cover slip, that coverslip should not be used for further experiments.
6. *If you wish to perform gene transfer, proceed to* **Subheading 3.6.** *at this time.*
7. Carefully place plates in incubator and incubate at 37°C with 5% CO_2 for 2 h. At the end of the incubation, add back 2 mL of DMEM + P/S.
8. Incubate at 37°C with 5% CO_2 until ready to use.

3.6. Viral Transduction

1. Incubate the plates for 2 h.
2. During the incubation period, prepare the virus. Aliquot 1.4 mL of DMEM + P/S into sterile microcentrifuge tubes. One tube is required for each plate.
3. Determine the desired multiplicity of infection (MOI) for the virus to be used. Then calculate the amount of virus needed for each 1.4 mL of media.

Example:

Take the viral concentration and convert from mL $\Rightarrow$ μL

$$1.42 \times 10^{10} \text{ pfu/mL} \Rightarrow 1.42 \times 10^7 \text{ pfu/μL}$$

Then multiply: MOI × number of cells/cover slip × number of cover slips

$$100 \times (2 \times 10^4)/\text{cs} \times 7 \text{ cs} = 1.4 \times 10^7 \text{ pfu}$$

Divide number of pfus needed/viral concentration:

$$\frac{1.4 \times 10^7 \text{ pfu}}{1.42 \times 10^7 \text{ pfu/μL}} = 0.99 \text{ μL for 1.4 mL DMEM + P/S}$$

Note: the calculation is based on 7 cs (200 μL/cs × 7 cs = 1.4 mL). This is used for one 6-well plate. We base the calculation on 7 cs to allow a margin for media that adheres to the tube or may spill.

4. Add the virus to the prewarmed DMEM + P/S just prior to the completion of the 2-h incubation period.
5. Aspirate the serum containing media off the cover slip with a Pasteur pipet, making sure to avoid the cells that are concentrated at the middle of the cover slip.
6. Replace the media with 200 μL/cover slip of the viral dilutions. Again, take care to maintain the bubble conformation so that the virus is concentrated directly on the attached cells. For control cells, replace with 200 μL/cover slip of serum-free media.

7. Carefully place the plates in the incubator so as to not disturb the cells. Incubate for 1 h.
8. After incubation, add back 2 mL of DMEM + P/S.
9. Incubate at 37°C with 5% CO_2 until ready to use.

3.7. Cell Culture

1. Maintain cells in serum-free DMEM + P/S.
2. Change the media after the initial 24 h and then every 48 h thereafter. Cells have been maintained in culture for 7 d.

4. Notes

1. The amount of phenobarbital required will vary between animals. Inject approximately half of the expected dose and assess the animal. The dog should receive enough phenobarbital so that all response to painful stimuli is abolished (toe pinch, corneal reflex); however, the heart should still be beating at the time of explantation, to minimize stasis in the coronaries and ischemic time prior to cooling of the myocardium.
2. When removing the heart, begin inferiorly by transecting the inferior vena cava followed by the pulmonary veins. This allows the heart to empty so that it is as relaxed as possible (giving improved yield and viability). Then transect the superior vena cava, pulmonary artery, and aorta. Pump the heart manually a few times to eject any residual blood and quickly place in the ice cold KHB-Ca^{2+} to minimize the warm ischemia time. Often the heart will still contract several times after explantation. Manually pump the heart again while it is in the KHB-Ca^{2+} to clear more blood.
3. The key to approximating the epicardium and endocardium is to occlude major perforators while still allowing adequate outflow from the tissue to prevent edema and elevated tissue pressure. The appropriate tension on the suture can take some work to perfect. The goal is to achieve a flow rate of about 20 mL/min without significant leaks from perforators. The purpose of the pursestring suture around the coronary ostia is twofold. First, after the catheter is advanced into the proximal portion of the LAD, the pursestring is tied down, thereby closing the ostia around the catheter. This will prevent the perfusate from backflowing out through the ostia. Second, leave the ends of the suture long. When mounting the heart to the perfusion apparatus, the catheter is attached to the stopcock, but the weight of the heart may allow it to fall off the catheter. Therefore, use the remaining long ends of suture from the pursestring to wrap around the stopcock to prevent the heart from slipping.
4. The purpose of the perfusion with KHB-Ca^{2+} is to flush the myocardium of residual blood and to warm the myocardium. Once the heart has begun to contract and the perfusate is running fairly clear, the perfusion can be changed to the MT. This usually takes 5–10 min. You do not want to allow the heart to contract for more than 1–2 min because this uses valuable cellular energy stores and reduces yield and viability.

5. If the flow rate is extremely fast or slow, it is possible to adjust to some degree. Carefully inspect the heart for any obvious leaks that could be suture-ligated while the heart is mounted. Ligation of major leaks can significantly slow the perfusion. If the perfusion is very slow, cutting one or two of the sutures at the apex of the specimen can increase the flow.
   Caution: the suture is continuous, so if you are too aggressive with cutting the suture, the whole suture line can open.

6. If the flow rate is very high (>25 mL/min) or very slow (<15 mL/min), you may opt to shorten or lengthen the time of enzyme perfusion by 5 min, respectively. The endocardial surface of the myocardium should have a slightly pale appearance and be somewhat spongy. If the enzyme perfusion is inadequate, extra digests will be needed to attain the desired yield. If the perfusion is excessive, the viability and yield will be diminished.

7. Prior to reuse, the tips of the iris scissors and forceps should be devoid of any residual EtOH because the EtOH will kill cells on contact. We use a small table-top heated instrument sterilizer.

8. The first two to three digests should be rather brief (the primary objective is to simply remove dead cells), approx 3 min. Then, depending on how well the tissue is digesting, further digests should be 3–5 min (very soft and falling apart nicely—3 min; firm and difficult to triturate—5 min). There is a tradeoff between the length of time that all the digests take and overall viability. The more digests the greater the yield, but if it takes a long time the viability will suffer, which affects long-term viability in culture and ability to stimulate the cells.

9. Passing cells through the cellector helps in isolating individual (i.e., nonclumped) cells and also improves the viability. The cellector can become clogged with debris and should be rinsed with sterile-filtered dH$_2$O between each digest.

10. If the tissue is not well digested when it is initially removed from the perfusion column or if overall yield is low, performing more digests may increase yield. As long as there is tissue remaining in the enzyme solution and a pellet is being isolated, you can continue with the digests.

11. If the viability appears to be less than 40% when the cells have been resuspended, it is helpful to do a quick (6-s) repeat spin to remove some of the dead cells and bring the viability up to around 50%. The cells will then need to be resuspended in fresh media as described in **Subheading 3.4.10.**

12. The laminin helps the cells to adhere to the cover slip. The larger the area covered with laminin, the larger the area available for the cells to attach. It is imperative that cells adhere in a monolayer if individual myocyte evaluation is desired (i.e., imaging, calcium transients, cell shortening).

13. Aspirate only one or two plates at a time to ensure cell resuspension when plating. The cells fall out of suspension quickly; therefore there is only enough time for two plates before the cells need to be resuspended.

12

Myofilament Protein Phosphorylation by PKC in Genetically Engineered Adult Cardiac Myocytes

Margaret V. Westfall

1. Introduction

Virus-based gene transfer results in the rapid and efficient expression of individual contractile proteins within the myofilaments of adult cardiac myocytes *(1–3)*. This ability to express genetically modified contractile proteins in myocytes now makes it possible to investigate the relative phosphorylation of a given contractile protein as it resides within the intact myofilament. Contractile proteins, including troponin I (TnI), troponin T (TnT), myosin light chain 2 (MLC$_2$), and myosin binding protein C (MyBPC) are in vitro targets for protein kinase C (PKC) phosphorylation *(4)*. Several protocols have been developed to detect contractile protein phosphorylation using ^{32}P-ATP and PKC preparations *(5–7)*. However, questions remain about whether these proteins are phosphorylated by agonist-activated PKC in intact adult cardiac myocytes *(5,8,9)*. Thus, there is a need to identify the relative phosphorylation of myofilament proteins in response to PKC activation in adult cardiac myocytes. This goal is accomplished by studying myofilament protein phosphorylation in genetically modified myocytes expressing contractile proteins with and without modified phosphorylation sites.

Phosphorylation of contractile proteins can be assayed using Western blot analysis with phosphospecific antibodies *(10)*, two-dimensional polyacrylamide gel electrophoresis (2D-PAGE) *(11)*, and/or radiolabeled phosphate incorporation *(4,8,9,12)*. Reliable phosphospecific antibodies are not commercially and/or readily available for each contractile phosphoprotein. The wide range of isoelectric points among the contractile proteins also makes 2D-PAGE difficult to utilize when one is analyzing phosphorylation of multiple contrac-

From: *Methods in Molecular Biology, vol. 219: Cardiac Cell and Gene Transfer*
Edited by: J. M. Metzger © Humana Press Inc., Totowa, NJ

tile protein targets for PKC. Radiolabeled phosphate incorporation can be difficult to interpret, owing to extensive phosphorylation of contractile proteins during the initial radiolabeling period. A detailed radiolabeled orthophosphate protocol designed to detect agonist-mediated, PKC-dependent phosphorylation and to minimize background phosphorylation during the labeling period is described here for use with adult rat cardiac myocytes. Steps for preparation of polyacrylamide gels, silver staining, and drying down of gels are also included in the protocol since phosphorylation is normalized to protein loading within each lane of the gel. A thorough gel electrophoresis protocol also is available in Giulian et al. *(13)*. The current protocol is used to analyze the myofilament proteins phosphorylated in response to the PKC agonist endothelin-1 in intact myocytes and could easily be adapted for other PKC agonists.

Prior to performing the phosphorylation assay described below, adult ventricular myocytes are isolated and collected from collagenase-digested rat hearts, as described in an earlier publication *(14)*. Phosphorylation can be assayed in myocytes cultured in serum-free media for 1–6 d post gene transfer. Myocyte morphology, sarcomere architecture, contractile protein stoichiometry, and isoform expression, along with tension generation, remain unchanged in cultured myocytes during this 6-d interval *(15)*, and recent evidence indicates that the stoichiometry and pattern of PKC isoform expression also does not change detectably. Thus, genetically modified adult myocytes expressing isoforms or mutants of a given contractile protein can be used for the protocol described below, to determine the relative phosphorylation of a given contractile protein in intact myofilaments.

2. Materials

2.1. Stock Solutions

1. M199 media++ = M199 media (Sigma, #M-2520; 500-mL aliquot) + 3.073 g glutathione (10 mM; Sigma, #G-6529), 0.2 mg/mL bovine serum albumin (Boerhringer Mannheim, #199 030).
2. 5 nM Endothelin-1 (ET) (Calbiochem, #05-23-3800) in M199++. To make 40 μM ET stock: add 0.5 mg to 5 mL deionized H_2O. ET is stored at –80°C as 40 μM stock. Dilute to 5 or 100 nM, as needed.
3. 10 μM Chelerythrine in M199++ (Calbiochem, #220285). 1 mM stock: 5 mg/13 mL dimethylsulfoxide (DMSO) = 1 mM stock. Store in 1-mL aliquots at –20°C. 180 μM Stock (make fresh for each experiment): 180 μL of 1 mM stock in 1 mL M199++.
4. Calyculin A (Calbiochem, #208851): 10 μg/400 μL ethanol = 25 ng/μL. Store at –20°C for no more than 2 wk.
5. ^{32}P-orthophosphate (Perkin Elmer Life Sciences, #NEX 053), 100 μCi/reaction.

6. Relaxing solution: 40 mL of 2.5 *M* KCl (100 m*M*), 20 mL of 0.5 *M* imidazole (pH 7.0, 10 m*M*), 20 mL 0.1 *M* EGTA (2 m*M*), 10 mL of 100 m*M* MgCl$_2$ (1 m*M*), 2.42 g Na$_2$ATP (4 m*M*). Adjust pH to 7.0 with KOH and dilute to 1.0 L.

7. Relaxing solution with 0.1% Triton X-100: 4 mL of 2.5 *M* KCl, 2 mL 0.5 *M* imidazole (pH 7.0), 2 mL 0.1 *M* EGTA, 1 mL 100 m*M* MgCl$_2$, 0.242 g Na$_2$ATP. Adjust to pH 7.0. Add 10 mL Pierce (#28314) Triton X-100 and dilute to 100 mL.

8. 12% Separating gel: 0.75 *M* Tris-H$_2$O, pH 9.3, 0.1% (w/v) sodium dodecyl sulfate (SDS; Bio-Rad, #161-001), 10% (v/v) glycerol (Sigma G7757), 0.028% (w/v) ammonium persulfate (Bio-Rad, #161-0700), 12% (w/v) acrylamide (Bio-Rad, #161-0101), 0.06% (w/v) piperazine diacrylamide (PDA; Bio-Rad, #161-0202), 0.14% (w/v) TEMED (Bio-Rad, #161-0800).

9. 3.5% stacking gel: 125 m*M* Tris-H$_2$O, pH 6.8, 0.1% (w/v) SDS, 10% (v/v) glycerol, 0.04% (w/v) ammonium persulfate, 3.5% (w/v) acrylamide, 0.17% (w/v) PDA, 0.3% (w/v) TEMED.

10. Electrode buffer, pH 8.4: 0.1% (w/v) SDS, 380 m*M* glycine (Bio-Rad, #161-0718), 50 m*M* Tris base.

11. Sample buffer: 62.5 m*M* Tris-H$_2$O, pH 6.8, 1% SDS, 15% (v/v) glycerol, 0.5 mg/mL leupeptin, 15 m*M* dithiothreitol (DTT; Sigma, #D9163), 7 mg/mL bromophenol blue (Bio-Rad, #161-0404). (*See* **Note 1**).

12. Silver stain reagents: *See* Methods for preparation of solutions.
    a. Fixative: 40% methanol, 10% acetic acid.
    b. Treatment solution: 12.5% ethanol.
    c. Silver staining solution: 14.25 m*M* silver nitrate (Sigma, #S6506), 50 m*M* NaOH, 0.375% (v/v) ammonium hydroxide (*see* **Note 2**).
    d. Developing solution: 11.9 m*M* citric acid, 0.025% formaldehyde.
    e. Stop solution: 1% acetic acid.

13. Reagents for drying down gels
    a. 0.5 *M* NaOH: 20 g in 1 L.
    b. 50% (v/v) glycerol: Dilute 500 mL of glycerol to 1 L with deionized H$_2$O.
    c. 20% (v/v) glycerol: Dilute 200 mL of glycerol to 1 L with deionized H$_2$O.

2.2. Supplies

1. Adult rat cardiac myocytes: 20,000 rod-shaped myocytes plated on each 18-mm^2 cover slip in 6-well plates. Isolated and cultured as previously described in detail by Westfall et al. *(14)*

2. Borosilicate glass micropipets (10-cm length) pulled to a tip diameter of 1.0 μm.

3. Microfuge tubes, 0.5 mL capacity.

4. Shielding: 3/4-in. plastic shields.

5. Bio-Rad Protean II vertical electrophoresis system: 16 × 16-cm glass plates, 0.75-m*M* spacers.

6. Pyrex dishes wrapped in PVC film.

7. Mylar and cellophane.

3. Methods

3.1. One Day Prior to the Experiment

1. Isolated adult cardiac myocytes plated on laminin-coated glass cover slips, and cultured for 1–6 d *(14)* are needed for the phosphorylation assay.
2. Prepare relaxing solution and store at 4°C. Make, store, and aliquot stock solutions for agonist, antagonist, and phosphatase inhibitor. Prepare gel and silver staining reagents.
3. Mix reagents for separating gel, degas for 10 min, and then cast gel. Overlay gel with 2% isobutanol, allow gel to polymerize for 30 min, and store at 4°C overnight.
4. Label 1.5-mL microfuge tubes for reagents and 0.5-mL microfuge tubes for samples undergoing phosphorylation.

3.2. Day of the Experiment

3.2.1. Preassay Preparations

1. Thaw sample buffer on ice and thaw the ^{32}P-orthophosphate in a shielded container at room temperature. Plexiglas shielding is needed for all solutions containing ^{32}P-orthophosphate.
2. Gel preparation: Siphon off butanol and rinse separating gel several times with deionized H_2O. Mix reagents for the stacking gel, degas for 15 min, and overlay stacking gel on polymerized separating gel. Place comb in stacking gel and polymerize for at least 30 min.
3. Prepare 4 L of electrode buffer while the stacking gel polymerizes.
4. Just prior to loading samples, remove comb from the polymerized stacking gel, wash the wells with deionized H_2O, aspirate, and replace the H_2O with electrode buffer.

3.2.2. ^{32}P-Orthophosphate Incorporation Assay in Adult Cardiac Myocytes

1. Prepare ^{32}P-orthophosphate labeling solution: Each cover slip will need 2 mL M199++ and 100 µCi ^{32}P-orthophosphate. Media used during the labeling interval is heated to 37°C prior to addition of ^{32}P. This solution is prepared by multiplying these volumes by the number of cover slips to be used for the phosphorylation assay (*see* **Note 3**).
2. Thoroughly aspirate unlabeled media off from each well and replace with 2 mL of ^{32}P-orthophosphate labeling solution. Each 6-well plate is placed inside a Plexiglas shielded box containing 6 holes (1/4-in. diameter), to allow for gas exchange. Shielded box containing 6-well plates is incubated in 37°C incubator with 95% O_2 and 5% CO_2 for 2 h.
3. Prepare PKC activating solutions. Each well will require 2 mL of M199++ media + 0.8 µL of 25 ng/mL calyculin A (10 n*M*). Calyculin A is included in each well to prevent dephosphorylation of proteins by phosphatase 2A. The treatment groups required for each assay include no added agonist (C),

endothelin (100 nM; ET), chelerythrine (10 µM; chel), and endothelin (100 nM) plus chelerythrine (10 µM; ET + chel). A 100 nM stock of ET is prepared by adding 5 µL of 40 µM stock to 2 mL M199++. A 10 µM stock of chelerythrine is prepared by adding 111 µL of 180 µM chelerythrine to 2 mL of M199++. These solutions are prepared by multiplying the volumes listed above by the number of cover slips used for each treatment group. Beakers (250 mL) containing relaxing solution and relaxing solution with 0.1% Triton X-100, respectively, are placed on ice for sample preparation after the phosphorylation assay.

4. Thoroughly remove the ^{32}P-orthophosphate labeling solution and discard in a shielded container. Add 2 mL of one of the PKC-activating solutions described above to individual wells containing myocytes. These phosphorylation reactions are carried out in the shielded Plexiglas box at 37°C with 95% O_2 and 5% CO_2 for 5–30 min.

5. Terminate the phosphorylation reaction by transferring the PKC-activating solution to a radioactive waste container and replacing with 2 mL of ice-cold relaxing solution.

6. Dip each cover slip in relaxing solution with 0.1% Triton X-100 for 30 s, and then dip 4 times in relaxing solution (no Triton X-100) (*see* **Note 4**).

7. Drain relaxing solution from each cover slip onto a Kimwipe.

3.2.3. Processing Samples and Loading onto Polyacrylamide Gel

1. Prepare samples processing and polyacrylamide gels the same day as the phosphorylation assay to maximize detection of myofilament protein phosphorylation. Scrape myocytes from two cover slips into a 0.5-mL microfuge tube along with 20 µL sample buffer using glass micropipets. Store each sample on ice and boil for 2 min to avoid the formation of multimeric complexes (*5*).

2. Add a second 10 µL aliquot of sample buffer to each tube, followed by brief centrifugation using a tabletop microfuge.

3. Sonicate each sample for 10 min at room temperature and briefly centrifuge for a second time.

4. Load samples onto the polyacrylamide gel using 10-µL gel loading tips. Position the gel behind plastic shielding during the loading and running periods.

5. Fill the upper and lower buffer chambers with the remaining electrode buffer, and run the gel at 20 mA for 4 h at room temperature.

3.2.4. Silver Stain Protocol for Protein Detection

Low protein concentrations are present in samples collected from cover slips. Silver-staining gels prior to phosphorimage analysis allows protein bands to be detected and quantified by densitometry after phosphorimage detection is complete.

1. Transfer the polyacrylamide gel to a film-wrapped Pyrex dish containing fixative solution for 20–30 min and then wash in deionized H_2O for 15 min.

2. Prepare treatment solution (200 mL), developer (400 mL), and stop solution (200 mL) during these time intervals.

3. Incubate each gel in treatment solution for 10 min and mix silver stain solution during this time interval. Silver stain solution is prepared by mixing refrigerated ammonium hydroxide (30% stock) with refrigerated silver nitrate stock solution (5% w/v), stirring, and then mixing with sodium hydroxide (1 M stock) and deionized H_2O just before use.

4. Incubate the gel in silver stain solution for 25 min and then wash 3 times at 5-min intervals in deionized H_2O.

5. Transfer the gel to 200 mL of developer for 1 min and transfer to fresh developer for 2–10 min. When protein bands are readily detectable with little background staining, immerse the gel in 200 mL of 1% acetic acid for 5 min.

6. Wash the gels 3 times at 5-min intervals in deionized H_2O.

3.2.5. Drying Polyacrylamide Gels in Preparation for Transfer to Phosphorimage Cassette

Polyacrylamide gels are dried prior to phosphorimaging to avoid damaging the phosphorimage cassette.

1. Soak gel in 20% glycerol, hydrate cellophane in 50% glycerol, and wet Mylar in 0.5 M NaOH for 20 min.

2. Immerse 71/2 × 91/2-in. rectangular plastic plate in deionized H_2O, and place Mylar sheet on top of plastic plate. Transfer plate with Mylar to a dry, flat surface.

3. Pour approx 1–2 mL of glycerol over Mylar, lay down gel on top of Mylar, and repeat application of glycerol.

4. Lay hydrated cellophane over gel and roll out air bubbles and excess glycerol with disposable 10-mL pipet. Tuck excess cellophane under Mylar.

5. Place plate containing Mylar, gel, and cellophane on an absorbent pad overnight.

3.3. Days 2–5

1. Remove excess glycerol from gel with Kimwipes, and trim away excess Mylar/cellophane. Heat-seal gel in a Kapak pouch and firmly tape down in a phosphorimage cassette (Bio-Rad) to prevent exposure of the cassette to moisture. Cassettes are exposed for 4 d prior to developing the phosphorimage in a Bio-Rad #G505 phosphorimager.

4. Notes

1. Preparation of bromophenol blue for sample buffer. Dissolve 1.25 g of bromophenol blue (Bio-Rad, #161-0404) in 5 mL of isopropyl alcohol; dilute to 50 mL with deionized H_2O. Aliquot 1 mL in 1.5-mL microfuge tubes and store at –80°C as one-use aliquots.

2. Silver stain reagents. The silver nitrate stock solution (5% w/v) should be stored at 4°C in an opaque brown bottle. Prior to discarding silver stain solution, add 5 mL of 1.0 M HCl to precipitate out silver chloride.

3. All solid and liquid waste collected beyond this point is radioactive and must be disposed of in appropriately shielded (3/4-in. Plexiglas) containers.
4. Samples should be rinsed and collected rapidly to prevent changes in myofilament protein phosphorylation.

References

1. Westfall, M. V., Albayya, F. P., and Metzger, J. M. (1999) Functional analysis of troponin I regulatory domains in the intact myofilament of adult single cardiac myocytes. *J. Biol. Chem.* **274**, 22,508–22,516.
2. Westfall, M. V., Albayya, F. P., Turner, I. I., and Metzger, J. M. (2000) Chimera analysis of troponin I domains that influence Ca^{2+}-activated myofilament tension in adult cardiac myocytes. *Circ. Res.* **86**, 470–477.
3. Westfall, M. V., Turner, I. I., Albayya, F., and Metzger, J. M. (2001) Troponin I chimera analysis of the cardiac myofilament tension response to protein kinase A. *Am. J. Physiol.* **280**, C324–C332.
4. Venema, R. and Kuo, J. F. (1993) PKC-mediated phosphorylation of troponin I and C-protein in isolated myocardial cells is associated with inhibition of myofibrillar actomyosin MgATPase. *J. Biol. Chem.* **268**, 2705–2711.
5. Edes, I. and Kranias, E. G. (1990) Phospholamban and troponin I are substrates for PKC in vitro but not in intact beating guinea pig hearts. *Circ. Res.* **67**, 394–400.
6. Katoh, N., Wise, B. C., and Kuo, J. F. (1983) Phosphorylation of cardiac troponin inhibitory subunit (troponin I) and tropomyosin binding subunit (troponin T) by cardiac phospholipid-sensitive Ca^{2+}-dependent protein kinase. *Biochem. J.* **209**, 189–195.
7. Noland, T. A., Jr. and Kuo, J. F. (1991) Protein kinase C phosphorylation of cardiac troponin I or troponin T inhibits Ca^{2+}-stimulted actomyosin MgATPase activity. *J. Biol. Chem.* **266**, 4974–4978.
8. Damron, D. S., Darvish, A., Murphy, L., Sweet, W., Moravec, C. S., and Bond, M. (1995) Arachidonic acid-dependent phosphorylation of troponin I and myosin light chain 2 in cardiac myocytes. *Circ. Res.* **76**, 1011–1019.
9. Huang, X. P., Pi, Y., Lokuta, A. J., Greaser, M. L., and Walker, J. L. (1997) Arachidonic acid stimulates protein kinase C- redistribution in heart cells. *J. Cell. Sci.* **110**, 1625–1634.
10. Bodor, G. S., Oakeley A. E, Allen, P. D., Crimmins, D. L., Ladenson, J. H., and Anderson, P. A. W. (1997) Troponin I phosphorylation in the normal and failing adult human heart. *Circulation* **96**, 1495–1500.
11. Foster D. B. and Van Eyk J. E. (1999) In search of the proteins that cause myocardial stunning. *Circ. Res.* **85**, 470–472.
12. Takeishi, Y., Chu, G., Kirkpatrick, D. M., et al. (1998) In vivo phosphorylation of cardiac troponin I by protein kinase C β_2 decreases cardiomyocyte calcium responsiveness and contractility in transgenic mouse hearts. *J. Clin. Invest.* **102**, 72–78.
13. Giulian, G. G., Moss, R. L., and Greaser, M. M. (1983) Improved methodology for analysis and quantitation of proteins on one-dimensional silver-stained slab gels. *Anal. Biochem.* **129**, 227–287.

14. Westfall, M. V., Rust, E. M., Albayya, F., and Metzger, J. M. (1997) Adenovirus-mediated myofilament gene transfer into adult cardiac myocytes. *Methods Cell. Biol.* **52,** 307–322.
15. Rust, E. M., Westfall, M. V., and Metzger, J. M. (1998) Stability of the contractile assembly and Ca^{2+}-activated tension in adenovirus infected adult cardiac myocytes. *Mol. Cell. Biochem.* **181,** 143–155.

IV

IN VIVO CARDIAC GENE TRANSFER

PROTOCOLS, APPLICATIONS,
AND PHYSIOLOGICAL ASSESSMENT

13

Embryonic and Neonatal Cardiac Gene Transfer In Vivo

Geir Christensen, Peter J. Gruber, Yibin Wang, and Kenneth R. Chien

1. Introduction

Gene transfer into the murine myocardium represents a powerful strategy for studying the mechanisms and potential treatments of cardiac disease. The mouse can be genetically engineered precisely, and cardiac function can be examined at both the organ and the cellular level *(1)*. Several mouse models have been developed that mimic features of acquired heart disease, such as hypertrophy, contractile dysfunction, or arrhythmias. Also, models of cardiac developmental defects as well as dilated and hypertrophic cardiomyopathy have been created by overexpression or deletion of specific genes. Gene transfer into the myocardium of such models of cardiac disease has already given insight into molecular mechanisms of cardiac dysfunction at the cellular level *(2)*. Furthermore, high-efficiency, long-term expression of foreign genes in the neonatal and embryonic heart is particularly valuable as a strategy for rescue of the various murine cardiac disease models. Finally, gene transfer to the myocardium may also allow genetic targeting of the heart prenatally and post-natally by virus-mediated delivery of Cre recombinase to mice with floxed alleles *(3)*.

Recombinant adenovirus is a useful vector for myocardial gene transfer because of the capacity for high-titer production, large insert capacity, and relatively low pathogenicity, as well as the ability to infect nondividing cells effectively. Moreover, adenovirus has several inherent advantages as a gene delivery vector for cardiac muscle, including high infectivity of cultured cardiac myocytes with preservation of relatively normal biologic function of the infected cells. However, the use of adenovirus-mediated gene transfer to

From: *Methods in Molecular Biology, vol. 219: Cardiac Cell and Gene Transfer*
Edited by: J. M. Metzger © Humana Press Inc., Totowa, NJ

the adult myocardium in vivo has been complicated by inflammatory reactions with only transient or low-efficiency gene expression. Here we describe a strategy for reproducible and efficient transduction of the embryonic and postnatal mouse myocardium with long-term gene expression and absence of inflammatory reaction.

For embryonic gene transfer, adenovirus was injected *in utero* into the ventricular cavity of living embryos using a microsurgical approach. Injected embryos were developed to term, and efficient expression of the transgene was detected in all cell types in the heart. For postnatal cardiac gene transfer, a solution containing adenovirus was injected into the cardiac ventricle of neonatal mice. Efficient expression of the transgene was observed several months after injection. Coinfection with adenoviral constructs harboring green fluorescent protein (GFP) allowed identification of infected isolated rod-shaped cardiomyocytes for functional assessments at the single-cell level.

2. Materials

2.1. Recombinant Adenoviruses

1. Recombinant human adenoviruses were constructed using the methods of Graham et al. *(4)*. An E1 deleted adenoviral shuttle vector, pacCMVpApL (gift from Dr. F. Gerard, McMaster University, Ontario, Canada), was linearized with *Bam*H1 (all restriction enzymes from Life Technologies, Gaithersberg, MD) and *Eco*R1. A *Bam*H1-*Eco*R1 fragment containing β-galactosidase cDNA from pSK-lacZ was inserted using standard techniques. Five micrograms of pacCMVlacZpApL was then cotransfected with 35 μg of pJM17 and 40 μg of carrier plasmid (pSK+ Bluescript II, Stratagene, La Jolla, CA) using calcium phosphate on 293 cells (ATCC, Rockville, MD). The cells were incubated until cytopathic effect was observed. All media for 293 cells culture was Dulbecco's modified Eagle's medium (DMEM)-high glucose (DMEM-HG) with 10% horse serum (HS; Life Technologies). The supernatant was aspirated and placed on new 293 cells followed by overlay with 1% agarose/DMEM-HG/2% HS. Cells were incubated before individual plaques were picked with sterile pipets, amplified on a third group of 293 cells before harvest. Similarly, the adenovirus-expressing GFP was generated using cDNAs from pEGFP (Clontech, Palo Alto, CA). Confirmation of appropriate structure was achieved by polymerase chain reaction (PCR).

2. High-titer preparation of confirmed adenovirus was performed by standard methods *(4)*. Briefly, 40 15-cm plates (Corning Costar, Acton, MA) of 293 cells at 60% confluency were incubated with plaque-purified adenovirus until early cytopathic effect was observed. Cells were harvested and lysed with 5 mL of 0.1% NP-40/PBS before 15-min centrifugation at 1500 rpm ($470g$) in an HS-4

tabletop centrifuge (Sorvall, Newtown, CT). The 4-mL supernatant was collected and layered on top of two 4-mL CsCl cushions (densities of 1.14 and 1.45 g/mL phosphate-buffered saline [PBS]$^{++}$; 10 mL 1 M CaCl$_2$, 10 mL MgCl$_2$, 980 mL PBS) before ultracentrifugation at 45,000 rpm (208,000g) for no less than 6 h (Beckman). The upper, adenoviral, band was aspirated using a 20-gauge needle and dialyzed in 0.2-µm Slide-a-Lyzer cassettes (Pierce, Rockford, IL) against PBS^{++} for 8 h before storage at –80°C in 50% HS/PBS^{++}. This preparation was titered using a variation of previously described methods (4).

2.2. Gene Transfer to the Embryonic Murine Heart

1. Pregnant dams at 10 d postcoitum.
2. Avertin (20 µL/g body weight) for anesthesia: 2.5 g 2,2,2-tribromoethanol, 5 mL 2-methyl-butanol (Sigma, St. Louis, MO), and 195 mL distilled, sterile H$_2$O.
3. Ethanol for cleansing of the abdomen of the pregnant dam: 70% ethanol in H$_2$O.
4. Tape for fixation of the extremities of the anesthetized animals.
5. Graefe surgical forceps, fine scissors, and Colibri retractor (Fine Science Tools, Vancouver, BC).
6. Eye cautery (Rumex, Miami, FL), pig fibrinogen (Sigma-Aldrich, St. Louis. MO), and sterile cotton applicator for hemostasis.
7. Cotton balls.
8. Sterile saline.
9. Lactated Ringer's solution (Baxter, Deerfield, IL).
10. Silk sutures, 7-0 (Ethicon).
11. Monofilament suture, 10-0 (Ethicon, Sommerville, NJ).
12. Glass capillary tubes (World Precision Instruments, New Haven, CT) for injection of solution containing adenovirus.
13. Model 730 pipet puller (David Kopf, Tujunga, CA) and model MF-79 microforge (Narishige, Sea Cliff, NY) for producing the glass capillary tube with side-hole.
14. Zeiss SV-6 stereo microscope (Carl Zeiss, Thornwood, NY).

2.3. Gene Transfer to the Postnatal Murine Heart

1. Neonatal mice, not older than 24 h.
2. Water and ice in isolated bucket for anesthesia.
3. Glass capillary tubes (World Precision Instruments) for injection of solution containing adenovirus.
4. Model 730 pipet puller (David Kopf) for producing a needle on the glass capillary tubes.
5. Rubber tubing, British Standard Softness 52, 800/010/125 (Portex, Hythe, Kent, England).
6. Syringe, 1 mL (Terumo Europe, Leuven, Belgium) and hypodermic needle, 18-gauge (B. Braun Melsungen, Melsungen, Germany).
7. Micromanipulator system (*see* **Fig. 1**).

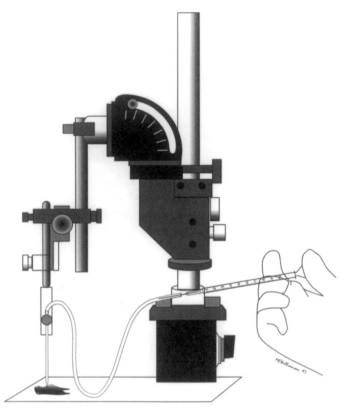

Fig. 1. Setup for injection of adenovirus into ventricular cavity of neonatal mice. A flame-stretched capillary tube was connected to rubber tubing and syringe. Capillary glass tube was mounted on a micromanipulator system for accurate positioning of the tip of the tube within the left ventricle.

3. Method

3.1. Adenovirus-Mediated Gene Transfer to the Embryonic Mouse Heart

3.1.1. Surgical Procedure

In utero manipulations were developed on the basis of methods described by Muneoka et al. *(5)* (*see* **Note 1**).

1. Anesthetize pregnant dams at 10 d post coitum with 20 µL/g body weight intraperitoneal avertin (2.5 g 2,2,2-tribromoethanol, 5 mL 2-methyl-butanol, and 195 mL distilled, sterile H_2O).
2. Cleanse the abdomen with 70% ethanol/H_2O and place the anesthetized animal in a supine position; secure the extremities in an extended position with tape.

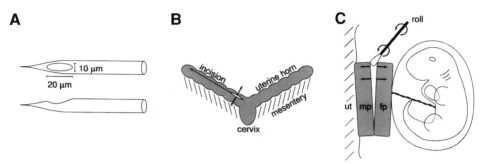

Fig. 2. *In utero* surgery. **(A)** Side-hole glass needles were specially crafted on a microforge such that the tip of the needle was sharp and closed. **(B)** Antimesenteric hysterotomy begun at the cervix and carried to the distal end of the uterine horn. **(C)** The proximal two (or more) embryos of the open uterine horn (ut) were removed by rolling a dry, sterile cotton applicator at the interface of maternal (mp) and fetal placentas (fp).

3. Perform a midline laparotomy using sharp scissors, taking care to stay on the linea alba and away from the inferior epigastric vessels. If bleeding is encountered at this or any subsequent stage of manipulations, achieve meticulous hemostasis utilizing either electrocautery, pig fibrinogen, or direct pressure using a dry, sterile cotton applicator.
4. Place an abdominal retractor and pack the bowel superiorly using sterile, saline-soaked cotton ball fragments.
5. Splay the uterine horns laterally, and perform bilateral, full-length, antimesenteric hysterotomies to expose the embryos (**Fig. 2B**).
6. Remove the two embryos closest to the cervix on each side by carefully rolling a dry, sterile cotton applicator at the interface of the maternal and fetal placenta (**Fig. 2C**). This allows the embryo, along with its corresponding placental surface, to be extracted from the uterus with minimal bleeding. Control any bleeding from the remaining maternal placenta with direct pressure.
7. Close the uterus loosely with interrupted 7-0 silk sutures.
8. Flood the abdomen with warm, lactated Ringer's solution, and position the distal uterus containing the remaining embryos in the right lateral decubitus position with sterile, saline-soaked cotton fragments.

3.1.2. Injection of Adenovirus

1. Develop crafted, pulled glass tubes with a pipet puller and a microforge using a method similar to that used in the injection of embryonic stem cells. A needle with a 10×20-μm side-hole was found to give the best results (**Fig. 2A**).
2. Under submersion, put a loosely placed 10-0 monofilament pursestring suture through the membranes, incorporating both the yolk sac and amnion. Make a small incision in the membranes within the limits of the suture.

3. Through this hole, introduce the needle containing the viral solution into the ventricular cavity of the embryo. Confirm the location of the side-hole of the needle by visual examination through a 10X Zeiss SV-6 stereomicroscope and by the observation of a retrograde flash of blood in the barrel of the needle.
4. Slowly inject approx 10^6 pfu of viral solution into the ventricular cavity as the needle is slowly withdrawn.
5. Gently approximate the preplaced pursestring suture without excessive strangulation of the embryonic membranes.
6. Copiously irrigate the abdominal cavity with sterile lactated Ringer's solution and make a final check for hemostasis. This part of the procedure is important since even small amounts of remaining intraperitoneal blood reduce the viability of the embryos (even those unmanipulated).
7. Close the abdomen with a running 7-0 silk suture, and allow the mother to recover in a warm area. Deliver embryos either by cesarean section or by maternal euthanasia and use of a foster mother.

3.1.3. Assessment of Transfection Efficiency

Assays for β-galactosidase of embryonic tissue were performed by a variation of standard techniques (*6*). Whole embryos were dissected such that communications were made throughout multiple body cavities, including the pleural, pericardial, intraventricular, and peritoneal spaces. The embryos were quickly rinsed twice in ice-cold PBS, permeabilized, and stained with X-galactosidase. Using the method presented, we were able to transduce the full thickness of the myocardium effectively when 10^6–10^8 pfu of viral particles were used. Moreover, we showed that all cell types in the heart could be effectively transduced, as determined by light microscopy. The success of the *in utero* viral transduction approach was confirmed in a series of 54 consecutive embryonic manipulations, resulting in an overall survival of 73%.

3.2. Adenovirus-Mediated Gene Transfer to the Neonatal Mouse Heart

3.2.1. Anesthesia

Before the suspension containing adenovirus was injected into the ventricular cavity, the animals were anesthetized by cooling in water at 4°C for 2 min. This method of anesthesia has previously been described (*7*) and suggested for general anesthesia in pre-weanling rodents. Rapid cooling is possible owing to the small body mass and lack of thermoregulatory capabilities. Neonatal mice can tolerate extended periods of a body temperature below 10°C, whereas after 2 wk of age such cooling may be lethal. By lowering the body temperature, we were able to arrest the heart temporarily, which prolonged the exposure of the heart to the virus.

3.2.2. Injection of Adenovirus into the Ventricular Cavity

1. Inject the suspension containing adenovirus using a flame-stretched capillary tube mounted on a micromanipulator system, as shown in **Fig. 1** (*see* **Note 2**). The capillary tube is connected by rubber tubing to a 1-mL syringe.
2. After the capillary tube is filled with 10-µL suspension, carry out injections by direct punctuation of the cardiac cavity through the chest wall on the left border of the sternum at the level of the axilla. Flashback of pulsatile blood into the glass tube indicates the intracavitary position of the needle. Dark-colored blood indicates positioning in the right ventricular chamber, and light-colored blood indicates positioning in the left chamber.
3. Slowly inject the suspension (10 µL/min), and ensure the right position of the glass tube at the end of injection by observing flashback of pulsatile blood.
4. Allow the mice to recover by rewarming. Approximately 1 out of 10 injected animals died immediately or within a day after intracardiac injection. The survivors developed normally compared with nonmanipulated littermates.

3.2.3. Gene Transfer Efficiency

We examined the efficiency of the described method by injecting 10^9 particles of adenovirus encoding β-galactosidase on the first, third, and fifth days after birth (*8*). Three days after injection, the hearts were excised, fixed, and subjected to β-galactosidase assay as described (*6*). Examination of hearts from mice injected on the first day after birth revealed that the entire outer layer of the myocardium expressed the transduced gene. Sections of the myocardium clearly demonstrated that the gene was expressed in cardiomyocytes. The most efficient expression was found in the outer layer of the myocardium, but cardiomyocytes in the trabecular network and the inner layer of the myocardium were also transfected. Myocytes in all parts of the atrial myocardium expressed β-galactosidase. When intracavitary injection of adenovirus was performed in a group of animals 3 or 5 d after birth, the infection was much less efficient. Our method also allows long-term expression, since efficient gene expression in cardiomyocytes was observed 3 and 6 wk after injection. After 6 mo, the β-galactosidase was still expressed in the transduced hearts. No inflammatory response was found in any of the sections from the atria or ventricles.

We also examined the efficiency of our method by isolating cardiac cells and counting cardiomyocytes from each heart of six animals 3 d after administration of adenovirus. In some animals 27% of the cardiomyocytes expressed β-galactosidase. The average percentage of cells expressing the gene was 10.9 ± 3.5%. Little expression of β-galactosidase was found in other organs except the liver, where numerous cells expressed the transduced gene.

3.2.4. Cotransfection with β-Galactosidase and GFP

Our method also allows coinfection of cardiomyocytes in vivo with a second virus by intracavitary injection of a mixture of adenovirus encoding GFP and adenovirus encoding β-galactosidase. We showed that almost all the cardiomyocytes identified by expression of GFP also expressed the β-galactosidase. When cardiomyocytes from six hearts were examined, 93% of the cells expressing GFP also expressed β-galactosidase.

3.2.5. Isolation and Identification of Viable Rod-Shaped Mouse Cardiomyocytes Expressing GFP

To allow physiologic assessment of infected cardiomyocytes, cells were isolated 3 wk after injection of adenovirus. Cardiomyocytes isolated 3 wk after birth were rod-shaped, and mechanical function, microfluorometry, and patch-clamp studies can be performed in cardiomyocytes expressing GFP. Noninfected cardiomyocytes were not visible when illuminated at 450 nm. We found in the adult noninfected mouse myocytes a shortening of $9.35 \pm 0.94\%$ and a shorting duration of 469 ± 29 ms. These functional parameters were not different from data obtained in infected cells, which were $9.84 \pm 1.46\%$ and 467 ± 34 ms, respectively.

The method presented was used in a subsequent study *(2)* to examine the effect of adenovirus-mediated delivery of phospholamban with a point mutation that disrupts the inhibitory effect on sarcoplasmic reticulum Ca^{2+} ATPase. Myocytes that overexpressed phospholamban with the point mutation displayed increased contractility, whereas myocytes that overexpressed the wild-type phospholamban exhibited decreased contractility compared with noninfected myocytes.

4. Notes

1. The most important aspect of embryonic cardiac injections is the preparation. All tools must be readily available so that time is not wasted searching for items (applicators, sutures, and so on) when rapid action is required. A few specific hints are given here.
   a. Use low eye point oculars on the dissecting scope to bring the field closer and be sure to rest one's forearms while operating.
   b. The scope must be adjusted to near perfect parfocality in order to maintain focus throughout the range of magnifications required throughout the operation.
   c. Have multiple syringes preloaded with warm irrigation solution. Keep these in a warm bath close at hand.
   d. Preload sutures before use.
   e. Address all bleeding immediately with pressure and patience. Occasionally cautery or application of fibrinogen is required.

f. Inhalation anesthetic can be used in place of injectable avertin. However, in our experience, abortion rates are higher with the use of inhalation anesthetics. Additionally, the titration of anesthetic by nosecone movement is cumbersome while one is attending to the surgical procedure.

g. Be sure to account for all packs placed in the abdomen before closure, as a retained pack will surely result in compromise of the pregnancy.

h. Closure of the hysterotomy is not required, but it helps to decrease secretions from the denuded maternal placenta. Be sure not to close the uterus over manipulated embryos.

i. Leaving Reichart's membrane intact enhances the stability of the embryo within the uterus. A small section can be scraped away to visualize the embryo.

2. A few hints that may be helpful to achieve right positioning of the tip of the capillary glass tube in the heart:

a. It is important to have a capillary glass tube with the right opening. We utilized a puller normally used for making patch-clamp pipets. We suggest starting with a relatively wide opening of the tip. Using a wide opening facilitates flashback of blood. However, later, when performing reproducible experiments, the size of the opening should be reduced to less than 6 µm to minimize bleeding. For injection in the neonates, we used a regular straight pulled pipet with the hole at the tip, not a side-hole. Right positioning of the tip of the glass tubing may be ensured by aspiration of a few microliters of blood using light suction, preferably both before and after injection of virus.

b. To find the right spot for penetration of the chest wall, it may be helpful to open a few neonates to observe their exact thoracic anatomy. It is also possible to see the heart by a light source placed under the neonate.

c. To perform reproducible intracavitary injections in neonates, it was necessary to mount the capillary glass tube on a micromanipulator system, as shown in **Fig. 1**. That system allowed correct positioning of the pipet. Even more important is that we were able to avoid penetration of the posterior wall of the heart. Since pressure must be applied to get through the chest wall, it is important to be careful at this point to avoid penetration of the whole heart.

d. We marked the glass tubes for 10 µL and filled them to the mark between each injection.

e. We used a warm bedding for rewarming of neonates after anesthesia and injection.

References

1. Christensen, G., Wang, Y., and Chien, K. R. (1997) Physiological assessment of complex cardiac phenotypes in genetically engineered mice. *Am. J. Physiol.* **272,** H2513–H2524.

2. Minamisawa, S., Hoshijima, M., Chu, G., et al. (1999) Chronic phospholamban-sarcoplasmic reticulum calcium ATPase interaction is the critical calcium cycling defect in dilated cardiomyopathy. *Cell* **99,** 313–322.

3. Rajewsky, K., Gu, H., Kuhn, R., et al. (1996) Conditional gene targeting. *J. Clin. Invest.* **98,** S51–S53.
4. Graham, F. L. and Prevec, L. (1995) Methods for construction of adenovirus vectors. *Mol. Biotechnol.* **3,** 207–220.
5. Muneoka, K., Wanek, N., and Bryant, S. V. (1986) Mouse embryos develop normally ex utero. *J. Exp. Zool.* **239,** 289–293.
6. Sanes, J. R., Rubenstein, J. L., and Nicolas, J. F. (1986) Use of a recombinant retrovirus to study post-implantation cell lineage in mouse embryos. *EMBO J.* **5,** 3133–3142.
7. Phifer, C. B. and Terry, L. M. (1986) Use of hypothermia for general anesthesia in preweanling rodents. *Physiol. Behav.* **38,** 887–890.
8. Christensen, G., Minamisawa, S., Gruber, P. J., Wang, Y., and Chien, K. R. (2000) High-efficiency, long-term cardiac expression of foreign genes in living mouse embryos and neonates. *Circulation* **101,** 178–184.

14

Efficient Viral Gene Transfer to Rodent Hearts In Vivo

Federica del Monte and Roger J. Hajjar

1. Introduction

Targeting genes to the heart through somatic gene transfer is allowing investigators to manipulate specific molecules and signal transduction pathways in both in vitro and in vivo models of cardiovascular disease *(1,2)*. This approach permits us to test the role of these molecules and pathways of disease pathogenesis and progression *(1)*.

Our understanding of both the technology of gene transfer and the biology of signal transduction, as it relates to cardiac dysfunction, has changed dramatically over the last few years *(3)*, during which significant advances have been made in both these areas. Earlier chapters have concentrated on vector developments. In this chapter, we review methods of gene delivery to the rodent heart and highlight the therapeutic targeting of calcium cycling proteins in a rodent model of heart failure *(4–7)*.

1.1. Somatic Gene Transfer

Somatic gene transfer into cells and tissues is performed through "naked DNA" (in a mammalian expression cassette) or packaged in association with a variety of vehicles or *vectors* designed to enhance gene transfer. These vectors are divided into nonviral vectors employing physical-chemical gene delivery and recombinant viral vectors in which the cDNA of interest has been incorporated into a virus, which is then used to infect the target cell and in the process conveys the exogenous cDNA. Quantification of the gene of interest is achieved based on two measurements: (1) the efficiency, and (2) the level of expression. *Efficiency* refers to the number of cells expressing the transgene as a function of the total number of cells in the tissue targeted. *Level of expression* indicates the total amount of exogenous protein expressed. Although these

From: *Methods in Molecular Biology, vol. 219: Cardiac Cell and Gene Transfer*
Edited by: J. M. Metzger © Humana Press Inc., Totowa, NJ

parameters are conceptually distinct, they are often related in practical terms. For example, the determined efficiency of gene transfer critically depends on the sensitivity of the assay employed to detect gene expression. Using a more sensitive assay, expression may be detectable in a higher percentage of the cell population even though the intrinsic efficiency of gene transfer has not changed. In addition, an increase in the level of expression, perhaps through use of a stronger promoter, will usually improve the calculated efficiency since transgene expression will now exceed the threshold necessary for detection in more cells.

1.2. Cardiac Gene Transfer

As systems for cardiovascular gene transfer are developed, *reporter genes* encoding proteins that are easily identified and/or quantitated are frequently employed. Generally these proteins have either enzymatic activity (e.g., β-galactosidase [β-gal], luciferase) or intrinsic fluorescent properties (e.g., green fluorescent protein [GFP]). Although reporter constructs have proved to be extremely useful in establishing and characterizing gene transfer models, it is important to realize that they are an imperfect model for the ultimate goal of such studies. First, the expressed reporter protein may itself have effects that confound experimental results *(7)*. For example, β-gal evokes a significant host immune response that can be difficult to distinguish from the response to the vector itself. Second, the level of expression detectable for a particular reporter gene depends on the sensitivity of the assay system and probably bears no relationship to a biologically relevant functional end point. The level of expression required of the relevant transgene to mediate a specific effect varies tremendously with the specific application and may be either grossly over- or underestimated by use of a reporter construct. Therefore the appropriate tools (vector, construct, delivery system) will also differ with the specific application. To test the ability of a particular gene transfer approach to modulate a particular biologic pathway, it is ultimately necessary to do just that without interposing a surrogate marker.

Although an exhaustive review of vector systems is beyond the scope of this chapter, certain general principles can be identified. Nonviral vectors have thus far had unacceptably low transfection efficiencies for in vivo applications that require transduction of a large proportion of myocytes. In contrast, applications that require only a low level of expression in a small percentage of cells may well be suitable for such approaches *(2,8,9)*. On the other hand, use of viral vectors significantly heightens biosafety concerns about possible contamination with replication-competent virus and the transgene-independent host response to the vector itself. Among viral vectors, retroviruses have been the most extensively studied and used clinically. However, retroviral vectors require an actively dividing host cell and are therefore not generally suitable for cardiac gene transfer. Recombinant adenoviral vectors, in contrast, can infect and transduce nonreplicating cells. Using these adenoviruses, many investigators have now demonstrated the feasibility of both in vitro and in vivo cardiac gene transfer, and these vectors are considered here in more detail.

2. Materials

2.1. Adenovirus

Materials and methods for adenoviral preparation are discussed in other chapters. It is, however, important to have an adenoviral solution with a high titer ($1-10 \times 10^{10}$) of plaque-forming units (PFU) per mL. The adenoviral solution is prepared and stored in a solution containing 10 mM Tris-HCl, pH 7.4, 1 mM MgCl$_2$, and 10% (v/v) glycerol stock solution (Sigma, St. Louis, MO). The viral solutions should be in aliquots of 50 μL and stored at –80°C. Prior to adenoviral gene delivery, the adenoviral solution should be placed at 37°C for 30 min.

2.2. Rats

Rats (150–250 g male or female) can be obtained from Taconic Farms (Germantown, NY) or Charles River (Cambridge, MA). The strains of animals can be Fisher 344, Brown Norway, Sprague-Dawley, or Wistar. It is important that the animals be acclimated for 2–3 d prior to surgery.

2.3 Ventilator

A rodent respiratory ventilator is necessary for the surgery (CWE, model SAR-830/AP, Ardmore, PA). The ventilator should be operated in volume-cycled, positive-pressure mode. To produce tidal volumes, a constant airflow is gated into the animal during inspiration. This *flow rate* multiplied by the *inspiratory time* gives the tidal volume. *Respiratory rate* is set independently. Typical settings for 150–250-g rats are: respiratory rate, 50 breaths/min; tidal volume, 2 mL; and inspiratory time, 0.5 s.

2.4 Surgical Instruments

All intruments are from WPI (Sarasota, FL) or Roboz (Gaithersburg, MD).
1. Two Dumont tweezers.
2. Two Adson forceps.
3. Two Kelly hemostatic forceps.
4. One surgical scissor, 14 cm.
5. One self-retaining retractor.

Table 1
Methods of Adenoviral Gene Transfer in Rats

Intracoronary injection
Intramyocardial injection
Intrapericardial injection
Clamping of the aorta
Crossclamping of the aorta and pulmonary artery
Ultrasound destruction of microbubbles combined with adenovirus

6. One micro-bulldog clamp 3 cm long.
7. 16–18-Gauge soft catheters (Angiocath, Becton-Dickinson, Sandy, UT).
8. 22-Gauge soft catheter.
9. One high-temperature cautery.
10. 4.0 Nylon sutures.
11. 7.0 Nylon sutures.

3. Methods

The feasibility of in vivo cardiac gene transfer by viral vectors has been consistently demonstrated in both large and smaller studies. Recombinant adenoviruses have been the most common vectors used in these initial studies, largely because of their flexible packaging constraints and their ability to transduce nonreplicating cells *(7)*. However, the robust immune response these vectors evoke suggests that clinical applications will probably require other vectors or further refined adenoviral systems.

A number of mechanical approaches have been used to achieve cardiac gene transfer, as shown in **Table 1**. These methods have been refined for rodent hearts and specifically for rat models. We explore here the methodologies for the different delivery approaches in the rat.

3.1. Preparation of the Rat

1. Obtain rats of different types of colonies (Fisher 344, Sprague-Dawley, Brown-Norway, or Wistar). Either all males or all females should be chosen for these studies. The rats should be free of antibody titers to a number of routinely tested rat viruses. In addition, the rats should be free of all endo- and ectoparasites and mycoplasma species.
2. Maintain the rats in a barrier room at $72 \pm 2°F$ with the relative humidity at $50 \pm 10\%$, and feed them a commercial laboratory diet and water *ad libitum*.
3. Set the room ventilation between 12 and 15 air changes per hour of 100% prefiltered outside air.

4. Control the light cycle period at 12 h of light and 12 h of dark with no twilight transition.
5. Have the institutional Animal Care and Use Committee approve the study.

3.2. Anesthesia

1. Anesthetize the rats with intraperitoneal pentobarbital (40–60 mg/kg).
2. Place a rectal temperature probe in the animal, and use a heating lamp to maintain body temperature while the animal lies dorsally.
3. Intubate the animals via the larynx by using a 16- or 18-gauge soft catheter (Angiocath, Becton-Dickinson, Sandy).
4. Place a small light source on the neck over the larynx, and lift the tongue. This allows the larynx to be clearly visualized, permitting the angiocath to be introduced accurately.
5. Ventilate the rats with tidal volumes of 2 mL at 50 cycles/min with an FiO_2 of 0.21 *(10)*.

3.3. Viral Preparation

1. Store adenoviruses stocks at $-70°C$, usually in glycerol-containing solutions. Since glycerol can be toxic to the lungs, we dilute our adenoviral solutions with phosphate-buffered saline (PBS) 1:1.
2. Thaw the solution and maintain at $37°C$.
3. Depending on the mode of gene delivery, deliver 100 to 200 µL of viral solution. For in vivo gene transfer, we try to achieve a multiplicity of infection of 100 pfu/cell. The rat heart has approx 10^7 cardiomyocytes. Therefore the viral solution should have a concentration of at least 10^{10} pfu/mL. Calculation:

$$\frac{0.1 \text{ ml } (100 \text{ µl}) \times 10^{10} \text{pfu/ml}}{10^7 \text{ cells}} = \text{pfu / cell}$$

3.4. Intracoronary Delivery

1. Shave the right neck of the animal, and make a 1-cm incision *(11)*.
2. Identify the right common carotid artery, place a 6-0 suture around it.
3. Insert a 5-cm 2-French flexible multipurpose catheter into the carotid artery and advance it down as shown in **Fig. 1**. Fluoroscopy helps to guide the catheter into the left main coronary artery or the right coronary artery. However if fluoroscopy is not available, the catheter should be connected to a pressure transducer, and once the catheter crosses the aortic valve, it should be pulled out a few millimeters. A slight rotation usually secures the catheter in the left main artery. These catheters have 0.2–0.5 mL of "dead space," which should be accounted for when delivering the solution of virus. Using this type of intracoronary catheter delivery of an adenovirus encoding β-gal achieved transduction of about 30% of the myocytes in the distribution of the coronary artery *(11)*.

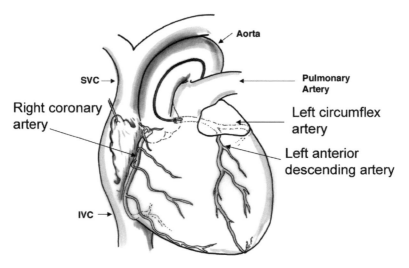

Fig. 1. Delivery of the viral solution directly into the left coronary artery. SVC, superior vena cava; IVC, inferior vena cava.

3.5. Direct Injection into the Ventricular Wall

Direct injection of adenovirus into the ventricular wall using an epicardial approach has also been shown to induce significant expression of reporter constructs *(12)* (**Fig. 2**). There are different approaches for this intervention. In an open-chested, ventilated animal, direct inspection of the heart is possible, and injection directly into the area of interest is possible *(12,13)*. Using a 30-gauge needle, the anterior, lateral, and inferoposterior walls can be readily penetrated. The interventricular septum can also be targeted by identifying the interventricular branch of the coronary artery and directing the needle parallel to that branch. For each it is important to introduce the needle only a few millimeters (since the walls are 1–3 mm thick). Angling the needle at 30–60° in relation to the ventricular wall yields the best results. Investigators have used volumes of 10–50 µL per injection. In this case, it is important to choose the solution in which the virus is placed judiciously. Solutions containing high concentrations can cause increased edema in the area of injection. Using the left anterior descending artery as a guide, investigators have injected directly around the vessel for optimal left ventricular gene transfer *(14)*. This has yielded excellent results in terms of functional effects. Coupled with needle injury, this method of injection induces focal expression within the myocardium. For global myocardial expression, this method has obvious shortcomings, but for local expression such as the various growth factors used for the blood vessel wall, this is an ideal approach.

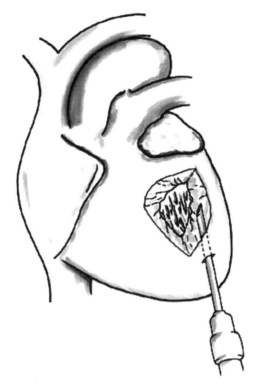

Fig. 2. Direct injection of the adenoviral solution into the myocardium.

Another approach is to inject the myocardium by echo-guidance using ultra-sound. This technique was used effectively for in vivo gene transfer of human endothelial cell nitric oxide synthase in cardiomyocytes using Sendai virus-coated liposomes *(15)*. With echo-guided techniques, gene delivery to the interventricular septum is most effective.

3.6. Pericardial Adenoviral Gene Transfer

1. For this procedure, make a small incision below the xyphoid in a transverse fash-ion after the animals are anesthetized as discussed earlier *(16)*.
2. Identify the pericardial sac and, using a 30-gauge needle, deliver adenovirus (100 µL) as shown in **Fig. 3**. This method has yielded mainly epicardial stain-ing. Collagenase and hyaluronic acid have been added to loosen the collagen fibers and allow further entry of the adenoviruses and greater transduction of the cardiomyo :ytes (up to 40%). A great deal of inflammation is present with this procedure, raising the concern that pericarditis and its sequelae may limit its usefulness.

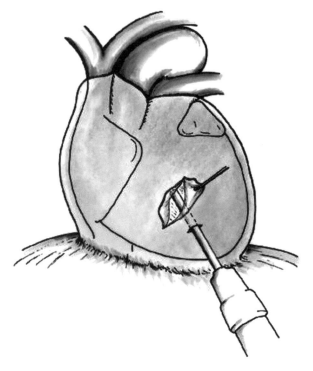

Fig. 3. Injection of the viral solution into the pericardial sac.

3.7. Crossclamping of the Aorta and Pulmonary Artery

1. In an open-chested rat (either by mid-sternotomy or through an incision from the left third intercostal space), open the pericardium, and place a 7-0 suture at the apex of the left ventricle *(5,17)*.
2. Identify the aorta and pulmonary artery.
3. Advance a 22- or 24-gauge catheter (depending on the size of the animal) containing 200 µL of adenovirus from the apex of the left ventricle to the aortic root. It is important either to feel or to visualize the catheter as it is advanced from the ventricular apex all the way to the aortic root.
3. Aortic clamping alone, as shown in **Fig. 4**, can be performed, but, as discussed later, expression with aortic clamping alone is low.
4. In another approach that has yielded better results, the aorta and pulmonary arteries are clamped distal to the site of the catheter and the solution injected as shown in **Fig. 5**. The clamp can be maintained for 10 up to 60 s while the heart is pumping against a closed system (isovolumically). This allows the solution that contains the adenovirus to circulate down the coronary arteries an 1 perfuse the heart without direct manipulation of the coronaries. In **Fig. 6**, meth,/lene blue was injected to evaluate the perfusion, and staining of the whole heart can be easily assessed. After 10–60 s, the clamp on the aorta and pulmonary artery is released.

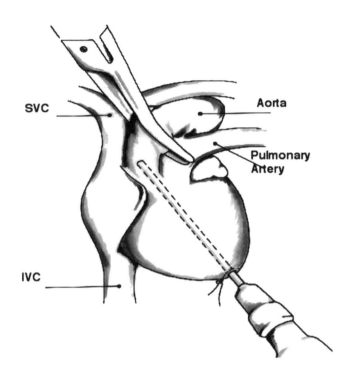

Fig. 4. Clamping of the aorta while injecting the viral solution within the aortic root.

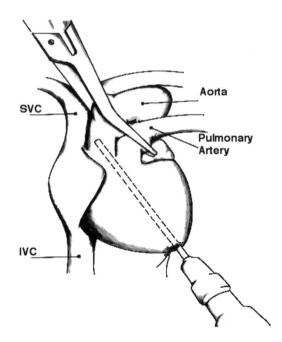

Fig. 5. Crossclamping of the aorta and pulmonary artery while injecting the viral solution within the aortic root.

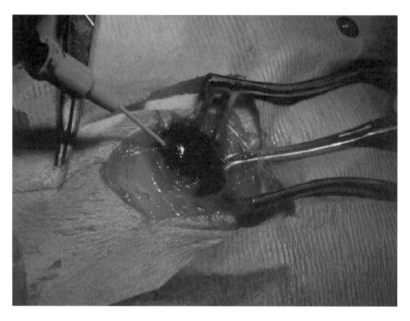

Fig. 6. Methylene blue is injected to evaluate the perfusion and staining of the whole heart while crossclamping the aorta and pulmonary artery.

During the period of crossclamping, the right and left ventricles become visibly pale as clear viral solution perfuses the myocardium through the coronary arteries. During the procedure, the heart rate decreases from ~300 to ~50 bpm but recovers to baseline within 30 s of clamp release. Ventricular pressure returns to baseline within 60 s.

5. Pretreatment of the animals with either adenosine or serotonin by injecting a solution containing 1–10 μ*M* into the inferior vena cava can also be used. This induces increased permeability of the capillaries, resulting in enhanced attachment of the viruses to myocardial cells. This method achieves grossly homogeneous transduction of cardiac myocytes throughout the left and right ventricles of the heart. More importantly, this technique can produce dramatic, transgene-specific physiologic effects on ventricular function in vivo. The success of this approach probably reflects in vivo optimization of the parameters previously shown to be important for ex vivo gene transfer, which are (1) the use of crystalloid solution as opposed to whole blood; (2) high coronary flow rate; (3) exposure time; (4) virus concentration; and (5) temperature. The high perfusion pressure presumably allows the opening of capillaries and optimizes the myocardial area of virus exposure *(18)*. By crossclamping both the pulmonary artery and the aorta, the left ventricular end-diastolic pressure does not increase since blood return to the left ventricle is minimal. This allows perfusion of the virus at a relatively low downstream pressure, and the endocardium can be efficiently infected.

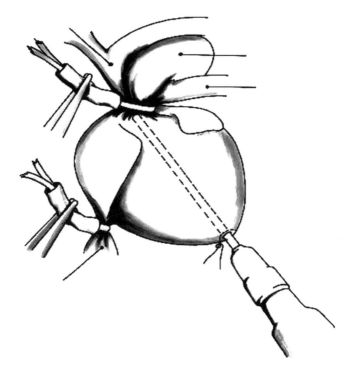

Fig. 7. Clamping of the aorta, pulmonary artery, and superior and inferior vena cava has been performed by tying the superior vena cava, pulmonary artery, and aorta with one 5-0 silk suture compressed with a small hollow tube. A similar compression is achieved for the inferior vena cava.

6. In a further refinement of this method, clamping of the aorta, pulmonary artery, and superior and inferior vena cava has been performed by tying the superior vena cava, pulmonary artery, and aorta with one 5-0 silk suture compressed with a small hollow tube. A similar compression is achieved for the inferior vena cava (**Fig. 7**). This totally isolates the heart, and injection in the aortic root enhances gene transfer as, evidenced by enhanced expression of transgene (**Fig. 8**).

3.8. Echo-Guided Albumin-Coated Approach

Using a novel approach, a group of investigators delivered adenovirus to rat myocardium by ultrasound-mediated microbubble destruction *(19)*. Microbubbles are formed in the following way:

1. Sonicate perfluoropropane-filled albumin containing 1% human serum albumin and 5% fructose along with 5 mL of perfluoropropane gas using a 20-kHz probe.
2. Discard the upper foam layer, freeze the lower suspension at −20°C overnight, and then lyophilize it for 28–30 h. Mean microbubble size and concentration are 3.0 μm and ~1 × 10^9 bubbles/mL, respectively.

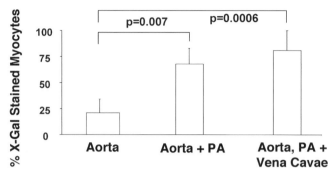

Fig. 8. Rat hearts were infected with adenoviruses E1-deleted carrying β-galactosi-dase at a concentration of 10^{10} pfu at 37°C using three different techniques of aortic clamping, crossclamping of the pulmonary artery (PA) and aorta, and clamping of aorta, pulmonary artery, and vena cava . The rats were euthanized and the cardiac cells isolated. The cells were then stained with X-gal overnight and counted. Hundred different areas were examined and the number of blue-staining cells quantified.

3. Prepare recombinant adenovirus containing the cDNA of interest or a reporter gene.
4. Add a 1-mL solution of adenovirus to a 1-mL microbubble suspension and mix for 2 h at 4°C. The mixture separates into two distinct layers. The upper layer consists of microbubbles with attached virus; the bottom layer, which contains unattached virus, is discarded. The concentration of microbubbles with attached adenovirus is usually 1×10^9 bubbles/mL.
5. Anesthetize rats as described earlier, and insert a 24-gauge catheter into the right jugular vein by cutdown.
6. Perform echocardiography with a transducer operating in second harmonic mode (transmit 1.3 MHz/receive 2.6 MHz) that has a mechanical index of 1.5 and a depth of 4 cm.
7. ECG-trigger the images to deliver a burst of 3 frames of ultrasound every 4–6 cardiac cycles. This burst eliminates all the microbubbles visible in the myocardium, and the triggering interval allows complete replenishment of the microbubbles before the next burst.
8. After infusion of microbubbles or control, tie off the jugular vein and close the skin.

The hearts of all rats that underwent ultrasound-mediated destruction of microbubbles containing virus showed nuclear staining with 5-bromo-4-chloro-3-indolyl-β-D-galactopyranoside substrate, indicating expression of the transgene. None of the control animals showed myocardial expression of the β-galactosidase transgene. By quantitative analysis, β-galactosidase activity was 10-fold higher in the treated group than in controls ($p < 0.0001$). This recently developed method is relatively noninvasive and may be easily translatable to human studies since microbubbles are routinely used in the clinic (*see* **Notes 1** and **2**).

4. Notes

1. Sarcoplasmic reticulum Ca^{2+} ATPase pump/phospholamban. The relative ratio of phospholamban/SERCA2a is an important determinant of sarcoplasmic reticulum function in cardiac myocytes *(1,5,20–22)*. Using adenoviral gene transfer, we have shown that increasing SERCA2a levels leads to an increase SR Ca^{2+} ATPase activity, a faster relaxation phase, an increase in the amount of Ca^{2+} released, and a decrease in diastolic Ca^{2+} *(1,5,20–22)*. An increased ratio of phospholamban/SERCA2a is an important characteristic of both human and experimental heart failure *(1,5,20–22)*. Both experimental and human heart failure are characterized by a prolonged calcium transient and impaired relaxation. Using adenoviral vectors, increasing levels of phospholamban relative to SERCA2a in isolated cardiac myocytes significantly altered intracellular calcium handling in the isolated cardiomyocytes by prolonging the relaxation phase of the Ca^{2+} transient, decreasing Ca^{2+} release, and increasing resting Ca^{2+} *(1,5,20–22)*. These results supported the hypothesis that altering the relative ratio of phospholamban to SERCA2a can account for the abnormalities in calcium handling observed in failing ventricular myocardium *(1,5,20–22)*. In our earlier studies, we showed that overexpressing SERCA2a can largely "rescue" the phenotype created by increasing the phospholamban to SERCA2a ratio *(1,5,20–22)*. This rescue effect by SERCA2a is especially encouraging since it suggests that restoring the normal phospholamban/SERCA2a ratio through somatic gene transfer could correct the abnormalities of calcium handling and contraction seen in failing hearts. In vivo, using methods of adenoviral gene transfer described earlier, we have shown that overexpressing phospholamban decreased developed pressure, increased the time course for relaxation, and significantly decreased-dP/dt *(1,5,20–22)*. These features reconstitute characteristic abnormalities of failing hearts in experimental models.

   More recently, we showed that overexpression of SERCA2a by gene transfer in failing human cardiomyocytes restored the function of these failing human hearts to normal. This was the first report of adenoviral gene transfer to human cardiomyocytes isolated from patients with end-stage heart failure. This study validated the premise that targeting SERCA2a by gene transfer may offer a new therapeutic modality in patients with heart failure *(1,5,20–22)*.

   We recently investigated whether increasing SERCA2a expression can improve ventricular function in a rat model of pressure-overload hypertrophy and failure. After 19–23 wk of banding, during the transition from compensated hypertrophy to heart failure, overexpression of SERCA2a restored both SERCA2a expression and ATPase activity to nonfailing levels. Furthermore, rats infected with Ad.SERCA2a had significant improvement in LVSP, +dP/dt, –dP/dt, and rate of isovolumic relaxation, normalizing them back to levels comparable to those of sham-operated rats. More recently, in the same animal model of heart failure, using E1 deleted adenovirus with the CMV promoter, we found that SERCA2a overexpression improved metabolic parameters and survival (at 28 d post gene transfer)*(1,5,20–22)*.

2. Future Directions. Although it is tempting to transfer the techniques used in rats directly to clinical applications, it is important to remember we are still very much in the early phases of a newly developing field. Although substantial progress has been made, before gene therapy can become a practical reality for cardiovascular disease, many hurdles need to be overcome. Newer vectors that provide prolonged, high-level, preferably cardiac-specific transgene expression, will need to be developed. Extensive in vivo testing of these will be necessary to clarify their effectiveness and safety. Although early human trials will probably rely on direct cardiac injection of vectors, minimally invasive delivery systems for either perfusion or injection of vectors will need to be developed to realize fully the potential of this therapeutic approach. However, the technologic promise will be empty if it is not founded on a solid understanding of disease pathogenesis, and this may represent the most challenging hurdle to gene therapy. Fortunately, it is also one of the most interesting aspects, and even the currently available gene transfer vectors can help in this regard. By using somatic gene transfer as an experimental tool, we can help elucidate the pathophysiology of cardiovascular diseases and explore the functional impact of modulating specific targets. Simultaneously, we can develop an appreciation of the power and limitations of specific vectors and delivery systems, as well as an understanding of how they interact with the host. All these elements will be necessary for somatic gene targeting to become a practical reality in cardiomyopathy.

References

1. Hajjar, R. J., del Monte, F., Matsui, T., and Rosenzweig, A. (2000) Prospects for gene therapy for heart failure. *Circ. Res.* **86,** 616–621.
2. Leiden, J. M. (2000) Human gene therapy: the good, the bad, and the ugly. *Circ. Res.* **86,** 923–925.
3. Graham, F. L. and Prevec, L. (1995) Methods for construction of adenovirus vectors. *Mol. Biotechnol.* **3,** 207–220.
4. Hajjar, R. J., Kang, J. X., Gwathmey, J. K., and Rosenzweig, A. (1997) Physiological effects of adenoviral gene transfer of sarcoplasmic reticulum calcium ATPase in isolated rat myocytes. *Circulation* **95,** 423–429.
5. Hajjar, R. J., Schmidt, U., Matsui, T., et al. (1998) Modulation of ventricular function through gene transfer in vivo. *Proc. Natl. Acad. Sci. USA* **95,** 5251–5256.
6. Hajjar, R. J., Muller, F. U., Schmitz, W., Schnabel, P., Bohm, M. (1998) Molecular aspects of adrenergic signal transduction in cardiac failure. *J. Mol. Med.* **76,** 747–755.
7. Kaji, E. H. and Leiden, J. M. (2001) Gene and stem cell therapies. *JAMA* **285,** 545–550.
8. Commander, H. (2000) Biotechnology industry responds to gene therapy death. *Nat. Med.* **6,**118.
9. Nyberg-Hoffman, C. and Aguilar-Cordova, E. (1999) Instability of adenoviral vectors during transport and its implication for clinical studies. *Nat. Med.* **5,** 955–957.

10. Kass, D. A., Hare, J. M., and Georgakopoulos, D. (1998) Murine cardiac function: a cautionary tail. *Circ. Res.* **82,** 519–522.
11. Barr, E., Carroll, J., Kalynych, A. M., et al. (1994) Efficient catheter-mediated gene transfer into the heart using replication-defective adenovirus. *Gene Ther.* **1,** 51–58.
12. Guzman, R. J., Lemarchand, P., Crystal, R. G., Epstein, S. E., and Finkel, T. (1993) Efficient gene transfer into myocardium by direct injection of adenovirus vectors. *Circ. Res.* **73,** 1202–1207.
13. Kirshenbaum, L. A., MacLennan. W., R., Mazur, W., French, B. A., Schneider, M. D. (1993) Highly efficient gene transfer into adult ventricular myocytes by recombinant adenovirus. *J. Clin. Invest.* **92,** 381–387.
14. Szatkowski, M. L., Westfall, M. V., Gomez, C. A., et al. (2001) In vivo acceleration of heart relaxation performance by parvalbumin gene delivery. *J. Clin. Invest.* **107,** 191–198.
15. Kawaguchi, H., Shin, W. S., Wang, Y., et al. (1997) In vivo gene transfection of human endothelial cell nitric oxide synthase in cardiomyocytes causes apoptosis-like cell death. Identification using Sendai virus-coated liposomes. *Circulation* **95,** 2441–2447.
16. Fromes Y, Salmon A, Wang X, et al. (1999) Gene delivery to the myocardium by intrapericardial injection. *Gene Ther.* **6,** 683–688.
17. Miyamoto, M. I., Guerrero, J. L., Schmidt, U., et al. (1998) Adenoviral gene transfer of SERCA2a improves LV function in aortic-banded rats in transition to heart failure. *Circulation* **98,** 736.
18. Donahue, J. K., Kikkawa, K., Thomas, A. D., Marban, E., and Lawrence, J. H. (1998) Acceleration of widespread adenoviral gene transfer to intact rabbit hearts by coronary perfusion with low calcium and serotonin. *Gene Ther.* **5,** 630–634.
19. Shohet, R. V., Chen, S., Zhou, Y. T., et al. (2000) Echocardiographic destruction of albumin microbubbles directs gene delivery to the myocardium. *Circulation* **101,** 2554–2556.
20. del Monte, F., Harding, S. E., Schmidt, U., et al. (1999) Restoration of contractile function in isolated cardiomyocytes from failing human hearts by gene transfer of SERCA2a. *Circulation* **100,** 2308–2311.
21. del Monte, F., Williams, E., Lebeche D., et al. (2001)Improvement in survival and cardiac metabolism following gene transfer of SERCA2a in a rat model of heart failure. *Circulation* **104,** 1424–1429.
22. Miyamoto, M. I., del Monte, F., Schmidt, U., et al. (2000) Adenoviral gene transfer of SERCA2a improves left ventricular function in aortic-banded rats in transition to heart failure. *Proc. Natl. Acad. Sci. USA* **97,**793–798.

15

Direct Gene Transfer
to the Adult Rodent Myocardium In Vivo

Michael L. Szatkowski, Margaret V. Westfall, and Joseph M. Metzger

1. Introduction

The objective of in vivo gene transfer is the expression of a specific gene product into a target cell population with the general intention of not altering other cell populations. Because of their ability to transduce nonreplicating cells, as well as their fairly large packaging capabilities, recombinant adenoviral vectors have frequently been utilized as a vector system. However, the immune response to recombinant adenoviral vectors utilized for gene transfer limits their clinical efficacy for certain applications. Adenovirus receptors are present on multiple cell populations, limiting the ability of systemic vector administration to target myocardial cells. Nonspecific gene transfer affects gene product expression in cell populations other than the population of interest. This alteration of nontargeted cell populations may interfere with cell homeostasis in multiple organs and may expand the immune response consequences. Thus, vector delivery techniques that optimize tissue specificity of delivery are advantageous.

The aim of this section is to describe an in vivo method for direct gene transfer to adult rodent myocardium. Attention is focused on techniques for optimizing the efficiency of vector delivery to the target population cells and the healthy recovery of the animal.

2. Materials
2.1. Environment

1. Desk with appropriate work area and chair.
2. Two or three lights with flexible optic necks.

From: *Methods in Molecular Biology, vol. 219: Cardiac Cell and Gene Transfer*
Edited by: J. M. Metzger © Humana Press Inc., Totowa, NJ

3. Heating pad.
4. Blue underpads (17 × 24 in.).
5. Gauze sponges (J & J, Steri-Pad [sterile], 4 × 4 in., 12 ply, #8519).
6. Q-tips.
7. Disposable surgical gloves.

2.2. Instruments and Solutions

1. Cautery.
2. Hair trimmers (Wahl ProSeries, #9550).
3. Scale and weight dishes (large enough to fit rodent).
4. Scalpel handle and blades (Bard-Parker Rib-Back carbon steel surgical blade, #10).
5. Rib spreaders.
6. Scissors.
7. Forceps.
8. Mosquito-tip hemostats.
9. Povo-iodine solution.
10. Ethyl alcohol 70%.
11. Sterile water.
12. Saline solution (bacteriostatic 0.9% sodium chloride; Abbott Labs, NDC#0074-1966-07).
13. Temperature probe (Barnant Thermocouple thermometer, Dual J-T-E-K, #600-1040).
14. Insulin syringe (B-D 1-mL Insulin syringe, U-100 28G1/2 needle, #309309).
15. Angiocath, 16-gauge.
16. 6-0 sutures (Ethicon 6-0 Ethilon black monofilament nylon with P-Prime needle, #697G.
17. 4-0 Sutures (Ethicon 4-0 silk with taper RB-1 needle, #K871H).
18. 25-Gauge needle (B-D PrecisionGlide, #305122).
19. Polyethylene tubing (B-D Clay Adams, Intramedic polyethylene tubing, ID 0.28 mm/OD 0.61 mm, B-D#427400).
20. 10-mL Syringe (B-D latex free, #309604).
21. Syringe automatic injector (Kent Scientific, #YA-12).

2.3. Anesthetics and Ventilator

1. Vaporizor (Matrx Medical, model MDS Matrx).
2. Isoflurane (Baxter AErrane 100 mL/btl, NDC#100190773-40).
3. Ventilator and oxygen source.
4. Isoflurane chamber.
5. Sodium pentobarbital, 30 mg/kg intraperitoneal.
6. Larygnoscope with #0 blade (Welch Allyn) and endotracheal tube (semirigid sterile tubing 1/16 in. inner diameter; electrical shrink tubing can be used).

3. Methods

3.1. Environment and Lighting

The environment is an essential consideration for the surgical procedure to facilitate the maintenance of homeostasis and limit morbidity and mortality. Aseptic environment and technique minimize the risk of infection. Animal body temperature should be monitored. Adequate space and lighting for the procedure limits surgeon fatigue and accommodates successful accomplishment of potentially difficult surgical manipulations.

1. The surgical table area should be cleaned. Wipe with alcohol-soaked gauze and allow to dry. Then place blue-pads to cover an adequate work area, overlapping the edges of the pads. Tape may be applied to overlapping pad edges, as well as to secure outer pad edges to the table area. This will be referred to as the work area and should be approx 2 × 3–4 ft. in dimensions.
2. Place the heating pad in the center of the work area, at the edge of the table, directly in front of the operator's chair, and cover with overlapping pads. This will be referred to as the surgical area and should be approx 1 × 2 ft. in dimensions. Turn on the heating pad to give adequate time to reach approximately body temperature.
3. Place two lights with flexible optic necks in the back of the surgical area, and adjust to illuminate the surgical area.

3.2. Anesthetics and Ventilator

1. To the left of the surgical area, place the ventilator with the tubing reaching to approximately where the rodent's head will rest.
2. If isoflurane is used, place a vaporizer and anesthetic induction chamber next to the ventilator and connect the appropriate tubing.
3. If a supplemental oxygen source is used, connect the tubing appropriately.

3.3. Instruments and Solutions

Place around the surgical area perimeter the following items at convenient locations:

1. Laryngoscope with endotracheal tube.
2. 500-mL Beaker with 70% ethyl alcohol to hold surgical instruments.
3. 500-mL Beaker with bleach for virus-contaminated waste.
4. 250-mL Beaker with 70% ethyl alcohol.
5. 250-mL Beaker with normal saline.
6. 250-mL Beaker with sterile water.
7. 250-mL Beaker to hold Q-tips.
8. Povo-iodine bottle.

9. 4 × 4 Gauze sponges.
10. 6.0 Suture.
11. 4.0 Suture.
12. Disposable surgical gloves.

Place the cautery at the perimeter of the surgical area.

3.4. Anesthesia and Ventilation

1. If pentobarbital is utilized, weigh the rodent and inject 30 mg/kg by the intraperitoneal route while properly restraining the animal. Allow approx 5–10 min for onset of anesthetic effect, and verify adequate depth of anesthesia.
2. If isoflurane is utilized, place rodent in breathing chamber, allow approx 5–10 min of breathing 5% isoflurane for onset of anesthetic effect, and verify depth of anesthesia.
3. When the animal is adequately anesthetized, perform direct laryngoscopy to visualize the vocal cords, and intubate the trachea with an appropriate diameter endotracheal tube of adequate length (0.06 × 3.5–4.0 in.) (*see* **Notes 1** and **2**) Connect the endotracheal tube to the ventilator circuit and observe for appropriate chest wall excursion. Verify that the gas source is correctly connected to the ventilator. Proper endotracheal tube placement is essential; if you are uncertain, remove the tube and repeat placement with direct laryngoscopy.

3.5. Surgical Preparation

1. Once proper endotracheal tube placement is verified by adequate chest wall excursion and pink tongue coloration, place the rodent on its right side and shave the area of the left chest from sternum to back, and from top of rib cage to bottom of rib cage (*see* **Notes 3**).
2. Remove residual hair, and then swab with povo-iodine-soaked gauze followed by alcohol-swabbed gauze.
3. Repeat the above swab sequence, and then dry with gauze.

3.6. Surgical Procedure

1. Identify the left third intercostal space and create a 2–3-cm-long skin incision with the scalpel. Utilize the cautery or hemostats to minimize bleeding.
2. Be careful to create a straight incision through the skin and intercostal muscles, which will facilitate approximation of tissue edges during suturing (*see* **Note 4**).
3. Subsequent layers of intercostal muscle are then blunt-dissected with mosquito-tipped hemostats. Once the chest wall opening is initiated, scissors can be used to lengthen the intercostal opening to 2–3-cm (*see* **Note 5**).
4. Once the intercostal opening has been established, wean the isoflurane from 5% to 1–2%. Next place the rib cage spreaders to allow adequate access to the thorax

through the third intercostal space. Sterile Q-tips or gauze are useful to clear blood from the thoracic space for improved visualization (*see* **Note 6**).

5. After ensuring adequate access to the heart, gently grasp the pericardium with forceps and mosquito hemostats. Avoid grasping the myocardium or coronary arteries. Expand the pericardial opening with the mosquito hemostats by blunt dissection, being careful not to injure the myocardium or coronary arteries.

6. With sterile Q-tips, properly position the heart with the apex directed upward toward the thoracotomy opening, and use needle holders to place a 6-0 suture at the apex. Avoid blood vessels during suture placement, with attention to placement of the suture superficially. Cut the suture to a total length of several centimeters, and hold the ends together with a hemostat. The purpose of this suture is to assist with positioning of the heart during the vector injection. If the suture is placed deep or too superficial, myocardial damage may occur (*see* **Note 7**).

3.7. Vector Injection

The aim of the vector injection is to achieve a wide area of distribution for gene expression with minimal myocardial trauma. Take strict care to avoid accidental contamination of the workplace with the viral vector, and wear appropriate protective apparel.

1. Draw up the desired amount of vector into a sterile tuberculin syringe. Carefully remove excess air bubbles by tapping the syringe while directing the needle tip upright. Be careful to prevent contamination of the work area while removing air bubbles. Only the vector fluid should occupy the space between the plunger and the tip of the needle (*see* **Note 8**).

2. Use the hemostats to grasp the suture at the apex of the heart and to position the heart for the vector injection. Identify the left anterior descending coronary artery and position this area of the heart in the opening of the third intercostal space. Sterile Q-tips may facilitate proper positioning.

3. Identify a potential myocardial injection tract to the anatomic left of the left anterior descending coronary artery extending from the apex to the base of the left ventricle. Advance the vector-containing needle into this tract as superficially as feasible while remaining within the myocardium. Be careful to avoid blood vessels or applying excess traction on the suture at the apex of the heart.

4. Simultaneously slowly withdraw the syringe needle while slowly advancing the syringe plunger. The goal is to deliver the vector along the entire needle tract as the needle is withdrawn. Larger areas of distribution may be achieved by multiple injections to expand the area of vector delivery.

5. During the injection process, if the needle tract is sufficiently superficial, a "blanching" or spread of the fluid may be visualized extending laterally from the tract along the left anterior descending artery.

6. When the needle is removed at the end of the injection, inspect the myocardial surface for areas of bleeding. Gentle application of pressure with a Q-tip may be necessary to control bleeding, especially if the coronary artery is affected.

3.8. Thoracotomy Closure

1. After the injection is completed, observe the heart for resolution of any bradycardia or blanching that may have occurred. Once the heart appears to be functioning appropriately, use sterile Q-tips to reposition the heart gently to its original position.
2. Remove the rib spreaders, and use a 4-0 suture needle with needle holders to close the intercostal muscle between the third and fourth ribs, starting from the top of the incision area, with a running suture. Place a 16-gauge angiocath between the ribs as they are sutured to act as a chest tube, and connect the catheter to a low suction source.
3. Next proceed to suture the inner muscle layer with a running 4.0 suture, while making sure the chest tube remains in proper position. Repeat the suturing of the outer muscle layer. Finally, approximate the skin edges with a running 4.0 suture.
4. Apply Vaseline to the incision area to minimize air leak potential. Time the rapid removal of the chest tube with the end of peak inflation/inhalation on the ventilator. Spread Vaseline to cover the exit site of the chest tube.

3.9. Removal from Ventilator

1. Wean the isoflurane to 0% and continue with mechanical ventilation while the anesthetic wears off. Observe for spontaneous respirations, and when spontaneous respirations appear regular in frequency and adequate in effort, disconnect the endotracheal tube from the ventilator.
2. If apnea or respiratory distress occurs, reinitiate mechanical ventilation and observe again for adequate respiratory effort before commencing another trial off the ventilator.
3. Continue to observe for adequate respiratory effort. When the rodent appears to be waking up or appears agitated by the breathing tube, remove the breathing tube. Observe for adequate respirations and pink tongue coloration.
4. Place the rodent on a clean cloth in a clean rodent recovery box and continue to observe for adequate respiratory effort. When the anesthetic wears off and the rodent is walking around, remove the cloth and make sure water and food pellets are easily accessible in the rodent box.

3.10. Convalescence

1. Place prophylactic antibiotics in the water bottles for a minimum of 3 d during recovery. Ensure an adequate water and food supply throughout the recovery period (*see* **Notes 9–12**).
2. Observe daily for adequate activity level and appearance of wound site. By using water bottles as the water source, fluid intake can be estimated by daily changes in water levels.

3. Recover rodents separately in individual boxes to eliminate the possibility of injury inflicted by other rodents.

3.11. Hemodynamic Assessment

1. At the appropriate interval after vector injection, to allow for gene expression, anesthetize and mechanically ventilate the rodent as described previously. Weigh the animal before proceeding. Set up and calibrate the pressure and/or conductance catheter and data acquisition equipment (e.g., Millar catheter, Millar Instruments, Houston TX) prior to anesthetizing the rodent. Monitor and maintain normal body temperature throughout the procedure.
2. Shave the area of the left ventral thorax from just below the left subcostal region to the neck, extending to the right of the sternum. Also shave the supracostal area above the jugular vein. Remove loose hair and prepare the skin with povo-iodine and alcohol and dry. Verify adequate anesthesia. (If using isoflurane, adjust to 5% for the duration of incision and thoracotomy.)
3. Incise the skin just left of the sternum and along the left sixth intercostal space anteriorly. Use the cautery to ensure hemostasis during incision and thoracotomy. Use scissors to incise the left sixth intercostal space, and extend the thoracotomy along the left sternal border. Avoid damaging blood vessels in the vicinity of the second and third intercostal space.
4. Decrease the isoflurane from 5% to approx 1.5–2% and adjust to ensure adequate anesthesia. Observe the myocardial contractility response to lower isoflurane levels, and adjust isoflurane levels sooner if myocardial depression is suspected (tongue less pink, extremities poorly perfused, and so on).
5. Incise the skin above the right jugular vein and with mosquito-tipped hemostats isolate the jugular vein by blunt dissection. Cannulate the jugular vein with a 25-gauge needle connected by polyethylene tubing to a 10-mL syringe containing 10% serum albumin. Infuse 200 µL/kg/min to maintain adequate intravascular hydration.
6. Open the thoracic cavity with rib spreaders to access the heart. Use forceps and hemostats to carefully open the pericardial sac. Direct the apex of the heart with saline-soaked Q-tips to place a 6-0 suture superficially at the apex of the heart.
7. Gently move the heart apex with the 6-0 suture and Q-tips to allow blunt dissection of the inferior vena cava (IVC) with hemostats, and place a suture or umbilical tape loosely around the IVC. Position both ends of the suture outside the thoracic cavity.
8. Elevate the apex of the heart with gentle tension on the 6-0 suture while inserting a 25-gauge needle into the left ventricle. Immediately upon removal of the needle, carefully insert an appropriately sized pressure catheter through the needle tract. Gently lower the heart back into the thoracic cavity. Adjust the position of the catheter to optimize the pressure and/or conductance signal obtained on the data acquisition system.
9. Acquire appropriate data according to established protocol. If conductance signals are acquired, transient IVC occlusion data can be obtained for subsequent

calibration by briefly pulling gently on the IVC suture to impede blood return to the heart. At the end of the experimental protocol, 20% hypertonic saline can be injected into the jugular vein to obtain parallel conductance parameters.

10. At the end of the experimental protocol, remove the left ventricular catheter and inject 1000 U/kg heparin ip. Allow sufficient time for heparinization, and then aspirate blood into a syringe. (If you are using a conductance catheter, this blood may be used to calibrate the conductance signal of wells of known volume.) Quickly remove the heart and place in appropriate physiologic solution. Weigh and process the heart to obtain desired specimen samples. Euthanize and properly dispose of the rodent.

4. Notes

1. Q-tips can facilitate visualization of the vocal cords during direct laryngoscopy by clearing excess fluids from interfering with the view.
2. Repeat isoflurane induction may be necessary when multiple intubation attempts are required.
3. Placing the rodent supine may facilitate the intubation procedure.
4. While performing the thoracotomy, cauterizing the larger blood vessels in the area of the third intercostal space can minimize bleeding.
5. When using the mosquito-tipped hemostats to initially enter the thorax in the third intercostal space, be careful to avoid excessive penetration into the cavity, which may result in the hemostats causing damage to the heart or blood vessels.
6. Adjust the isoflurane during the procedure to ensure adequate anesthesia while avoiding excessive levels, which can result in cardiovascular side effects such as bradycardia and decreased inotropy.
7. Saline-soaked gauze can be placed over the thoracotomy to minimize fluid evaporative losses if the thoracotomy is left open for a short period.
8. Aspirate sterile water into a tuberculin syringe and manipulate the plunger to allow for a smooth injection without sudden excess movements of the plunger during injection.
9. Use of clean rodent boxes with clean bedding for recovery may help to minimize the risk of wound infection during recovery.
10. Place food pellets on the rodent bedding to ease access to nourishment during recovery.
11. Use brown water bottles for light-sensitive antibiotics to impede inactivation of the antibiotic.
12. Avoid water bottles that appear prone to leaking.

16

Adenovirus-Mediated Gene Transfer to Cardiac Myocytes In Vivo Using Catheter-Based Procedures

Damien Logeart and Jean-Jacques Mercadier

1. Introduction

It is now expected that gene transfer to somatic cells will offer, in the future, a new therapeutic approach to correct various pathogenic processes, including those responsible for common acquired or degenerative diseases such as heart failure. Indeed, a number of recent studies have shown that adenovirus-mediated gene transfer to cardiac myocytes can improve cardiac contractility *(1–4)*. However, a number of methodologic obstacles still need to be overcome regarding, for instance, vector safety and infection efficiency, cardiac restriction and regulation of transgene expression, and, especially in terms of myocardial gene therapy, vector delivery procedures. Indeed, gene transfer to the myocardium should be as diffuse and homogeneous as possible, especially in heart failure therapy.

Various vector delivery methods have been put forward with variable results. Direct transpericardial or transendocardial injection into the ventricular wall *(5–8)* resulted in gene transfer restricted to the injection sites. Injection into the pericardial sac *(9,10)* improved the efficiency and distribution of gene expression, but experiments were done mainly in newborn animals. Efficient gene transfer to cardiac myocytes using intracoronary delivery has also been obtained, but using surgical procedures poorly compatible with the clinical setting, such as aortic clamping *(11,12)*, or ex vivo procedures with transient cardioplegic arrest *(13)*, or coronary recirculation of vectors *(14)*.

Using isolated perfused hearts, we and others have shown that coronary pretreatment with agents such as serotonin, bradykinin *(13)*, and histamine *(15)*

From: *Methods in Molecular Biology, vol. 219: Cardiac Cell and Gene Transfer*
Edited by: J. M. Metzger © Humana Press Inc., Totowa, NJ

increases gene transfer to explanted hearts. In addition, we found that, even when the endothelial barrier permeability has been increased by histamine pretreatment, a brief interruption of adenovirus-containing coronary flow is mandatory for significant gene transfer to cardiac myocytes *(15)*. This prompted us to develop a percutaneous catheter-based approach and selective intracoronary artery delivery in adult rabbits, which allowed us to test various procedures to optimize adenovirus-mediated gene transfer efficiency. The present chapter summarizes the various methodologies we used as well as their relative efficiencies.

2. Materials

2.1. Adenoviruses

Ad.CMV.luc and Ad.CMV.lacZ are recombinant, replication-defective adenoviruses derived from human adenovirus type 5. They contain, respectively, a luciferase gene or a nuclear-targeted β-galactosidase gene, driven by the cytomegalovirus (CMV) promoter. Titers of virus stocks are determined by plaque titration on the 293 cell line as described elsewhere *(16)* and are expressed as plaque-forming units (pfu). Virus stocks are aliquoted in small volumes and stored in phosphate-buffered saline (PBS) with 10% glycerol at –80°C until use. To allow comparison between the various delivery procedures, it is important that all experiments be carried out using aliquots of the same virus stock.

2.2. Animals

Animals used are adult New Zealand rabbits weighing 3.5–4 kg, i.e., a size compatible with percutaneous selective coronary catheterism. Rabbits are homed in single cages and treated in accordance with the local recommendations for Laboratory Animal Care. Because of adenovirus use, specific rooms are required for homing, as for experimental procedures, in accordance with national regulations.

2.3. Surgical Materials

A typical surgical box should contain the following:

1. Scalpel.
2. Blunt scissors for dissection.
3. Hemostatic forceps.
4. Microdissection and tissue forceps.
5. Microscissors for arteriotomy.
6. Yarns for skin suture and vessel ligation.
7. Compresses.

2.4. Catheters

For catheterization of the venous coronary sinus, the following equipment is needed:

1. A Judkins Right 4 coronary catheter (JR4, Cordis) is cut to shorten its length to 20 cm.
2. A 19-gauge needle is inserted into the proximal cut tip. The shape of the JR4 distal tip can be accentuated to obtain a 90° angle using boiling water steam if necessary.
3. A standard 200-cm-long and 0.014-in. diameter wire (Guidant ACS, Temecula, CA) is used to allow the exchange of the JR4-derived catheter by a 75-cm 5-F Swan-Ganz catheter (Baxter, Irvine, CA).

For coronary artery catheterization, two types of catheters are used:

1. The JR4-derived catheter previously described results in its occlusive engagement in the left coronary artery and is too large for the right coronary artery. Therefore, for a nonocclusive catheterization of both right and left coronary arteries, a 3-F infusion catheter (Cook, Denmark) is used, and the distal tip is hand-modified using steam to obtain a 1-cm-long tip exhibiting a 70° angle with the main axis of the catheter.
2. The proximal tip is also cut to shorten its length to 20 cm, and, last, a 23-gauge needle is introduced into it.
3. Catheters are carefully rinsed with sterilized water and cleaned after each procedure.

2.5. Monitoring and Fluoroscopic System

1. Electrocardiographic monitoring is obtained with three electrodes placed on well-shaved skin: one on the left anterior paw, the second on the right anterior paw, and the third on the right side of the thorax.
2. The PowerLab system (ADinstruments) allows monitoring of the electrocardiogram (ECG) and arterial pressure during the whole procedure.
3. Finally, a fluoroscopic system allowing an anteroposterior view is required.

3. Methods

3.1. Carotid and Jugular Catheterization

1. First tranquilize the rabbit is with acepromazine (20 mg im) (*see* **Note 1**).
2. Approximately 20 min later, perfuse a large superficial vein of the ear with a 14-gauge needle, and sedate the animal with pentobarbital (10 mg/kg iv), which is infused very slowly over 10 min in order to avoid respiratory failure and the use of mechanical ventilation. A relatively slight but sufficient sedation is obtained over 1–2 h.
3. Carefully shave the front of the neck, and place the rabbit on its back.

4. Administer local anesthesia of the neck skin with 10 mL of lidocaine 1% and a 25-gauge needle.
5. Make a 3–4-cm-long vertical incision in the middle of the neck, and cut the underlying layer through the same lane.
6. Carefully dissect tissues to expose the right carotid artery and jugular vein.
7. Carefully dissect, isolate, and slightly hold out the jugular vein with two nylon yarns.
8. Ligate the jugular vein, and make a small incision just below.
9. Introduce a 6-F sheath (Terumo) over 3–4 cm, and fix with a yarn around the vein.
10. Rinse this sheath with saline and use it to inject heparin (200 U/kg) and lidocaine (1 mg/kg).
11. Dissect the right carotid artery and also slightly hold it with two nylon yarns rounding the artery.
12. Ligate the carotid artery at its distal part.
13. Make a small incision just below the ligature while blood flow is stopped upstream by holding the artery with the second yarn.
14. Immediately introduce a 4-F sheath (Terumo) into the carotid artery over 3–4 cm.
15. Rinse the sheath with saline.

3.2. Coronary Catheterization

1. Maintain the rabbit on its back, and perform selective catheterization of the coronary venous sinus and coronary artery under fluoroscopic guidance.
2. First catheterize the coronary venous sinus with the 4-F JR4 derived-catheter (Cordis), and check its appropriate position by injecting 1–2 mL of contrast agent Hexabrix(r) (Guerbet, France) diluted with sterile water (v/v) under fluoroscopy.
3. Introduce the 0.014-in. wide wire into the catheter, and position its end 3 cm downstream of the tip of the catheter.
4. Remove the catheter while the wire is carefully maintained in the coronary sinus under fluoroscopy.
5. Introduce the 4-F Swan-Ganz catheter over the wire and advance it into the coronary sinus under fluoroscopic guidance. The wire can be left in the Swan-Ganz catheter, which is then infused through a shut-off.
6. Carefully adjust the position of the catheter in order to place its distal tip and balloon exactly in the ostium of the coronary venous sinus.
7. Fill the balloon with 0.5 mL of air to occlude the coronary sinus, and infuse 1 mL of diluted contrast agent downstream, i.e., against the venous flow, under fluoroscopy. When the coronary sinus is actually occluded, the contrast agent is retained in the sinus upstream of the balloon and does not wash out (**Fig. 1A**).
8. Catheterize the selective coronary artery with either the 3-F coronary catheter using the hand-made tip or the 4-F JR4-derived coronary catheter as described above (*see* **Note 2**), which is placed into the left circumflex (*see* **Note 3**) or right coronary artery under fluoroscopic guidance. Nonocclusive engagement of the catheter into the coronary artery is ensured by both spontaneous backflow of blood out of the catheter and the absence of any ECG change.

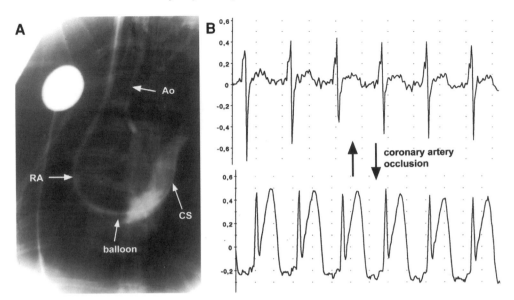

Fig. 1. (**A**) Chest radiogram illustrating the percutaneous catheter-mediated procedure: a catheter with a hand-made tip is placed in the ostium of the left coronary artery via the carotid artery, and a fluid-filled balloon catheter is placed in the coronary venous sinus via the jugular vein and checked by Hexabrix(r) retroinfusion. Ao, aorta; RA, right atrium; CS, coronary venous sinus. (**B**) Continuous electrocardiographic monitoring during adenovirus delivery: a transient ST-segment elevation was consistently observed during coronary artery occlusion.

9. Check the position of the catheter by injecting 1 mL of diluted Hexabrix(r) under fluoroscopy. Occlusive engagement results in an ECG change (ST-segment elevation) approx 15 s following coronary artery occlusion (**Fig. 1B**).

3.3. Adenoviruses Delivery

1. Thaw the adenovirus-containing aliquot just before the in vivo delivery.
2. Dilute the aliquot with 500 µL of saline buffer and draw up into a 1-mL glass syringe. Carefully chase out any air bubbles.
3. When the appropriate catheter position into the coronary artery has been carefully registered several times under fluoroscopy with contrast agent injection as described above, disengage the catheter from the coronary artery to avoid unintended occlusion.
4. Adjust the adenovirus-containing syringe to the catheter, which is then promptly replaced into the coronary artery under fluoroscopy without additional contrast injection, and deliver the adenoviruses into the coronary artery.
5. Various adenovirus delivery procedures can be used:

a. Vector delivery as a 5–10-s bolus after ensuring the nonocclusive engagement of the catheter into the coronary artery (spontaneous backflow of blood and no electrocardiographic change).

b. Coronary flow interruption for 30–60 s after occlusive engagement of the catheter into the coronary artery and downstream vector delivery. (In our experience, efficient adenovirus-mediated gene transfer required such a transient artery occlusion and delivery downstream; **Fig. 2**.) Occlusive engagement into the main stem of left coronary artery for more than 30 s results in frequent severe arrhythmia.

c. Vector delivery 5 min after pharmacologic pretreatment of the coronary vessels in order to increase vessel permeability; such a pretreatment consists of the intracoronary delivery of 2 mL of saline containing 10^{-5} M histamine (Sigma), or 10^{-5} M bradykinin (Sigma), or 10^{-5} M serotonin (Sigma), or 2.4 μg of vascular endothelial growth factor (VEGF)165 (a gift from Dr. J. Plouet, Toulouse, France) for 1 min.

d. Pressure increase in the coronary artery by infusion of a 3-mL vector-containing bolus for 4–8 s.

e. Combined catheter-mediated occlusion of the arterial side and retroinfusion of saline buffer upstream of the occlusive balloon into the coronary venous sinus in order to increase pressure into postcapillary veinules, which are probably the main site for adenovirus transfer out of vessels. The saline buffer infusion into the coronary venous sinus should start 5–10 s before delivery of the adenovirus into the coronary artery, and it requires around 3–4 mL for 60 s to achieve a pressure increase such as 60 mmHg.

6. **Figure 2** shows the transfer efficiency results we obtained with these various procedures. In our experience, the best results were obtained with procedure.

7. At the end of adenovirus delivery, carefully remove catheters and sheaths, and ligate the vessels.

8. After verifying the absence of any bleeding, disinfect and suture the cervical incision. Allow the rabbit to recover in the cage only when it is fully awakened.

3.4. Gene Transfer Efficiency

1. Seventy-two hours after virus injection, study the gene transfer efficiency.

2. Perfuse an ear vein again with a 14-gauge catheter, heparinize the rabbit (200 U/kg), and deeply anesthetize it with a pentobarbital infusion.

3. Before respiratory failure, incise the skin and quickly perform a sternotomy using large scissors.

4. Locate the beating heart and aorta through the sternum incision, and open the pericardium with scissors.

5. Cut the aortic root and the stem of the pulmonary artery 1 cm above the heart, and also cut the pulmonary veins behind the heart.

6. Immediately immerse the heart into ice-cold PBS, where the last spontaneous cardiac contractions flush the blood out of the ventricular cavities.

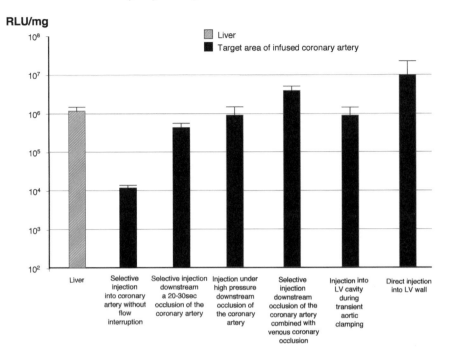

Fig. 2. Comparison of delivery procedures. The figure shows luciferase activity(relative light units [RLU]) in the liver and in the target region of the infused circumflex coronary artery 3 d after adenovirus delivery. The figure also shows a comparison with surgery-based procedures. LV, left ventricle.

7. Adjust a 50-mL ice-cold PBS-containing syringe to the aortic root and carefully fixate it with yarn to wash the myocardium by coronary perfusion with PBS (around 1 mL/s).
8. After any blood has been totally chased out, cut the right and left ventricles and separate them from the atria.
9. Dissect, blot dry, freeze in liquid nitrogen, and store at –80°C until analysis the right ventricular wall, left ventricular septum, and anterior and inferolateral walls.
10. Also sample, wash, freeze, and store at –80°C, pieces of liver (*see* **Note 4**), lung, and kidney as controls for gene transfer.
11. To assess luciferase gene transfer efficiency, pulverize pieces of ventricles, liver, lung, and kidney in liquid nitrogen and incubate them on ice with 2 vol of 1X cell culture lysis reagent (Promega).
12. Centrifuge the resulting homogenates at 10,000g for 2 min.
13. Add the luciferase assay reagent containing D-luciferin (Promega) to cleared supernatants, and measure peak light emission at 25°C for 10 s using a luminometer (Berthold Bioluminat 9501, Wildbad, Germany).

14. Subtract background values (lysis reagent only) from total light units per sample.
15. Determine total protein content from an aliquot for each sample supernatant (DC Protein Assay, Bio-Rad), and express luciferase activity as relative light units (RLU)/mg protein. As the liver is the peripheral organ that traps most of the circulating virus, consistently leading to RLU values around 1×10^6 RLU/mg of protein ($1.1 \pm 0.1 \times 10^6$ RLU/mg of protein) whatever the procedure performed, it is used as the standard to which each sample is compared.
16. LacZ gene expression is determined by histochemical staining for β-galactosidase activity in heart sections.
17. After washing by perfusing the aortic root with 50 mL of ice-cold PBS, fix the heart by perfusing with 50 mL of 0.5% glutaraldehyde/1% formaldehyde-containing PBS and then with 50 mL of X-Gal-containing buffer (K-ferrocyanide 4 mM, K-ferricyanide 4 mM, MgCl$_2$ 2 mM, X-Gal 0.4 mg/mL, 0.02% NP40 in PBS) via the aortic root.
18. Cut the heart into 2–3-mm transverse sections.
19. Immerse the sections in the X-Gal solution for 3–4 h, rinse, embed in paraffin, and counterstain with hematoxylin and eosin.
20. Determine the percentage of myocytes positive for β-galactosidase staining in each ventricular segment by examining 10 randomly selected high-power microscope fields, i.e., 300–400 myocytes.
21. To assess catheterization procedure-mediated or adenovirus-mediated cardiac damage, check for the presence of ventricular necrosis by microscopic examination of the heart sections.

4. Notes

1. The time following acepromazine injection is usefully used to prepare the various pharmacologic agents and materials, such as: (1) the 22-gauge venous catheter and pentobarbital; (2) the sodium heparin-containing 10-mL syringe; (3) the 1% lidocaine-containing 10-mL syringe and 25-gauge needle; (4) five 4–5-cm-long pieces of silk yarn; (5) surgical materials including compresses; (6) the 4-F and 6-F sheaths; and (7) catheters.
2. Occlusion of the main stem of left coronary artery with the 4-F catheter results in severe ventricular arrhythmia 30–60 s later. Distal occlusion into the circumflex branch using distal engagement with the 3-F catheter is usually better tolerated without arrhythmia for as long as 1 or 2 min.
3. The coronary arteries of an adult New Zealand rabbit consist of a dominant left coronary artery, which consists of a short main stem, a small left anterior descending artery, and a large circumflex artery, which is the main coronary artery branch. Selective catheterization of the left coronary artery results in nearly constant engagement into the circumflex branch, whereas selective engagement in the left anterior descending branch is difficult. Using a 4-F catheter, engagement into the circumflex artery is often occlusive from the main stem. Using a 3-F catheter, nonocclusive engagement of the circumflex artery can be performed.

4. The liver traps most of the circulating virus, consistently leading to a constant level of transgene expression whatever the delivery procedure used. Thus the level of transgene expression into the liver is used as the standard with which each sample of myocardium or other organ is compared.

References

1. Miyamoto, M. I., del Monte, F., Schmidt, U., et al. (2000) Adenoviral gene transfer of SERCA2a improves left-ventricular function in aortic-banded rats in transition to heart failure. *Proc. Natl. Acad. Sci. USA* **97,** 793–798.

2. Shah, A. S., Lilly, E., Kypson, A. P., et al. (2000) Intracoronary adenovirus-mediated delivery and overexpression of the β2-adrenergic receptor in the heart. *Circulation* **101,** 408–414.

3. Schmidt, U., del Monte, F., Miyamoto, M. I., et al. (2000). Restoration of diastolic function in senescent rat hearts through adenoviral gene transfer of sarcoplasmic reticulum Ca^{2+}-ATPase. *Circulation* **101,** 790–796.

4. Weig, H. J., Laugwitz, K. L., Moretti, A., et al. (2000) Enhanced cardiac contractility after gene transfer of V2 vasopressin receptors in vivo by ultrasound-guided injection or transcoronary delivery. *Circulation* **101,** 1578–1585.

5. Guzman, R. J., Lemarchand, P., Crystal, R. G., Epstein, S. E., Finkel, T. (1993) Efficient gene transfer into myocardium by direct injection of adenovirus vectors. *Circ. Res.* **73,** 1202–1207.

6. French, B. A., Mazur, W., Geske, R. S., Boll, R. (1994) Direct in vivo gene transfer into myocardium using replicant-deficient adenoviral vectors. *Circulation* **90,** 2414–2424.

7. Leor, J., Quinones, M. J., Patterson, M., Kedes, L., Kloner, R. A. (1996) Adenovirus-mediated gene transfer into infarcted myocardium: feasibility, timing and location of expression. *J. Mol. Cell. Cardiol.* **28,** 2057–2067.

8. Lamping, K. G., Rios, C. D. D., Chun, J. A., Ooboshi, H., Davidson, B. L., Heistad, D. D. (1997) Intrapericardial administration of adenovirus for gene transfer. *Am. J. Physiol.* **272,** H310–H317.

9. Fromes, Y., Salmon, A., Wang, A., et al. (1999) Gene delivery to the myocardium by intrapericardial injection. *Gene. Ther.* **6,** 683–688.

10. Hajjar, R. J., Schmidt, U., Matsui, T., et al. (1998) Modulation of ventricular function through gene transfer in vivo. *Proc. Natl. Acad. Sci. USA* **95,** 5251–5256.

11. Maurice, J. P., Hata, J. A., Shah, J. A., et al. (1999) Enhancement of cardiac function after adenoviral-mediated in vivo intracoronary β2-adrenergic receptor gene delivery. *J. Clin. Invest.* **104,** 21–29.

12. Kypson, A. P., Hendrickson, S. C., Wilson, K., et al. (1999) Adenovirus-mediated gene transfer of the $β_2$-adrenergic receptor to donor hearts enhances cardiac function. *Gene Ther.* **6,** 1298–1304.

13. Donahue, J. K., Kikkawa, K., Thomas, A. D., Marban, E., Lawrence, J. H. (1998) Acceleration of widespread adenoviral gene transfer to intact rabbit hearts by coronary perfusion with low calcium and serotonin. *Gene Ther.* **5,** 630–634.

14. Logeart, D., Hatem, S. N., Rücker-Martin, C., et al. (2000) Highly efficient adenovirus-mediated gene transfer to the myocardium following single-pass coronary delivery. *Hum. Gene Ther.* **11,** 1015–1022.

15. Logeart, D., Hatem, S. N., Heimburger, M., Le Roux, A., Michel, J. B., and Mercadier, J. J. (2001) How to optimise in vivo gene transfer to cardiac myocytes: mechanical or pharmacological procedures? *Hum. Gene Ther.* **12,** 1601–1610.

16. Graham, F. L., Smiley, J., Russell, W. C., and Nairn, R. (1977) Characteristics of a human cell line transformed by DNA from human adenovirus type 5. *J. Gen. Virol.* **36,** 59–74.

17

Coronary Perfusion Cocktails
for In Vivo Gene Transfer

Stephan E. Lehnart and J. Kevin Donahue

1. Introduction

Gene therapy has tremendous potential as a treatment option for heart disease. Before successful implementation of gene transfer strategies, however, several problems need to be addressed. These include: increased efficiency and homogeneity of delivery to cardiac myocytes; dosage minimization to limit untoward effects; delivery localization to avoid nonspecific gene transfer; and simplification of delivery techniques to broaden applicability of the intervention. To address the problem of efficient and homogeneous delivery, we studied adenovirus behavior in a variety of in vivo, ex vivo, and in vitro models *(1–3)*. We found that the adenovirus behavior was characterized by a diffusional component and a receptor-ligand interaction. The percentage of cells infected by the vector varied with coronary flow rate, virus contact time, and virus concentration. A significant improvement in gene transfer efficiency was noted with modulation of microvascular permeability. The focus of this chapter is on improving in vivo delivery by increasing microvascular permeability.

A variety of inflammatory mediators and growth factors can increase microvascular permeability. Serotonin, bradykinin, histamine, substance P, and vascular endothelial growth factor (VEGF) are a few examples of the agents that have proved to increase permeability at the capillary or postcapillary venular level. The intracellular mechanism for this effect appears to be similar for all of these compounds. Receptor binding by the permeability factor initiates a cascade of reactions **(Fig. 1)**, including activation of phospholipase Cγ, protein kinase Cα, constitutive nitric oxide synthase, guanylate cyclase, and cyclic GMP-dependent protein kinases *(4–8)*. Since the permeability signaling

From: *Methods in Molecular Biology, vol. 219: Cardiac Cell and Gene Transfer*
Edited by: J. M. Metzger © Humana Press Inc., Totowa, NJ

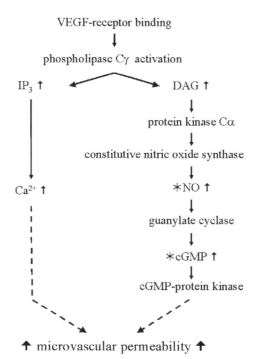

Fig 1. Diagram of the intracellular pathways responsible for vascular endothelial growth factor (VEGF)-mediated increases in vascular permeability. Many of the steps shown in this diagram for VEGF have also been demonstrated for substance P, serotonin, histamine, and bradykinin. ✳ denotes specific points of the pathway that have been modulated to increase permeability to adenoviral vectors: nitric oxide (NO) donors like nitroglycerin, cyclic guanosine monophosphate (cGMP) donors like 8-Br-cGMP, slowing of cGMP breakdown by phosphodiesterase 5 inhibition with sildenafil. DAG, diacylglycerol. (Modified from **ref. 3**.)

cascade includes nitric oxide and cyclic GMP, exposure to nitric oxide donors or cyclic GMP analogs potentiates the effect of the permeability factors. Further enhancement of microvascular permeability can be achieved by exposure to phosphodiesterase V inhibitors, slowing the breakdown of cyclic GMP *(3)*.

In our experience, the best tolerated and most efficient increase in permeability occurs with sildenafil pretreatment followed by VEGF and nitroglycerin exposure *(9)*. Unfortunately, VEGF is also the most expensive agent of those listed above. Substance P has the fastest onset of action, but toxicity limits its utility. Relative to VEGF or substance P, longer exposures to serotonin, histamine, and bradykinin are required to achieve similar levels of permeability.

2. Materials

All solutions are prepared in double-distilled water and filter-sterilized with 0.22-μm membrane filters.

1. Crystalloid, HEPES-buffered Krebs' solution is prepared within 1 d of the experiment by dilution of a 10X Krebs' stock solution and addition of 2.7 g/L glucose and 1 mL of 1 M CaCl$_2$ stock solution. The pH is adjusted to 7.4 using 10 N NaOH. The solution is kept refrigerated until use. The 10X stock solution is prepared as needed with 80.06 g NaCl, 4.03 g KCl, 2.96 g MgSO$_4$, 3.22 g Na$_2$HPO$_4$, and 47.66 g HEPES. The stock solution does not require refrigeration, although it should be used within a few weeks of preparation.
2. We use the 165-amino acid splice variant of VEGF (R & D Systems, Minneapolis, MN). The lyophilized powder is reconstituted in sterile phosphate-buffered saline with 0.1 mg/mL albumin. The resulting solution is divided into 5-μg aliquots and frozen at –70°C until needed. Aliquots should be used within 3 mo of reconstitution.
3. Nitroglycerin, 5 mg/mL (American Regent Laboratories, Shirley, NY), is diluted at the time of use. Nitroglycerin is heat- and light-sensitive, so we use it immediately after dilution. We have found that special tubing and light shielding are unnecessary if the nitroglycerin is used immediately.

3. Methods
3.1. Adenoviral Ex Vivo Heart Perfusion and Transplantation

1. Give adult New Zealand white rabbits (2–3 kg) heparin anticoagulation (1000 IU iv) prior to pentobarbital euthanasia (50 mg/kg iv). Immediately excise the heart with intact sections of the vena cavae, pulmonary veins, and great vessels and rinse twice in ice-cold Krebs' solution saturated with O$_2$.
2. Cannulate the aorta and suspend the heart in an insulated chamber at 37°C (**Fig. 2**). Perfusion with oxygenated Krebs' solution occurs by retrograde flow from the cannula in the ascending aorta to the coronary arteries at 30–35 mL/min by gravity flow.
3. After an initial perfusion with Krebs' solution for 2–3 min to wash out the remaining blood, perfuse the heart for 2 min with 1 nM VEGF and 90 μM nitroglycerin in Krebs' solution at 30–35 mL/min by gravity flow (*see* **Notes 1** and **2**).
4. Following pretreatment, infect the heart with 2×10^9 pfu/mL recombinant adenovirus in 20 mL of Krebs' solution containing 1 nM VEGF and 90 μM nitroglycerin. Coronary flow rate during infection is 30 mL/min, which is controlled by a peristaltic pump (Masterflex, Cole-Parmer). Collect the perfusate and recirculate it in order to conserve the amount of virus and VEGF used in each experiment (*see* **Notes 3** and **4**).
5. After infection, perfuse the heart with 10 mL of Krebs' solution to wash out virus or permeability factor remaining in the coronary circulation. Decannulate the heart and transplant it into a recipient animal. To study the heart in a protected

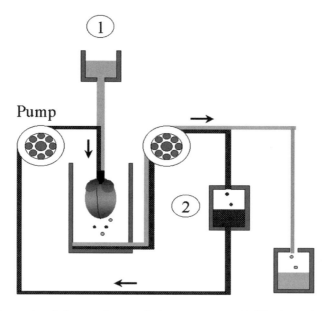

Fig 2. Schematic of the ex vivo perfusion apparatus. 1, The heart is perfused with non-recirculating Krebs' solution with or without vascular permeability agents (shaded in light gray). 2, The permeability agent and recombinant adenovirus in Krebs' solution are recirculated to conserve virus and VEGF (shaded in dark with dots). At the end of infection, the heart is again perfused with non-recirculating Krebs' solution to wash out the virus and permeability agent.

environment, heterotopic intraabdominal heart transplantation may be performed using a technique previously described by Ono and Lindsey for rats *(10)*. In brief, the infrarenal aorta and vena cava are exposed via a midline abdominal incision. Anastomosis between recipient and donor aortas and vena cava with pulmonary artery is performed. During the surgical procedure, the donor heart is wrapped in gauze and kept at approx 4°C through use of topical iced saline solution.

3.2. Adenoviral In Vivo Heart Perfusion

1. Immediately before catheterization, give domestic pigs (30–40 kg) 180 mg diltiazem, 325 mg aspirin, and 25 mg sildenafil orally (*see* **Note 5**), and a mixture of 400 mg ketamine and 10 mg acepromazine intramuscularly. Diltiazem and aspirin are used to prevent coronary spasm and thrombosis; sildenafil potentiates vascular permeability, and both ketamine and acepromazine are sedatives.
2. After sedation, induce anesthesia with 5–10 mL of intravenous sodium pentothal 2.5% solution and maintain with inhaled isoflurane 2% in oxygen.
3. Expose the right carotid or femoral artery and insert a 7-F introducer sheath into the vessel.
4. Cannulate the selected coronary artery with the 7-F guiding angioplasty catheter under fluoroscopic guidance. Select a terminal branch of the coronary artery with

a 0.014 in. guidewire, and advance a 2.7-F infusion catheter into the terminal vessel (*see* **Note 5**).

5. Infuse through the infusion catheter 10 mL normal saline containing 5 µg VEGF-165 and 200 µg nitroglycerin over 3 min, followed by a 30 s-infusion of 1 mL normal saline containing 7.5×10^9 pfu/mL adenovirus Adβgal and 20 µg nitroglycerin, and 2 mL of normal saline over 30 s (*see* **Notes 2, 6,** and **7**).

6. Following virus delivery, remove the catheters and sheaths. Repair the vessel with a running 7-0 silk suture or ligate with a 2-0 silk tie. Close the subcutaneous tissue with 2-0 silk suture, and close the skin with 3-0 vicryl suture.

4. Notes

1. Elimination of blood and radiographic contrast media during virus perfusion and delivery of pretreatment and virus at 37°C are necessary for optimal results.

2. Interruptions in pretreatment or virus delivery reduce the efficacy of gene transfer. The best possible strategy is 2 min of exposure to VEGF followed by 2 min of exposure to VEGF and virus.

3. The importance of accurate quality control of the recombinant adenovirus stock cannot be overemphasized. Contamination with wild type or mutants with decreased biological activity resulted in substantially decreased gene transfer efficiency.

4. In the ex vivo perfusion model, pulsatile flow from a peristaltic pump resulted in better gene transfer efficacy than continuous flow by hand push. The reason for this finding is not readily apparent, but it is reproducible.

5. Oral sildenafil must be given approx 1 h before perfusion to give adequate time for adsorption.

6. In the in vivo intracoronary perfusion model, infusion volume and coronary flow rate were limited to avoid efflux of the adenoviral vectors from the target vessel. Using balloon catheters rather than perfusion catheters will eliminate the risk of flow down nontarget vessels, but balloon catheters tend to have smaller internal diameters, reducing the potential flow rate.

7. Longer pretreatment times are definitely better than shorter times. Physiologic limitations from ischemia or reduced cardiac output are usually reached before adequate time for pretreatment and virus delivery. A compromise between gene transfer outcome and test subject well-being is usually required.

References

1. Donahue, J. K., Kikkawa, K., Johns, D., Marban, E., and Lawrence, J. (1997) Ultrarapid, highly efficient viral gene transfer to the heart. *Proc. Natl. Acad. Sci. USA* **94,** 4664–4668.

2. Donahue, J. K., Kikkawa, K., Thomas, A., Marban, E., and Lawrence, J. (1998) Acceleration of widespread adenoviral gene transfer to intact rabbit hearts by coronary perfusion vith low calcium and serotonin. *Gene Ther.* **5,** 630–634.

3. Nagata, K., Marban, E., Lawrence, J., and Donahue, J. K. (2001) Phosphodiesterase inhibitor-mediated potentiation of adenovirus delivery to myocardium. *J. Mol. Cell. Cardiol.* **33,** 575–580.

4. Xia, P., Aiello, L., Ishii, H., et al. (1996) Characterization of vascular endothelial growth factor's effect on the activation of protein kinase C, its isoforms, and endothelial cell growth. *J. Clin. Invest.* **98,** 2018–2026.

5. Wu, H., Yuan, Y., Zawieja, D., Tinsley, J., and Granger, H. (1999) Role of phospholipase C, proetin kinase C, and calcium in VEGF-induced venular hyperpermeability. *Am. J. Physiol.* **276,** H535–H542.

6. Wu, H. M., Huang, Q., Yuan, Y., and Granger, H. J. (1996) VEGF induces NO-dependent hyperpermeability in coronary venules. *Am. J. Physiol.* **271,** H2735–H2739.

7. Kubes, P. and Granger, D. N. (1992) Nitric oxide modulates microvascular permeability. *Am. J. Physiol.* **262,** H611–H615.

8. van Hinsbergh, V. (1997) Endothelial permeability for macromolecules. *Arterioscler. Thromb.* **17,** 1018–1023

9. Donahue, J. K., Heldman, A., Fraser, H., et al. (2000) Focal modification of electrical conduction in the heart by viral gene transfer. *Nat. Med.* **6,** 1395–1398.

10. Ono, K. and Lindsey, E. (1969) Improved technique of heart transplantation in rats. *J. Thorac. Cardiovasc. Surg.* **57,** 225–229.

18

Modification of In Vivo Cardiac Performance by Intracoronary Gene Transfer of β-Adrenergic Receptor Signaling Components

Hendrik T. Tevaearai and Walter J. Koch

1. Introduction

Alterations in β-adrenergic receptor (βAR) signaling typically occur in cardiomyocytes from hearts progressing toward failure *(1)*. Regulation of G-protein-coupled βARs mostly involves phosphorylation of agonist-occupied receptors by a βAR kinase (βARK1), leading to desensitization. This process also requires a second protein, β-arrestin, which binds to phosphorylated receptors and sterically interdicts further coupling. βARK1, also known as GRK2, is primarily a cytosolic enzyme that must translocate to the membrane in order to phosphorylate its receptor substrate. This is accomplished through a direct physical interaction between the GRK and the βγ-subunits of G-proteins ($G_{\beta\gamma}$) *(2,3)*. The $G_{\beta\gamma}$-binding site on βARK1 has been mapped to a region located toward the carboxyl terminus of the enzyme, and a peptide derived from this region (βARKct) can act as an effective in vivo βARK1 inhibitor. The βARKct represents the last 194 amino acids of βARK1 containing the $G_{\beta\gamma}$-binding domain *(2)* and has been utilized in transgenic mice to inhibit the in vivo activity of βARK1 *(4)*. Moreover, these mice present with enhanced cardiac contractility that has led to the rescue of several mouse models of cardiomyopathy *(4,5)*.

In addition to the functional improvement in βARKct transgenic mice, the myocardial-targeted transgenic overexpression of β_2ARs also results in a mouse model of hypercontractility *(6)*. In fact, several different lines of mice overexpressing the β_2AR have been generated, with all these lines having enhanced contractility *(5–8)*. The overexpression of β_2ARs in the hearts of

From: *Methods in Molecular Biology, vol. 219: Cardiac Cell and Gene Transfer*
Edited by: J. M. Metzger © Humana Press Inc., Totowa, NJ

these transgenic mice ranges from 15 to 350-fold *(6–8)*. Interestingly, with up to 150-fold overexpression, there is enhanced contractility with no pathology. Mice with >150-fold overexpression do present with cardiac fibrosis and pathology in the form of cardiomyopathy later in life *(7)*. However, more modest overexpression (~60-fold) has led to a phenotype of enhanced function that reversed the pathology seen in a mouse model of cardiomyopathy *(8)*. In stark contrast to β_2AR overexpression in the hearts of transgenic mice, minimal overexpression of β_1AR (5–15-fold) induces early pathology in the form of cardiomyopathy and premature death *(9,10)*. Other findings in vitro have shown that β_1AR overexpression can cause myocyte apoptosis, whereas β_2AR overexpression does not and can even protect against the β_1AR-mediated toxicity *(10)*. Thus, these studies have demonstrated the potential for targeted overexpression of β_2ARs or $\beta ARKct$ as representing novel therapeutic strategies for improving the function of the failing heart *(10)*.

Accordingly, our laboratory has been investigating genetic modulation of the myocardial βAR signaling pathway in larger animals in an attempt to restore the biochemical and functional alterations observed during acute and chronic heart failure. We have been employing adenoviral vectors for this purpose. Gene transfer using adenoviral vectors in animal models of heart failure can be done by direct injection into the left ventricular (LV) free wall. However, this technique provokes significant local damage and does not allow global myocardial expression. Intracoronary delivery of adenoviral transgenes has been shown in our hands, as well as others, to provide consistent gene expression using various transgenes. As described above, our laboratory is focusing on the myocardial gene delivery of the β_2AR and $\beta ARKct$ to improve cardiac function. In addition to these potentially therapeutic transgenes, we have also used the marker transgenes β-galactosidase and green fluorescent protein (GFP). These marker genes provide an understanding of the area and volume of global transgene expression in the myocardium using intracoronary delivery techniques. Importantly, we have been successful in improving the cardiac function of rabbits with three separate intracoronary delivery techniques using the β_2AR transgene or the $\beta ARKct$ transgene *(11–14)*. This includes the functional reversal of heart failure in rabbits using the $\beta ARKct$ transgene *(13,14)*. We have also demonstrated successful global gene transfer in transplanted rat and rabbit hearts using the β_2AR or β_2ARKct transgene *(15–17)*. In this chapter, we describe three different approaches for intracoronary adenovirus-mediated myocardial gene transfer.

The first technique consists of global intracoronary gene delivery in vivo. The principle consists of clamping the ascending aorta while the gene solution is injected into the LV cavity *(11,13)*. This way, the solution mixes with oxygenated blood incoming from the lungs and is forced into the coronaries. The aortic cross-clamping time is the key element of the technique. On the one hand, the longer time the aorta is clamped, the more the coronaries are exposed to the virus and consequently, the more time the virus has to infiltrate the myocardial interstitium and infect cardiomyocytes. On the other hand, clamping the aorta provokes a sudden pressure overload, adding to the myocardial ischemia, which may result in ventricular fibrillation or myocardial stunning if prolonged. Importantly, however, this technique allows consistent global myocardial gene transfer without affecting mid- and long-term ventricular function.

With the second technique, a specific rabbit coronary is selectively catheterized, allowing selective gene delivery into a specific myocardial territory *(12,14)*. This technique offers the major advantage that the animal does not require a thoracotomy and consequently, there is no cardiac manipulation that may affect the immediate postoperative myocardial function. However, the risk for coronary dissection is not null, and the risk of ventricular fibrillation is higher than for the previous technique.

Finally, an alternative method for global myocardial gene transfer in rats or rabbits is to perfuse the heart ex vivo before transplanting it into a recipient animal *(15–17)*. Although the donor heart has been arrested with cold cardioplegic solution, this technique allows longer myocardial exposure, which lasts as long as the heart is not reperfused, and subsequently gene expression is increased compared with both other techniques.

Obviously, these three techniques target different objectives, and one may choose the most appropriate according to the specific design of the study.

2. Materials

2.1. Technique 1: Global Intracoronary Gene Delivery In Vivo

1. Heat pump and pad (Gaymar, Orchard Park, NY).
2. Animal hair clipper.
3. Small animal ventilator set at 30×20 mL/kg/min (Harvard, #683).
4. Sterile Drapes (Barrier™, Johnson & Johnson, Arlington, TX).
5. Scrub solution (chlorhexidine).
6. Isopropyl rubbing alcohol 70%.
7. Vein catheter 24-gauge (Insyte-N™, Becton Dickinson, Franklin Lakes, NJ).
8. Perfusion tubing (Piggyback Microdrip®, Abbott Laboratories, North Chicago, IL).
9. Cuffed 3.0-mm tracheal tube (Intermediate Hi-Lo®, Mallinckrodt, St. Louis, MO).
10. Oxygen.
11. 2-0 (3.0 metric) silk surgical suture (Sherwood, Davis & Geck, St. Louis, MO).
12. 3-0 (2.0 metric) silk 30 in. RB-1 (Ethicon™, Somerville, NJ).
13. 3-0 (2.0 metric) 27", FS-2 Coated Vicryl suture (Ethicon).
14. Three-way stopcock with male Luer slip adapter (Baxter, Deerfield, IL).

15. 1 mL Syringe (Tuberculin syringe, Becton Dickinson).
16. 2 × 3-mL syringe Luer-lo™, Becton Dickinson).
17. Butterfly 23 × 12 3/4 in. Tubing infusion set (Butterfly®, Abbott Laboratories).
18. Sterilized surgical tray: surgical blade #15, (Becton Dickinson) mounted on a knife handle, Finochietto-deBakey infant rib retractor, pickup, scissors, right-angle forceps, atraumatic vascular clamp, 4 × 4-cm gauze.
19. Drugs and solutions:
    a. Ketamine 100 mg/mL (Ketaflo™, Abbott Laboratories).
    b. Acepromazine maleate 10 mg/mL (PromAce®, Fort Dodge Animal Health, Fort Dodge, IA).
    c. Butorphenol tartrate 10 mg/mL (Torbugesic®, Fort Dodge Animal Health).
    d. Adenosine 3 mg/mL (Adenocard®, Fujisawa, Deerfield, IL).
    e. Phosphate-buffered saline (PBS).
    f. NaCl 0.9%.
20. Quik-Cath® Chest tube (Baxter).

2.2. Technique 2: Selective Coronary Gene Delivery

1. Drugs and solutions:
    a. Ketamine 100 mg/mL (Ketaflo™, Abbott Laboratories).
    b. Acepromazine maleate 10 mg/mL (PromAce®, Fort Dodge Animal Health).
    c. Lidocaine HCl (Abbot Laboratories).
    d. Contrast liquid (Renografin®-60, Bracco Diagnostics, Princeton NJ).
    e. Heparin (Elkins-Sinn, Cherry Hill, NJ).
2. Surgical instruments: surgical blade #15 (Becton Dickinson) mounted on a knife handle, scissors, pickup, right-angle forceps, atraumatic bulldog clamp.
3. 2-0 (3.0 metric) silk surgical suture (Sherwood, Davis & Geck).
4. 3-0 (2.0 metric) 27 in., FS-2 Coated Vicryl suture (Ethicon).
5. Fluoroscopy system.
6. 4-F Introducer (Cook, Bloomington, IN).
7. 3-F Angled tip access catheter (Cook).
8. Infusion pump.
9. 3-mL Tubing (made out of a Universal administration set, Baxter fluven 0153/C; 26 in. contain 3 mL).
10. 2X three-way stopcock with male Luer slip adapter (Baxter).

2.3. Technique 3: Ex Vivo Global Gene Delivery

The same as in **Subheading 2.1.** plus:

1. University of Wisconsin cardioplegic solution.
2. Heparin (Elkins-Sinn).
3. Lidocaine (Abbot Laboratories).
4. Dexamethasone sodium phosphate 4 mg/mL (American Regent Laboratories, Shirley, NY).
5. Sterile saline slush.

6. Add to the surgical tray: microdissecting scissors, microsuturing needle holder, atraumatic vascular tissue forceps, four microvessel clips.
7. Suction system.
8. 7-0 (0.5 metric) 24 in. BV-1 polypropylene suture (Ethicon).

3. Methods

3.1. Technique 1: Global Intracoronary Gene Delivery In Vivo

3.1.1. Anesthesia and Preparation

1. Anesthetize the rabbit with ketamine (60 mg/kg im) and acepromazine (1.0 mg/kg im).
2. Shave the left thoracic area. Also shave the back of one ear for venous access.
3. Install an iv catheter inside the dorsal ear vein of one ear and perfuse the animal with ~25 mL/h of saline 0.9%.
4. Intubate the animal with the endotracheal tube, slightly inflate the cuff, and tape the tube to the animal. Ventilate the animal with oxygen-enriched air (2 L/min).
5. Administer butorphenol (0.25 mg/kg iv).
6. If necessary, adjust the level of anesthesia with ketamine (10 mg) so that the animal is easily ventilated.
7. Install the animal on the heating pad, on its right side, extending the upper and lower right legs.
8. Scrub the shaved left thoracic area with chlorhexidine followed by ethanol.

3.1.2. Cardiac Access

1. Drape and leave exposed only the area comprising the midportion of the right thorax (*see* **Notes 1** and **2**).
2. Perform a vertical cutaneous incision of about 5 cm approx 3 cm above the lower edge of the most inferior rib.
3. Cut two muscle layers following the same direction until you have reached the ribs (*see* **Note 3**).
4. Palpate the thoracic cage with the index finger and count the intercostal spaces. Open the chest into the fourth intercostal space, paying special attention not to injure the lung.
5. Position the retractor and open it progressively.
6. With a 4 × 4-cm gauze, carefully move the left lung lobes out of the field.
7. Open the pericardial layer longitudinally until the apex of the heart and up as far as possible to give access to the great vessels **(Fig. 1A)**.
8. With the right-angle forceps, turn around the pulmonary arch to isolate it from the ascending aorta. Pass a 2-0 silk suture around it. Gently pull on this suture to facilitate access to the underlying ascending aorta. Using the right-angle forceps, turn around the aorta and pass a second 2-0 silk suture, to individualize it from the adjacent structures. These two sutures will help in clamping the aorta quickly during the next step of the procedure **(Fig. 1B)**.

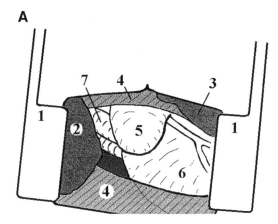

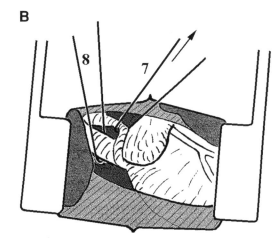

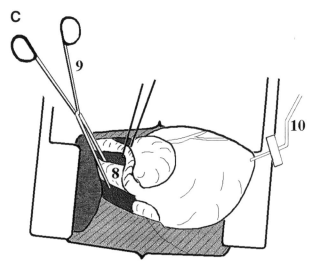

3.1.3. Gene Preparation

1. Connect a 3-mL syringe filled with PBS to the three-way stop cock and carefully purge the system of any bubble.
2. Thaw the gene solution and dilute it with PBS to a final volume of 2.0 mL using a 3-mL syringe.
3. Connect the gene syringe to the second entry of the three-way stopcock. Connect the stopcock to the butterfly tubing and purge it with PBS, taking care to purge it carefully of air bubbles. Switch the stopcock to the gene syringe position, and inject 0.6 mL of the gene solution into the line of the butterfly tubing to purge it with the gene solution (0.6 mL corresponds to the volume of the butterfly tubing line).

3.1.4. Gene Delivery

1. Inject 1.2 mg of aenosine into the right ventricle with a tuberculin syringe connected to a 30-gauge needle (*see* **Note 4**).
2. Clamp the aorta and simultaneously start the timer.
3. Quickly lift the heart to have access to the apex of the left ventricle. Insert the needle of the butterfly tubing into the LV cavity through the apex (**Fig. 1C**). Quickly inject the rest of the gene solution (1.4 mL), switch the stopcock to the PBS syringe, and purge the line off the gene solution with 0.6 mL of PBS. Remove the needle from the LV (*see* **Notes 5–7**).
4. After 45 s of aortic crossclamping, remove the clamp (*see* **Note 8**).
5. Remove the gauze and allow the left lung lobes to reinflate by occluding the exhaust of the ventilator for 3–5 s.

3.1.5. Thoracic Closure

1. Place three pericostal sutures using the 3-0 silk.
2. Insert a Quik-Cath catheter through the skin approx 1 cm below the cutaneous incision and direct its tip through the muscular layers and then through the thoracic incision. Remove the needle and keep the catheter in the thoracic cavity to be further used as a thoracic vent.

Fig. 1. (*Opposite page*) Global intracoronary gene delivery technique in vivo (rabbits). (**A**) After having performed a right thoracotomy through the fourth intercostal space, the retractor (1) is positioned and spread. The thymus (2) is moved toward the head, and a gauze (3) is placed to move the right lung lobes out of the field. The pericardium (4) is opened longitudinally. This lets the left atrium (5), the ventricles (6), and the pulmonary artery (7) appear. (**B**) A 2-0 silk suture is passed around the pulmonary artery (7) and pulled to expose the ascending aorta (8), which is also dissected free and isolated with a 2-0 silk suture. (**C**) After the adenosine is injected directly into the right ventricle, the ascending aorta (8) is occluded using a vascular clamp (9), the heart is quickly lifted up, and the needle of the butterfly catheter (10) is inserted into the apex of the left ventricle and the gene solution is delivered.

3. Tie the three sutures to close the thoracic cage.
4. Close the muscle layers with a single running 3-0 silk suture.
5. Close the skin with a running 3-0 vicryl suture.
6. Using a 10-mL syringe with a stopcock, aspirate the air from the pleural space via the transthoracic catheter before removing it while keeping a suction force.
7. Disconnect the animal from the ventilator and wait for spontaneous respiration before removing the tracheal tube.
8. Keep the animal in a warm area with oxygen by its nose until recovery is complete.

3.2. Technique 2: Selective Coronary Gene Delivery

3.2.1. Catheterization Technique

1. Anesthetize the rabbit with ketamine (60 mg/kg im) and acepromazine (1.0 mg/kg im). Shave the anterior neck area. Place a vein catheter into the ear vein, and inject 300 IU heparin. Position the animal on the back with a small pad under the upper back to extend the head up and thus expose the anterior neck.
2. Scrub and drape.
3. Prepare the infusion system (**Fig. 2A**): Fill the 30-mL syringe with saline containing 20 IU/mL heparin and connect successively to a stopcock, the 3-mL tubing, a second stopcock, and then the coronary catheter. Flush the entire system and check for the absence of residual bubbles. Prepare the introducer and flush it also with heparinized saline solution. Fill a 10-mL syringe with contrast (8.0 mL) mixed with heparin (2.0 mL). Connect the contrast syringe to the distal stopcock.
4. Infiltrate the incisional area with approx 2.0 mL lidocaine 1%. Perform a left paramedial longitudinal cutaneous incision, incise the plathysma muscle longitudinally, and isolate the carotid artery between the sternocleidomastoideus and the pretracheal muscles.
5. Ligate the carotid artery distally with a 2-0 silk suture, and place a Potz loop 2-0 silk suture proximally.
6. Clamp the artery proximally before performing a small arteriotomy. Insert the introducer and remove the inner guide.
7. Insert the coronary catheter into the introducer and conduct its tip under fluoroscopic assistance and intermittent push delivery of contrast liquid until it enters the desired (right or left) coronary artery. Confirm the position with injection of contrast liquid and fluoroscopic vision (*see* **Note 9**).

3.2.3. Gene Delivery

1. Thaw the gene solution and mix with PBS (warmed at 37°C) to a final volume of 3.0 mL.
2. Slowly infuse the solution into the 3-mL tubing via the proximal stopcock (**Fig. 2B**). This way, the solution still remains in the tubing before being injected at a controlled speed and pressure rate by means of the pump.

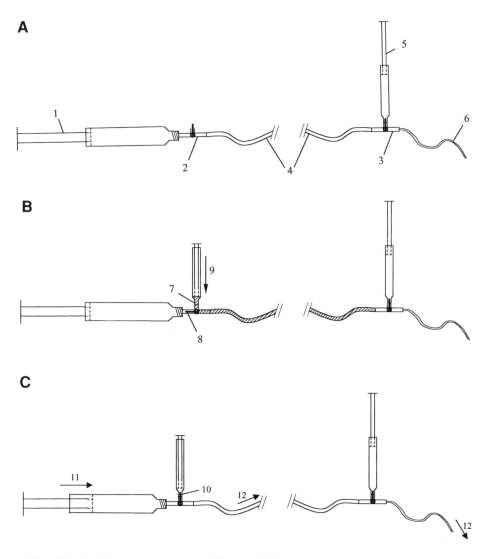

Fig. 2. Selective coronary gene delivery. (**A**) Preparation of the infusion set, which includes the 30-mL syringe (1) filled with heparinized saline, proximal (2) and distal (3) three-way stopcocks, 3-mL tubing (4), the contrast syringe (5), and the coronary catheter (6). (**B**) After the coronary catheter has been positioned correctly into the coronary artery, the syringe containing the adenoviral solution is connected to the proximal stopcock (7). The stopcock is switched (8), and the adenoviral solution is gently pushed (9) in order to fill the 3-mL tubing. (**C**) The coronary catheter is then slightly pushed into the coronary artery and its position checked by mean of the contrast liquid, making sure there is no backflow into the ascending aorta. The proximal stopcock is switched back (10), and the pump is then turned on (11) in order to deliver the adenoviral solution (12) at a rate of 10 mL/min for a total delivery of 3.0 mL.

3. Slightly move the coronary catheter forward until you feel resistance. Confirm the wedge position of the catheter by injecting ~1 mL of contrast. The coronary artery should be easily visualized and, importantly, no backflow in the aorta should be observed.

4. Drive the pump at 10 mL/min (if in the right coronary; 20 mL/min if in the left circumflex coronary artery) for a total injectate volume of 3.0 mL (**Fig. 2C**) (*see* **Notes 10** and **11**).

5. Slowly remove the coronary catheter.

6. Remove the introducer, and ligate the coronary artery using the Potz loop suture.

7. Close the skin with a running 3-0 vicryl suture.

3.3. Technique 3: Ex Vivo Global Gene Delivery

3.3.1. Donor Heart Harvesting

1. Anesthetize the rabbit with ketamine (90 mg/kg im) and acepromazine (1.5 mg/kg im). Widely shave the anterior thoracic area. Install a vein catheter into the ear vein. Intubate and ventilate as in **Subheading 3.1.1.** Administer butorphenol (0.5 mg/kg iv). Position the animal on the back. Use ropes to spread the upper and lower legs. Scrub and drape the anterior thoracic area.

2. Infiltrate the incisional area (sc and im) with approx 5 mL lidocaine 1% before performing a clamshell thoracotomy. Pull the thoracic cage up with a heavy forceps. Eventually clamp the right and left mammary artery, which may bleed abundantly.

3. Open the pericardium to expose the heart and the major vessels widely. Isolate the pulmonary artery and the ascending aorta with a 2-0 silk suture. Isolate the inferior vena cava with a 2-0 silk suture.

4. Anticoagulate the animal with 3000 IU heparin.

5. Fill a 30-mL syringe with cold University of Wisconsin cardioplegic solution and connect the syringe to the 23 in. butterfly needle. Purge the system of any bubbles.

6. Back to the rabbit, partially section the inferior vena cava and allow partial exsanguination. Aspirate blood with the suction system to allow unloading of the heart.

7. Clamp the ascending aorta and immediately stick the butterfly needle into the LV cavity through its apex. Inject the cardioplegic solution over approx 1 min. This usually allows cardiac arrest within about 10 s.

8. Remove the needle. Ligate the inferior vena cava and complete its section. Remove the aortic clamp and section successively the pulmonary artery and ascending aorta, both as far as possible from their cardiac emergence.

9. Lift the heart up and ligate *en bloc* the remaining vessels (superior vena cava and pulmonary veins). Section these vessels and transfer the heart into cold saline solution at 4°C.

3.3.2. Gene Delivery

1. Mix the gene solution with PBS to a final volume of 2.0 mL in a 3-mL syringe. Connect the syringe to a buttoned needle. Insert the tip of that needle into the ascending aorta of the freshly harvested heart and tighten it with a 2-0 silk suture. Gently inject the solution into the aortic root. Lift the syringe/needle to pull the heart up and facilitate dripping into the coronaries.

3.3.3. Transplantation Technique

1. Anesthetize the recipient rabbit with ketamine (60 mg/kg im) and acepromazine (1.0 mg/kg im). Shave the anterior neck area. Place a vein catheter into the ear vein and inject 300 IU heparin. Position the animal on the back with a small pad under the upper back to extend the head up and thus expose the anterior neck.
2. Scrub and drape.
3. Infiltrate the incisional area with approx 2.0 mL lidocaine 1%. Perform a left paramedial longitudinal incision over 4 cm. Longitudinally incise the plathysma muscle and dissect the jugular vein free. Isolate the carotid artery between the sternocleidomastodeus and the pretracheal muscles.
4. Clamp the carotid artery up and down to isolate a segment of approx 1.5–2.0 cm. Perform a longitudinal arteriotomy over approx 7–8 mm. Do the anastomoses between the donor ascending aorta and the recipient carotid artery using a running 7-0 polypropylene suture (*see* **Note 12**).
5. Administer steroids iv (dexamethasone 4 mg/kg iv).
6. Clamp and isolate the jugular vein over a similar segment and perform a longitudinal veinotomy over approx 1.2 cm Do the terminolateral anastomoses using a running 7-0 polypropylene suture (*see* **Note 13**).
7. Unclamp the venous side first and verify hemostasis. Then progressively open the upper arterial clamp and verify hemostasis. If necessary, replace the clamp to correct hemostasis. Remove the lower arterial clamp and wait for spontaneous heart beating. (It takes about 15–60 s to start; usually the heart beats vigorously within 2–3 min after reperfusion) (*see* **Note 14**).
8. Close the skin over the transplanted heart with a running 3-0 vicryl suture.
9. Keep the animal in a warm area with oxygen by its nose until recovery is complete.

3.3.4. Postoperative Care

1. Administer steroids daily (dexamethasone 4 mg/kg iv).
2. Observe and palpate the heart daily.

4. Notes

1. The left thoracic access is proposed, as it gives a nice exposure to the LV free wall and particularly the left circumflex artery with its marginal branches, as

well as the left anterior descending artery. In some experiments, the investigator can take the opportunity of this access to induce an infarction, with subsequent development of LV dysfunction. The combination of gene delivery and creation of a myocardial infarction is particularly appropriate to study the role of a specific gene during the initial evolution and progression of heart failure *(7)*.

2. The same procedure can be performed via a right thoracotomy through the fourth intercostal space. From this side, it is not necessary to turn around the pulmonary artery, as the ascending aorta can be reached directly.

3. Bleeding is usually not a problem if the operator pays attention to the thoracic subcutaneous veins, which are visible through the skin. In addition, the thoracic opening needs to respect the mammary artery and vein, which run close to the sternum. In case of bleeding, compression for a few minutes is usually sufficient, and an electrocautery system is usually never necessary.

4. Adenosine has been proposed to slow down the cardiac rhythm while the adenoviral solution is injected; 0.1 mL/kg is administered in the right ventricle immediately before the aorta is clamped, and the adenoviral transgene is delivered.

5. Since there are only a few seconds to deliver the adenoviral transgene, the needle of the butterfly needs to be positioned rapidly and correctly. Sometimes it is not easy to lift the heart to give access to its apex. The operator may want to use a gauze previously positioned under the heart so that, by pulling on it, the apex is rapidly lifted up. Another way to lift the heart is to use a teaspoon, which can quickly and easily be sliced under the heart before pulling it up.

6. A pulsating red backflow into the tubing of the butterfly confirms the good positioning of the needle into the LV cavity and should be seen before injecting the adenoviral transgene.

7. This technique or a similar one can also be employed in rats *(18)*. The major difference for rats is that it is difficult to separate the aorta from the pulmonary artery. However, both arteries can be clamped together before administering the adenoviral transgene into the LV cavity. In rats, it is important to pay attention to the lungs, as they are much more delicate compared with rabbits. In addition, no thoracic drain is used before chest closure. However, increasing the ventilation pressure for a few seconds allows lung hyperinflation and should be done immediately before chest closure.

8. Because of the pulmonary volume overload during the 45 s of aortic cross-clamping, the rabbit may react by coughing violently after unclamping. Just wait and protect the lung from being excavated out of the thoracic cavity by occluding the thoracic opening with gauze.

9. In rabbits, selective catheterization can only be performed safely into the right and left circumflex coronary arteries. In piglets, we have found that selective catheterization can be done in these two plus the left anterior descending coronary artery (unpublished data).

10. After coronary gene delivery, wait approx 30 min for an eventual hypotensive reaction, which is common after this technique of gene delivery. An easy way to record arterial pressure continuously is to insert a catheter connected to a pres-

sure transducer into the carotid introducer instead of the coronary catheter. In case of hypotension, place the animal in a Trendelenbug position (lift the legs) to optimize venous blood mobilization. In worst cases, volume replacement by infusion of saline solution may be necessary.

11. Infusion speed rate depends on the mass of perfused territory. As a general rule, we propose in rabbits a perfusion rate of 10 mL/min for the right coronary artery and 20 mL/min for the left circumflex coronary artery. In piglets, a perfusion of 80 mL/min permits optimal gene expression.

12. Try to maintain the graft in wet gauze with ice slush.

13. Do not pull extensively on the venous suture as it may provoke a pursestring effect and occlude the venous drainage.

14. Purge the graft aorta of air using a 27-gauge needle immediately before unclamping. Massive bubbles and coronary artery emboli may alter LV function of the freshly transplanted heart.

References

1. Brodde, O. E. (1993) Beta-adrenoceptors in cardiac disease. *Pharmacol. Ther.* **60,** 405–430.

2. Koch, W. J., Inglese, J., Stone, W. C., and Lefkowitz, R. J. (1993) The binding site for the βγsubunits of heterotrimeric G proteins on the β-adrenergic receptor kinase. *J. Biol. Chem.* **268,** 8256–8260.

3. Pitcher, J. A., Inglese, J., Higgins, J. B., et al. (1992) Role of βγ-subunits of G proteins in targeting the β-adrenergic receptor kinase to membrane-bound receptors. *Science* **257,** 1264–1267.

4. Koch, W. J., Rockman, H. A., Samama, P., et al. (1995) Cardiac function in mice overexpressing the β-adrenergic receptor kinase or a βARK inhibitor. *Science* **268,** 1350–1353.

5. Koch, W. J., Lefkowitz, R. J., and Rockman, H. A. (2000) Functional consequences of altering myocardial adrenergic receptor signaling. *Annu. Rev. Physiol.* **62,** 237–260.

6. Milano, C. A., Allen, L. F., Rockman, H. A., et al. (1994) Enhanced myocardial function in transgenic mice overexpressing the β_2-adrenergic receptor. *Science* **264,** 582–586.

7. Liggett, S. B., Tepe, N. M., Lorenz, J. N., et al. (2000) Early and delayed consequences of β_2-adrenergic receptor overexpression in mouse hearts: critical role for expression level. *Circulation* **101,** 1707–1714.

8. Dorn, G. W. 2nd, Tepe, N. M., Lorenz, J. N., Koch, W. J., and Ligett, S. B. (1999) Low- and high-level transgenic expression of β_2-adrenergic receptor differentially affect cardiac hypertrophy and function in Galphaq-overexpressing mice. *Proc. Natl. Acad. Sci. USA* **96,** 6400–6405.

9. Engelhardt, S., Hein, L., Wiesmann, F., and Lohse, M. J. (1999) Progressive hypertrophy and heart failure in β_1-adrenergic receptor transgenic mice. *Proc. Natl. Acad. Sci. USA* **96,** 7059–7064.

10. Lefkowitz, R. J., Rockmann, H. A., and Koch, W. J. (2000) Catecholamines, cardiac β-adrenergic receptors, and heart failure. *Circulation* **101,** 1707–1714.

11. Maurice, J. P., Hata, J. A., Shah, A. S., et al. (1999) Enhancement of cardiac function after adenoviral-mediated in vivo intracoronary β_2-adrenergic receptor gene delivery. *J. Clin. Invest.* **104,** 21–29.

12. Shah, A. S., Lilly, R. E., Kypson, A. P., et al. (2000) Intracoronary adenovirus-mediated delivery and overexpression of the β_2-adrenergic receptor in the heart: prospects for molecular ventricular assistance. *Circulation* **101,** 408–414.

13. White, D. C., Hata, J. A., Shah, A. S., Glower, D. D., Lefkowitz, R. J., and Koch, W. J. (2000) Preservation of myocardial β-adrenergic receptor signaling delays the development of heart failure following myocardial infarction. *Proc. Natl. Acad. Sci. USA* **97,** 5428–5433.

14. Shah, A. S., White, D. C., Emani, S., et al. (2001) In vivo ventricular gene delivery of a β-adrenergic receptor kinase inhibitor to the failing heart reverses cardiac dysfunction. *Circulation* **103,** 1311–1316.

15. Kypson, A. P., Peppel, K., Akhter, S. A., et al. (1998) Ex vivo adenoviral-mediated gene transfer to the transplanted adult rat heart. *J. Thorac. Cardiovasc. Surg.* **115,** 623–630.

16. Kypson, A. P., Hendrickson, S. C., Akhter, S. A., et al. (1999) Adenoviral-mediated gene transfer of the β_2-adrenergic receptor to donor hearts enhances cardiac function. *Gene Ther.* **6,** 1298–1284.

17. Shah, A. S., White, D. C., Tai, O., et al. (2000) Adenovirus-mediated genetic manipulation of the myocardial β-adrenergic signaling system in transplanted hearts. *J. Thorac. Cardiovasc. Surg.* **120,** 581–588.

18. Hajjar, R. J., Schmidt, U., Matsui, T., et al. (1998) Modulation of ventricular function through gene transfer in vivo. *Proc. Natl. Acad. Sci. USA* **95,** 5251–5256.

19

Protocols for Hemodynamic Assessment of Transgenic Mice In Vivo

Dimitrios Georgakopoulos and David A. Kass

1. Introduction

In the past few years there has been an explosive growth in the development of animal models of cardiovascular disease based on transgenic and gene-targeted strategies *(1)*. Almost exclusively, the mouse has been the animal model employed in these studies owing to the relative ease with which its genome may be manipulated, short reproductive cycle, and low cost. Further advances now provide the ability to control gene expression in a temporal manner in the postnatal mouse heart *(2)* and, as described in other chapters of this monograph, the potential for assessing the feasibility and effectiveness of treating cardiovascular disease at the molecular genetic level through the use of gene therapy. Phenotypic analysis in the mouse though, has generally lagged behind the rapid advances in molecular biology owing to the unique challenges posed by the small size of the mouse heart (<6 mm length) and rapid heart rate (550–650 beats/min).

Nearly two decades ago, the pioneering studies by Suga, Sagawa, and colleagues *(3)*, using an isolated canine heart preparation and a physiologic loading system, developed a framework for analysis of cardiac function through the use of pressure-volume relations. Obtaining pressure-volume loops in real time at steady state and at varying preloads (by obstructing inflow to the heart), subsequent studies in larger mammals *(4)* and humans *(5)* have established this method as the most comprehensive in describing the pumping ability of the heart separately from its primary determinants: preload, afterload, contractility, relaxation, and heart rate. Obtaining pressure-volume relations in vivo requires invasive catheterization of the left (or right) ventricle. Although measurement of pressure is quite common, measurement of instantaneous and continuous

From: *Methods in Molecular Biology, vol. 219: Cardiac Cell and Gene Transfer*
Edited by: J. M. Metzger © Humana Press Inc., Totowa, NJ

volumes has historically been very difficult. A technique by Baan and colleagues *(6)* was developed that correlates the change in ventricular volume to a change in electrical resistance of the chamber. Briefly, a multielectrode catheter (conductance catheter) is placed along the long axis of the ventricle, and a high-frequency (20-kHz) constant current (20–30 µA) electric field is established between the base and apex. A time-varying voltage is then measured across a pair(s) of intervening electrodes. Since the current is constant, the voltage change is proportional to the change in resistance inside the ventricle. Theoretically, ventricular volume is proportional to the inverse of resistance (conductance) so that the inverse of the voltage is actually determined.

Although conversion of conductance to absolute volume is theoretically possible, calibration of the raw signal is usually accomplished empirically by an independent measure of cardiac output (e.g., flow probe) from which stroke volume is obtained, which is then used to derive the gain of the signal, defined as: gain = flow probe stroke volume/conductance stroke volume. In addition, since the ventricular cavity is not a perfect insulator, a portion of the current leaks outside the cavity, resulting in an offset that must be subtracted to obtain absolute volume. This offset is usually estimated by the hypertonic saline dilution method *(5)*.

Recently, miniaturization techniques have resulted in the development and application of the pressure-volume catheter to the mouse heart *(7,8)*. Although the methodology is invasive and provides information at one time point, complete characterization of systolic and diastolic properties, coupling to the arterial system, and mechanical efficiency can all be obtained, thereby providing the ability to translate the effects of specific molecular alterations to the complex function of the intact heart and animal. Although echocardiography can be used to assess ventricular function noninvasively and serially over time, resolution is still limited in mice. Functional analysis is limited to cavity volumes and fractional shortening (ejection fraction), which can be greatly influenced by loading conditions without changes in ventricular properties, thus making interpretation of systolic function difficult or impossible. Preliminary studies are under way in our lab to develop a chronically instrumented model allowing measurement of pressure-volume relations in conscious mice. The application of the pressure-volume approach to the mouse used in our laboratory is described in detail in this chapter.

2. Materials

1. Dissecting microscope with boom stand and fiberoptic ring light. A 0.5× objective lens attachment is recommended to allow for sufficient operating space (World Precision Instruments, Sarasota, FL).

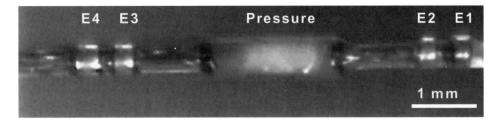

Fig. 1. Pressure-volume catheter used in the mouse. Electrodes E1 and E4 are positioned at the base and apex of the heart, respectively. Current is injected between electrodes E1 and E4, and the potential difference is measured across electrodes E2 and E3.

2. A constant flow rodent ventilator (Harvard Apparatus, Holliston, MA) (*see* **Note 1**).
3. Pressure-volume catheter (SPR-719, Millar Instruments, Houston TX) (**Fig. 1**) and constant current signal conditioner/pressure module (Aria, Millar Instruments). This system also contains a PC computer for data acquisition and analysis of pressure-volume signals.
4. Ultrasound flow meter (T106, Transonic, Ithaca NY) and perivascular flow probe (1RB, Transonics).
5. Methoxyflurane (*see* **Note 2**), urethane (Sigma, St. Louis, MO) dissolved in saline (300 mg/mL), etomidate (2 mg/mL), morphine (10 mg/mL), fentanyl (0.05 mg/mL), 2% lidocaine gel (Astra Pharmaceuticals). These last four anesthetic agents are readily available through the hospital supply pharmacy.
6. 25% human albumin solution (Red Cross, Switzerland). This may also be obtained from the hospital pharmacy supply.
7. Battery-operated high-temperature cautery (#500389) and high temperature tips (#500394) (World Precision Instruments).
8. Polyethylene tubing (PE-10) and 30-gauge needles (Thomas Scientific, Swedesboro, NJ).
9. Water recirculating heating pad (Baxter Pharmaceuticals, Valencia, CA) and water bath.

3. Methods

3.1. Anesthesia and Ventilation

1. Place the mouse in an anesthetic chamber containing gauze pads soaked with methoxyflurane for approx 1 min. (Times will vary depending on the strength of the anesthesia.) Careful monitoring of the animal is required, and the mouse should be removed as soon as there is no response to tail pinch.
2. After removing the animal, deliver an intraperitoneal injection of urethane (800–1000 mg/kg), etomidate (5–10 mg/kg) and morphine (1–2 mg/kg). If the animal

shows signs of waking before this mixture has reached effect, it may be trans-ferred back to the anesthesia chamber or, alternatively, a Falcon tube containing methoxyflurane-soaked gauze pads may be placed over the nose. Caution should be taken so as not to have any liquid methoxyflurane come into contact with the animal, as this is very toxic.

3. Once the animal is asleep, transfer to a heating pad with the water temperature set to 40°C. This higher temperature compensates for ambient heat loss.

4. Position the animal so that the head is pointing toward the investigator. Tape down the front paws to the heating pad, place a thin piece of tape across the tip of the snout, and tape this down as well. This pulls the head back slightly, creating traction on the trachea. Care should be taken not to obstruct the nostrils since mice are obligate nose breathers.

5. Manually palpate over the neck region to localize the trachea by feeling the ridges from the cartilage rings. Pull the skin away from the underlying muscles and cut this part off. Where the muscles on either side of the neck insert into the midline, pull these away gently with forceps, exposing the surface of the trachea. Blunt dissect the around and underneath the trachea to free it away from the tissue. Care should be taken not to tear the carotid arteries, which run along both sides of the trachea.

6. Pass a 4-0 silk suture underneath the proximal end of the trachea and make a small cut onto the surface of the trachea. Insert a blunt end (this is accomplished by smoothing the end of the needle on a grinding wheel) 19-gauge needle half of its length into the trachea and tie down with the suture.

7. Turn the animal so that it is now facing away from the investigator, connect the needle to the ventilator, and initiate ventilation with 100% oxygen delivered from a tank with the gauge pressure set to 40 psi. This initial high pressure setting is used to provide constant flow into the animal. Ventilation settings are set to deliver a tidal volume of 200 μL at a rate of 120 breaths/min (*see* **Note 3**). Monitoring of airway pressure from a side port in the tracheal cannula can be done to ensure adequate ventilation. Peak inspiratory pressures in the mouse are the same as in other mammals and range between 5 and 10 cmH$_2$O. The expiratory vent is usually to atmosphere; however, tubing from the expiratory port may be placed in a beaker of water to provide positive end-expiratory pressure if the lungs appear to be collapsing.

8. Depth of anesthesia should be assessed regularly by monitoring the response to tail pinch. If required, anesthesia may be supplemented with an intraperitoneal injection of 50 μL fentanyl.

3.2. Left Ventricular Catheterization

1. Make a superficial incision to the right of the trachea to expose a large salivary gland. Place some lidocaine gel over this area to minimize any discomfort. Under the dissecting microscope, gently pull the gland to the side to expose the external jugular vein. This vessel is relatively large and very superficial. By blunt dissection, remove some of the tissue away from the vein.

2. Dilute the human albumin solution with saline to 12.5% and withdraw into a 5-mL syringe attached to a 30-gauge needle via PE-10 tubing. Under the microscope, pull on the distal end of the vein to provide traction; the vein is directly cannulated by directly inserting the 30-gauge needle. Place the syringe into an infusion pump and infuse 150–180 µL at a rate of 25 µL/min. Slow the infusion rate to 5 µL/min. and continue for the duration of the experiment. This volume loading is required to obtain physiologic blood pressures and replace fluid loss from surgery and respiration.

3. Make an incision over the xyphoid. Blunt dissect laterally on both sides of the incision, separating the skin from the chest wall. Using the heat cautery, cauterize the blood vessels in the skin, running along both sides of the incision. Cut the skin out laterally on both sides beginning from the incision. Apply lidocaine gel to the exposed chest wall. Beginning at the xyphoid, use the heat cautery to cut through the chest wall laterally on both sides. Continue until the diaphragm is clearly visible from beneath. In a semicircular fashion, cut through the diaphragm to expose the apex of the heart.

4. Insert a 25-gauge needle approx 1.5 mm into the apex of the left ventricle and slowly remove. In the same hole, insert the pressure-volume catheter along the long axis toward the aortic root until the bottom electrode (E4; **Fig. 1**) is just inside the endocardium. The position of the catheter can then be adjusted to obtain rectangular-shaped pressure-volume loops.

5. Following stabilization, data can be collected at steady state and by varying preload by direct manual compression of the inferior vena cava. The latter procedure is used to derive the end-systolic pressure-volume relationship (ESPVR) and other indices of systolic function *(9)*. During data collection, respiration should be suspended to minimize lung motion artifact. An L-shaped device constructed from thin metal (e.g., small paper clip) can be placed underneath the inferior vena cava and esophagus and used to compress the thoracic aorta, providing an increase in load on the heart and an alternate means of generating the ESPVR.

3.3. Conductance Catheter Calibration

Following collection of data, the conductance signal needs to be calibrated to convert it to absolute volume units of microliters. This is accomplished by two procedures.

1. To calibrate for offset, rapidly inject manually a 10-µL bolus of hypertonic saline (35%) into the jugular vein. Analyze the subsequent perturbation of the signal to estimate the offset or parallel conductance (**Fig. 2**). This procedure may be repeated to obtain a second estimate. Care should be taken in hemodynamically compromised animals since hypertonic saline is a potent negative inotrope. No more than two saline calibrations should be performed since this may cause an alteration in blood conductivity that will influence the conductance signal irrespective of a change in ventricular volume *(10)*.

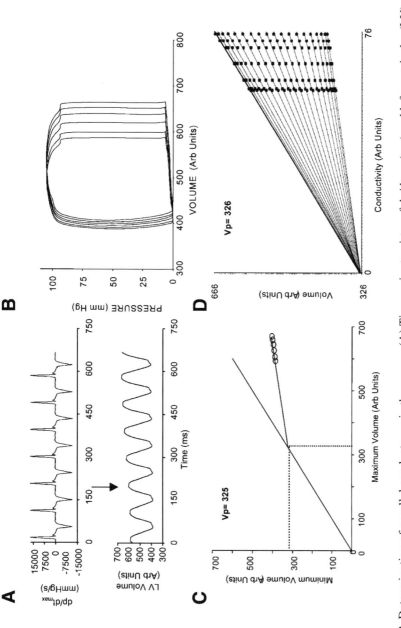

Fig. 2. Determination of parallel conductance in the mouse. (A) Time series tracings of dp/dt$_{max}$ (top) and left ventricular (LV) volume (bottom). Arrow indicates the onset of hypertonic saline washin with subsequent change in the position and stroke volume of the conductance signal owing to the increased blood conductivity. Lack of change in dp/dt$_{max}$ indicates no alteration in contractility or LV volume. (B) Pressure-volume loops during the saline washin. (C) Regression of maximum and minimum conductance from the transient in A; the intersection with the line of identity is used to determine the parallel conductance (Vp), 325 in this example. (D) Same data analyzed by the method of Lankford et. al. (11) whereby the volume signal is divided into equal segments and each is individually regressed. The value of Vp is in perfect agreement with the method in C, indicating the constancy of the parallel conductance throughout the cardiac cycle.

238

2. Then turn the animal onto its left side, taking care not to perturb the volume signal. Make a lateral thoracotomy between T3 and T5 to create a small window. Under the microscope, the thoracic aorta may be visualized running parallel to the spinal column. Gently dissect a small portion free from the spinal column, and place a perivascular flow probe around it. Obtain optimal signals when the probe and aorta are parallel. Flow probe and conductance signals can be recorded at steady state and during multiple loading cycles (**Fig. 3**) to assess the linearity of the signal over a broad loading range *(7)*. The width of the pressure-volume loops should be the same in moving the animal from its back onto its side. If this is not possible, then once a flow signal is obtained, the animal can be immediately placed on its back and the conductance stroke volume recorded. This stroke volume should then be matched to the flow probe-derived stroke volume to determine the gain.

With proper calibration, the pressure-volume approach provides a powerful means of assessing the different types of cardiomyopathy (**Fig. 4**). As a reference, we have provided the hemodynamic indices derived from pressure-volume relations with our protocol (**Tables 1** and **2**) along with the corresponding human values. Note the similarity between human and mouse when the values are normalized for heart rate or volume.

4. Notes

1. The ventilator referenced here is based on a pressurized design rather than the conventional piston-driven ventilators. We have found that the former minimizes dead space and provides more uniform ventilation. The ventilator used in our lab has been custom designed and is currently available for purchase. For further inquiries, please contact Dr. Wayne Mitzner, wmitzner@jhsph.edu.
2. As of the time of this writing, methoxyflurane is no longer commercially available in North America. It is available from a drug company in Australia, Medical Developments Australia Pty Ltd., at a cost of US $367.50 per 120-mL bottle. Please contact the company for more information. As a substitute, we have had good success with mixing 1.5 mL isoflurane (A.J. Buck, Owings Mills, MD) with 8.5 mL light paraffin oil. This mixture may then be used in a manner similar to methoxyflurane
3. To simply estimate the minute ventilation, a glass 10-mL syringe with plunger may be connected to the ventilator, and the volume of air delivered can be measured over a specified time period. The glass offers minimal resistance to air flow.

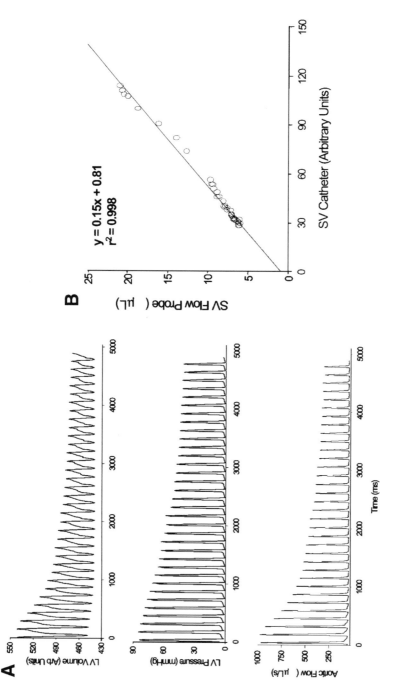

Fig. 3. (**A**) Time series tracings of left ventricular (LV) volume, LV pressure, and thoracic aortic flow during inferior vena caval occlusion. (**B**) Comparison of beat-to-beat stroke volume determined by flow probe and conductance catheter. The two variables are highly correlated and the gain in this example is 0.15.

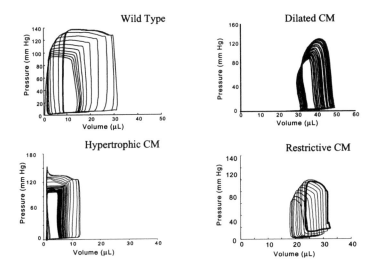

Fig. 4. Pressure-volume relations for normal and diseased ventricles in mice. Dilated cardiomyopathy is associated with high end-diastolic volumes, a shallow ESPVR, and reduced ejection fraction. Hypertrophic cardiomyopathy is characterized by a leftward shift and steep slope of the ESPVR and reduced chamber volumes. Restrictive cardiomyopathy displays a rightward shifted and shallow ESPVR and a very steep diastolic relationship with end-diastolic pressures in excess of 30 mmHg.

Table 1
Hemodynamic Parameters Derived in the Mouse
from Pressure-Volume Relations

Parameter	Mouse	Human[a]	Mouse/human
Heart rate (min⁻¹)	597 ± 58	71	8.4
Systole (% of cardiac cycle)	36.4 ± 3.5	35	1
Diastole (% of cardiac cycle)	63.6 ± 3.5	65	1
End-diastolic pressure (mmHg)	5.73 ± 2.1	12.5	2.0
End-systolic pressure (mmHg)	117.5 ± 10.1	121	1
End-diastolic volume (μL)	29.3 ± 3.1	108.1×10^3	1/3700
End-systolic volume (μL)	6.1 ± 4.1	43.9×10^3	1/7200
Stroke volume (μL)	23.2 ± 2.6	64.9×10^3	1/2800
Cardiac output (mL/min)	13.8 ± 2.5	4.6×10^3	1/333
Arterial elastance (Ea) (mmHg/μL)	4.8 ± 0.91	2.3×10^{-3}	2100
Body mass (g)	25.3 ± 4.6	70×10^3	1/2800
Heart mass (mg)	118.4 ± 18.3	325×10^{3b}	1/2800
LV mass (mg)	95.4 ± 9.6	$130 \times 10^{3\,b}$	1/1400
Heart mass/body mass (mg/g)	4.3 ± 0.42	4.6	1
End-diastolic volume/LV wall volume	0.31 ± 0.04	$0.8–1^c$	0.31
Cardiac output/body mass (mL/min · kg)	533.6 ± 23.4	65.7	8.1

[a]All human data from Liu et al. (12) except for [b]Little et al. (13) and [c]Mirsky et al. (14).

Table 2
Indices of Systolic and Diastolic Function Derived
from Pressure-Volume Relations

Parameter	Mouse	Human[a]	Mouse/human
Diastole			
Diastolic compliance (β^{-1}) (μL/mmHg)	11.1 ± 5.4	5.1×10^3	NA
Peak filling rate/end-diastolic volume (s^{-1})	31.5 ± 6.8	3.6	8.75
Time to peak filling rate (ms)	25.1 ± 4.4	200^b	1/8
Pressure half time (ms)	3.1 ± 0.73	26^b	1/8.4
Tau (Ln) (ms)	3.9 ± 0.96	38^b	1/9.7
Tau (G) (ms)	6.53 ± 1.2	45^b	1/7
Tau (L) (ms)	3.01 ± 0.76	21^b	1/7
Tau (N) (ms)	6.37 ± 0.18	46^b	1/7.2
Peak early/peak late filling (E/A ratio)	No late filling	$1.5–15^b$	NA
dP/dt_{min} (mmHg/s)	-15432 ± 2189	-1900	8.1
Systole			
Ejection fraction (%)	80 ± 6.8	61	1.3
Stroke work (SW) (mmHg $\times$ μL)	2732 ± 289.7	9.6×10^6	1/3500
dP/dt_{max} (mmHg/s)	$16,894 \pm 2132$	2100	8
dP/dt_{max}/pressure at dP/dt_{max} (s^{-1})	251.6 ± 39.5	35	7.2
Power$_{MAX}$/end-diastolic volume (mmHg/s $\times$ 100)	44.5 ± 9.9	6.3	7.1
End-Systolic elastance (Ees) (mmHg/μL)	10.1 ± 4.3	2.1×10^{-3}	1/4800
Ea/Ees	$0.48 \pm .06$	0.5–1	0.5–1.0
Stroke work/end-diastolic Vol. relation (mmHg)	100.5 ± 29.1	82	1.2
dP/dt_{max} - end diastolic vol. relation (mmHg/s/mL)	610 ± 178.2	20×10^{-3}	30×10^3
Efficiency (SW/pressure-volume area) (%)	81.3 ± 3.5	80^c	1
Peak stress (σ) (g/cm^2)	298.4 ± 54.2	280^d	1.1
End-systolic stress-strain relation (g/cm^2)	1210 ± 270	1100^d	1.1

[a]All human data from Liu et al. (12) except for [b]Little et al. (13) and [c]Mirsky et al. (14).

References

1. Dalloz, F., Osinska, H., and Robbins, J. (2001). Manipulating the contractile apparatus: genetically defined animal models of cardiovascular disease. *J. Mol. Cell Cardiol.* **33**, 9–25.

2. Minamino, T., Gaussin, V., Demayo, F. J., and Schneider, M. D. (2001). Inducible gene targeting in post-natal myocardium by cardiac-specific expression of a hormone activated cre fusion protein. *Circ. Res.* **88**, 587–592.

3. Sagawa, K., Maughan, W. L., Suga, H., and Sunagawa, K. (1988). *Cardiac Contraction and the Pressure-Volume Relationship.* Oxford University Press, New York.

4. Little, W. C. and Cheng, C. P. (1993). Effect of exercise on left ventricular-arterial coupling assessed in the pressure-volume plane. *Am. J. Physiol.* **264,** H1629–H1633

5. Kass, D. A., Midei, M., Graves, W., Brinker, J. A., and Maughan, W. L. (1988). Use of a conductance (volume) catheter and transient inferior vena caval occlusion for rapid determination of pressure-volume relationships in man. *Cathet. Cardiovasc. Diagn.* **15**, 192–202.

6. Baan, J., Van Der Velde, E. T., De Bruin, H. G., et al. (1984). Continuous measurement of left ventricular volume in animals and humans by conductance catheter. *Circulation* **70**, 812–823.

7. Georgakopoulos, D., Mitzner, W. A., Chen, C. H., et al. (1998). In vivo murine left ventricular pressure-volume relations by miniaturized conductance micromanometry. *Am. J. Physiol.* **274**, H1416–H1422

8. Georgakopoulos, D., Christe, M. E., Giewat, M., Seidman, C. M., Seidman, J. G., and Kass, D. A. (1999). The pathogenesis of familial hypertrophic cardiomyopathy: early and evolving effects from an alpha-cardiac myosin heavy chain missense mutation [see comments]. *Nat. Med.* **5**, 327–330.

9. Little, W. C., Cheng, C. P., Mumma, M., Igarashi, Y., Vinten-Johansen, J., and Johnston, W. E. (1989). Comparison of measures of left ventricular contractile performance derived from pressure-volume loops in conscious dogs. *Circulation* **80**, 1378–1387.

10. Georgakopoulos, D. and Kass, D. A. (2000). Estimation of parallel conductance by dual frequency conductance catheter in Mice. *Am. J. Physiol.* **279**, 443–450.

11. Lankford, E. B., Kass, D. A., Maughan, W. L. and Shoukas, A. A. (1990). Does volume catheter parallel conductance vary during a cardiac cycle? *Am. J. Physiol.* **258**, H1933–H1942

12. Liu, C. P., Ting, C. T., Lawrence, W., Maughan, W. L., Chang, M. S. and Kass, D. A. (1993). Diminished contractile response to increased heart rate in intact human left ventricular hypertrophy. Systolic versus diastolic determinants. *Circulation* **88**, 1893–1906.

13. Little, W. C. and Downes, T. R. (1990). Clinical evaluation of left ventricular diastolic performance. *Prog. Cardiovasc. Dis.* **32**, 273–290.

14. Mirsky, I., Cohn, P. F., Levine, J. A., et al. (1974). Assessment of left ventricular stiffness in primary myocardial disease and coronary artery disease. *Circulation* **50**, 128–136.

Index

A

AAV vectors, *see* Adeno-associated
  virus vectors
Adeno-associated virus (AAV)
  vectors,
    advantages in myocardial gene
      transfer, 29, 136
    animal model studies, 29, 30
    packing capacity expansion with
      dual vectors,
    cell culture, 32, 33, 46
    materials, 32-34, 46, 47
    overlapping vector generation,
      construction for any gene,
        42, 43, 47
      design, 42
      LacZ overlapping vector
        construction, 42, 47
      overview, 40, 41, 45, 46
      proviral plasmid cloning, 42
    recombinant virus production
      and purification, 34, 43-
      45, 47, 48
    trans-splicing vector design
      and cloning,
      cloning strategy, 37
      proviral plasmid construction,
        33, 34, 37-40
      splicing signal selection, 35
      splicing site selection, 35
      trans-splicing vs overlapping
        approaches, 30-32, 45,
        46

Adenoviral vectors,
  catheter-based gene transfer, *see*
    Catheter-based adenoviral
    gene transfer, cardiomyocytes
    in rabbit
  cell culture passage and
    maintenance, 4, 7, 16
  characteristics, 19
  coronary perfusion cocktails for
    gene transfer, *see* Perfusion
    cocktails, coronary
    adenoviral gene transfer
  cotransfection, 4, 7, 8
  cytotoxicity, 53, 137
  DNA isolation, 4, 5, 8, 9, 16
  embryonic/neonatal cardiac gene
    transfer, *see* Embryonic/neo-
    natal cardiac gene transfer
  gutted vectors,
    amplification through serial
      passages, 23, 26
    genome construction in
      plasmid backbones, 20
    helper virus role, 20
    materials for construction, 21, 22
    overview, 19, 20
    preparation principles, 20, 21
    purification, 24-26
    rescue by cotransfection, 22,
      23, 26
    titering,
      colorimetric assay for
        transducing units, 25, 26

245